PLACE IN RETURN BOX to remove this checkout from your record.
TO AVOID FINES return on or before date due.
MAY BE RECALLED with earlier due date if requested.

DATE DUE	DATE DUE	DATE DUE
MAR 7 2000		
MAR 2005		
3 9 1 90 9		

Stress Physiology in Animals

Sheffield Biological Sciences

A series which provides an accessible source of information at research and professional level in chosen sectors of the biological sciences.

Series Editors

Professor Peter N.R. Usherwood
Head of Division of Molecular Toxicology
School of Biological Sciences
University of Nottingham

and

Dr Jeremy A. Roberts
Reader in Plant Biology
School of Biological Sciences
University of Nottingham

Stress Physiology in Animals

Edited by

PAUL H.M. BALM
Department of Animal Physiology
University of Nijmegen
The Netherlands

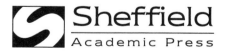

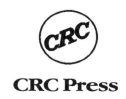

CRC Press

First published 1999
Copyright © 1999 Sheffield Academic Press

Published by
Sheffield Academic Press Ltd
Mansion House, 19 Kingfield Road
Sheffield S11 9AS, England

ISBN 1-85075-908-1

Published in the U.S.A. and Canada (only) by
CRC Press LLC
2000 Corporate Blvd., N.W.
Boca Raton, FL 33431, U.S.A.
Orders from the U.S.A. and Canada (only) to CRC Press LLC

U.S.A. and Canada only:
ISBN 0-8493-9741-3

This book contains information obtained from authentic and highly regarded sources. Reprinted
material is quoted with permission, and sources are indicated. Reasonable efforts have been
made to publish reliable data and information, but the author and the publisher cannot assume
responsibility for the validity of all materials or for the consequences of their use.

Trademark Notice: Product or corporate names may be trademarks or registered trademarks,
and are used only for identification and explanation, without intent to infringe.
No claim to original U.S.A. Government works.

Printed on acid-free paper in Great Britain by
Bookcraft Ltd, Midsomer Norton, Bath

British Library Cataloguing-in-Publication Data:
A catalogue record for this book is available from the British Library

Library of Congress Cataloging-in-Publication Data:
A catalog record for this book is available from the Library of Congress

Preface

The concept of stress was formulated during the first half of the twentieth century by W.B. Cannon ('fight or flight response') and H.A. Selye (the General Adaptation Syndrome). Until relatively recently, Selye's ideas were regarded highly only by psychologists, while scientists from other disciplines, such as (patho)physiology, regarded his concept of little significance. Following the discovery of novel immunological and neuroendocrine principles, it became possible to describe the state of stress in physiological terms, and to approach the underlying mechanisms experimentally.

The past decade has seen a disproportionate increase in the number of 'stress' studies published (the annual total has almost doubled in the biological sciences). This results partly from an increase in the number of biological disciplines studying stress, but also from the recognition that the concept of stress can be applied to all levels of organisation—from ecosystems to the molecular level—and that the relevant physiological mechanisms evolved at least 400 million years ago.

Over the years, researchers have been puzzled by what may appear to be inconsistencies of stress, such as the specificity/aspecificity of the stress response and the adaptive/maladaptive character of the stressed state. Some of these enigmas may in part be explained by temporal aspects of the development of stress, but others are far from a solution. One of these concerns is the paradox of the function of corticosteroids, which resembles the relationship between oxygen and aerobic life ('oxygen stress').

By and large, overviews of stress have focused on specific animal groups, and mammals in particular. A second category of publications has addressed specific levels of organisation. The present volume aims to provide an overview of stress physiology in animals from a comparative point of view. It contains chapters which compare the impact of stress on behaviour, metabolism, reproduction, histopathology, immune-endocrine interactions and toxicology between animal groups. In particular, because the physiological mechanisms underlying stress have evolved with the vertebrates (and probably even earlier), a comparative approach may develop further the unifying character of the stress concept. A comparative approach will facilitate research into fundamental aspects of stress (i.e. identification of specific messenger molecules), but it will also prove useful in applied research (animal husbandry).

I wish to thank the authors of the individual chapters for their contributions, and Dr G. MacKintosh at Sheffield Academic Press for his collaboration.

Paul H.M. Balm

Contributors

Dr P.H.M. Balm

Department of Animal Physiology, University of Nijmegen, Toernooiveld 1, 6525 ED Nijmegen, The Netherlands

Dr S.F. de Boer

Department of Animal Physiology, University of Groningen, P.O. Box 14, 9750 AA Haren, The Netherlands

Dr Malin Celander

Göteborg University, Department of Zoology, Zoophysiology, Box 463, SE 405 30 Göteborg, Sweden

Dr Kathleen M. Gilmour

Department of Biology, Carleton University, 1125 Colonel By Drive, Ottawa, Ontario K1S 5B6, Canada

Dr Alec G. Maule

USGS-Biological Resources Division, Western Fisheries Research Center, Columbia River Research Laboratory, 5501A Cook-Underwood Rd., Cook, WA 98605, USA

Professor Steve F. Perry

Department of Biology, University of Ottawa, 30 Marie Curie Street, PO Box 450, Stn. A, Ottawa, Ontario K1N 6N5, Canada

Dr Tom G. Pottinger

The NERC Institute of Freshwater Ecology, Windermere Laboratory, The Ferry House, Far Sawrey, Ambleside, Cumbria LA22 OLP, UK

Dr Marilyn Ramenofsky

Department of Zoology, Box 351800, University of Washington, Seattle, WA 98195, USA

Professor A.B. Steffens

Department of Animal Physiology, University of Groningen, P.O. Box 14, 9750 AA Haren, The Netherlands

Mr Scott P. VanderKooi

USGS-Biological Resources Division, Western Fisheries Research Center, Columbia River Research Laboratory, 5501A Cook-Underwood Rd., Cook, WA 98605, USA

Professor S.E. Wendelaar Bonga

Department of Animal Physiology, University of Nijmegen, Toernooiveld 1, 6525 ED Nijmegen, The Netherlands

Professor John C. Wingfield

Department of Zoology, Box 351800, University of Washington, Seattle, WA 98195, USA

Contents

7   Impact of stress on animal toxicology   246
M. CELANDER

1 Hormones and the behavioral ecology of stress

John C. Wingfield and Marilyn Ramenofsky

1.1 Introduction

'Climate' may be defined as the overall average environmental conditions that may be expected over the year at any one location. All climatic conditions, even the most severe, are predictable and organisms prepare for future changes in environment. 'Weather', on the other hand, denotes the minute-to-minute environmental conditions at any time, and may or may not have any bearing on the predicted 'climate' for that locality. Thus, organisms not only prepare for predictable changes of climate, but must also be able to respond in an adaptive way to unpredictable weather conditions, or other environmental perturbations, at short notice. The case of weather versus climate raises the concepts of predictability and unpredictability in both the physical and social environments that are be the focus of this chapter. We will argue that 'stress' tends to occur during unpredictable perturbations of the environment and not as a result of the predictable changes that occur during the course of, for example, a day, high tide, low tide, or the seasons. It is important to bear in mind that although most people consider climates with long cold winters or equally long hot summers as generally 'stressful', they are nonetheless predictable allowing organisms to anticipate the phenology of a particular climate and thus avoid stress. Also, we often use phrases such as 'the stress of reproduction' or 'the stress of migration'. Again, we feel that such statements are inaccurate, because these processes occur on predictable schedules and an individual can make necessary preparations. They may be energetically demanding, but are not necessarily stressful (see Wingfield et al., 1998).

Virtually no habitat on earth is static (except, perhaps, thermal vents in the deep ocean), and organisms must anticipate environmental change and respond appropriately (e.g. L.F. Jacobs, 1996). There is a highly predictable component to environmental conditions, no matter how severe, that allows organisms to modify their morphology, physiology and behavior accordingly and thus reduce the potential for stress. Many organisms adjust their phenotype to maximize fitness in any given habitat (called phenotypic plasticity, e.g. West-Eberhard, 1989). This is especially true if predictable changes occur between generations as in many invertebrates. However, predictable changes in environmental conditions occur within generations in longer lived organisms such as vertebrates (e.g. Stephens, 1991). In these cases a single phenotype must be able to change its physiology, morphology and behavior as environmental conditions fluctuate–i.e. analogous to a genotype expressing different phenotypes at the population level. In other words, a single phenotype in a predictably oscillating environment must express several phenotypic stages that maximize fitness throughout the organism's lifetime. These have been described as a series of life-history stages (LHS) such as non-breeding, migration, breeding, molt, etc. (J.D. Jacobs, 1996).

A crucial factor that is often overlooked is that day-to-day conditions can also have a highly unpredictable component that has great potential to be stressful. In addition to the predictable series of LHSs within an organism's life cycle, there is growing evidence for an 'emergency life history stage' (ELHS) that is triggered by unpredictable events in the environment termed modifying factors or labile perturbation factors (LPFs, J.D. Jacobs, 1996; Wingfield et al., 1998). LPFs trigger facultative behavioral and physiological responses that make up the ELHS. These appear to be mediated by increases in glucocorticosteroid secretion (Wingfield et al., 1998).

There are several components to the ELHS (Wingfield and Ramenofsky, 1997). Firstly the current LHS must be deactivated (e.g. territorial behavior, abandonment of current reproductive effort, etc.). Secondly, there are two, possibly three strategies that may be adopted in an ELHS: (a) movements away from the source of the LPF ('leave-it' strategy); (b) if the individual remains it will seek a refuge ('take-it' strategy); (c) seek a refuge first and then move away if conditions do not improve ('take-it' at first and then 'leave-it' strategy). For example, many species from all five major vertebrate classes are relatively sedentary and would likely seek a refuge. Others, however, being more mobile, may leave the area in search of a refuge or temporary alternate habitat. Some variants of these strategies include facultative developmental changes. In western spadefoot toads, *Scaphiopus hammondi*, premature drying of ponds results in facultative metamorphosis. This can be accelerated experimentally by artificially lowering the water level in captive conditions (Denver, 1998) and is accompanied by precocial increases in whole body contents of T3, T4 and corticosterone in tadpoles. Injections of corticotropin-releasing factor (CRF) activate both thyroid hormone and corticosterone secretion that in turn precipitate facultative metamorphosis (Denver, 1997). Crowding, limited resources, predation as well as habitat desiccation may also trigger this (reviewed in Denver, 1997; see also Hayes, 1997). Similarly, crowding, stress, etc. may increase corticosterone levels and precipitate premature metamorphosis in the toad *Bufo boreas* so the animal can leave the pond (Hayes, 1997).

The third component of an ELHS involves mobilization of stored energy sources such as fat and perhaps protein to fuel movement away from the source of the LPF, or to provide energy while sheltering in a refuge. Fourth, if the animal leaves its habitat, then a suitable alternate habitat must be sought, or movement will continue until the perturbation passes. Finally, the organism must settle in an alternate habitat once an appropriate site is identified, or return to the original site and resume the normal sequence of LHSs (Wingfield and Ramenofsky, 1997).

Very rapid responses to some LPFs, for example the 'fight-or-flight' reactions to predators or dominant conspecifics, trigger immediate avoidance behavior and self-defense. These responses are generally too rapid to activate an ELHS as described above (Wingfield and Ramenofsky, 1997). More chronic LPFs such as periods of inclement weather, increased predation pressure in general, social subordinance, human disturbance, etc. trigger the ELHS via increased secretion of glucocorticosteroids from adrenocortical tissue (Wingfield and Ramenofsky, 1997; Wingfield *et al.*, 1998). The ELHS is temporary (hours to days) and maximizes the likelihood of survival in the face of direct LPFs. Most, if not all vertebrates respond in a similar manner, suggesting that there has been strong selection for mechanisms that trigger an ELHS over a long period of evolutionary history. Hormones of the hypothalamo–pituitary–adrenocortical axis (HPA), which may play a major role in regulating the ELHS, have also been largely conserved throughout the vertebrate classes. Evidence for this will be summarized next.

1.2 The hypothalamo–pituitary–adrenal axis in comparative context

Glucocorticosteroids and catecholamines provide the front-line defense for mammals and other vertebrates under stress conditions (e.g. Greenberg and Wingfield, 1987; Francis *et al.*, 1996). In teleost fish, and all tetrapods, LPFs in the environment result in the release of adrenocorticotropin (ACTH) from the precursor molecule pro-opiomelanocortin in the anterior pituitary (Hadley, 1996; Norris, 1997). Other peptides such as beta-endorphin and alpha-melanocyte-stimulating hormone may also be involved in some aspects of a stress response (e.g. Axelrod and Reisine, 1984) although this is much less well known in non-mammalian vertebrates. However, in male domestic ganders (*Anser anser*), ether stress results in an increase in both ACTH and beta-endorphin (Barna *et al.*, 1998). ACTH release is stimulated by corticotropin-releasing factor (CRF) arginine vasopressin (AVP, or arginine vasotocin (AVT) in non-mammalian tetrapods) and oxytocin (OT or mesotocin (MT) in many non-mammalian tetrapods), although these peptides vary in their potency as secretogogues of ACTH (Hadley, 1996; Norris, 1997). ACTH acts primarily on the adrenal cortex of mammals and the adrenocortical homologue (interrenal tissue) in other vertebrates to promote synthesis and secretion of glucocorticosteroids. These are primarily corticosterone in non-mammalian tetrapods, cortisol in teleost fish, and cortisol, corticosterone or both in various mammalian taxa (Idler, 1972). The HPA axis of vertebrates, particularly aves, has many of the same feedback controls as in mammals (Carsia, 1990; Norris, 1997). Thus, although there may be minor differences in the HPA axis across vertebrate taxa, overall function and also responses to a wide spectrum of stresses (see below) appear to be identical.

1.2.1   Actions of glucocorticosteroids during stress

Responses of the HPA axis to stress are widespread in vertebrates (Greenberg and Wingfield, 1987), and involve a broad spectrum of unpredictable environmental perturbations, e.g. mammals (Walker, 1994), birds (Wingfield, 1988, 1994), reptiles (Lance, 1994; Tyrrell and Cree, 1998), amphibians (Yon et al., 1994) and teleost fish (Pickering and Fryer, 1994; Sumpter et al., 1994). There is growing evidence that glucocorticosteroids play a major role in orchestrating the ELHS in response to unpredictable events such as LPFs. However, these relatively short-term effects of glucocorticosteroids (hours to a day or so) are less well known than marked deleterious effects if glucocorticosteroid secretion is prolonged over periods of days to weeks (e.g. Axelrod and Reisine, 1994; Sapolsky, 1987, 1996). Chronic high levels of circulating glucocorticosteroids (days to weeks) can inhibit gonadotropin secretion resulting in gonadal involution and delay of puberty onset, suppression of growth hormone secretion (plus insulin-like growth factors) to inhibit growth, metabolic exhaustion from breakdown of skeletal muscle, suppression of T lymphocyte activity resulting in an increase in susceptibility to disease, decreased arachidonic acid formation which disrupts cell processes, and neuron death in the hippocampus (Axelrod and Reisine, 1984; Greenberg and Wingfield, 1987; Sapolsky, 1987, 1996). It is difficult to conceive that any of these effects of glucocorticosteroids typical of severe stress have any adaptive value for a free-living organism. An individual under natural conditions would be moribund and close to death under the influence of chronically high glucocorticosteroids. The effects of glucocorticosteroids in the short-term, however, appear to be far more adaptive in that they trigger physiological and behavioral responses that function to re-direct an individual away from the current LHS into a 'survival mode'–i.e. the ELHS (Wingfield, 1994; Wingfield et al., 1998). This is not to diminish the fact that the chronic effects of high circulating concentrations of glucocorticosteroids are important in biomedical and agricultural contexts; they are treated elsewhere in this volume. The short-term effects of glucocorticosteroids and the experimental evidence for them are the focus here.

1.2.2 The emergency life history stage (ELHS) and short-term effects of glucocorticosteroids

1.2.2.1 Suppression of reproductive and territorial behavior

Experimentally elevated levels of corticosterone reduce territorial aggression in free-living male song sparrows, *Melospiza melodia* (Wingfield and Silverin, 1986). These observations are consistent with abandonment of a breeding territory or winter range in search of a refuge or alternative resources. Corticosterone treatment results in reduced home range in side-blotched lizards, *Uta stansburiana* (DeNardo and Sinervo, 1994a). Furthermore, this effect remains despite simultaneous implants of testosterone, suggesting that corticosterone acts directly rather than indirectly through inhibition of testosterone secretion (DeNardo and Licht, 1993; DeNardo and Sinervo, 1994b). Older evidence indicates that corticosterone also suppresses both sexual and parental behavior in birds (Deviche, 1983), and implants of corticosterone into breeding pied flycatchers, *Ficedula hypoleuca*, decreases parental behavior in both sexes (Silverin, 1986). In the latter study, young are provisioned less frequently, nestlings weigh less and fewer young fledge from the nest than in controls. Larger doses of corticosterone result in abandonment of nests and territories and complete reproductive failure. In amphibians, clasping (a sexual behavior involved in mating) of male rough skinned newts, *Taricha granulosa*, is suppressed by injections of corticosterone (Moore and Miller, 1984). The net results of these actions of glucocorticosteroids are to inhibit expression of the current LHS (i.e. deactivate it) so that the ELHS can be expressed. In the examples given here, reproductive behaviors are suppressed without inhibiting the reproductive system. Thus breeding can resume immediately once the LPF passes and glucocorticosteroid concentrations subside (see Wingfield et al., 1998).

1.2.2.2 Facilitate foraging behavior and increase gluconeogenesis

One obvious adaptive response to LPFs would be to enhance foraging behavior and food intake to combat potential stress. This may be an integral component of the ELHS closely linked to gluconeogenesis. Elevated corticosteroid levels have been shown to facilitate food intake (Tempel and Leibowitz, 1989) and affect circadian activity patterns in mammals (Iuvone and Van Hartesveldt, 1977; Micco et al., 1980). Additional effects include enhanced exploratory behavior (Veldhuis et al., 1982), avoidance behavior (Moyer and Leshner, 1976), and learning retention (Bohus and De Kloet, 1981), all of which may combine to orchestrate a behavioral response to LPFs. There is also an intimate interaction of glucocorticosteroids with insulin and feeding. Corticosterone can both antagonize and synergize with insulin effects on metabolism and with insulin secretion. Corticosterone stimulates feeding at low doses and inhibits it at high doses (Dallman *et al.*, 1993). Implants of corticosterone also tend to elevate foraging behavior in white-crowned sparrows, *Zonotrichia leucophrys*, and song sparrows, *Melospiza melodia*, although there is variation in this response (Astheimer *et al.*, 1992; Wingfield, 1994). Moreover, in chickens and dark-eyed juncos, *Junco hyemalis*, corticosterone administered in the diet did not affect food intake (Davidson *et al.*, 1983; Gray *et al.*, 1990). This may be explained by a possible role for glucocorticosteroids to facilitate promotion of food intake and foraging behavior, possibly in conjunction with peptides such as ACTH and CRF (Deviche and Delius, 1981; Vergoni *et al.*, 1986; Maney and Wingfield, 1998).

In addition to facilitating foraging behavior and food intake, glucocorticosteroids decrease hepatic glucose output, increase fat and protein degradation to produce glucose, elevate gluconeogenic enzyme activity, and potentiate the action of catecholamines and glucagon on fat catabolism and glucose formation (e.g. Chester Jones *et al.*, 1972; McMahon *et al.*, 1988). Corticosterone can both antagonize and synergize with insulin effects as well as insulin secretion. In general, although corticosterone can stimulate feeding at low doses and inhibit it at high doses (i.e. central actions, Dallman *et al.*, 1993), actions in the periphery are catabolic causing mobilization of energy (Dallman *et al.*, 1995). Chronic stress and glucocorticosteroid treatment result in an increase in circulating corticosterone and insulin but with the normal ratio maintained between them. This results in remodeling of body energy stores away from muscle stores toward fat depots (Dallman *et al.*, 1995). In adrenalectomized rats given streptozotocin to lower circulating insulin and thus induce diabetes, corticosterone treatment stimulates whereas insulin administration inhibits mRNA for NPY in the hypothalamus and food intake (Strack *et al.*, 1995a). This suggests that at the central level corticosterone and insulin are antagonistic, long-term regulators of energy balance. At the non-central level, other recent evidence suggests that cortisol may act primarily on substrate delivery for hepatic gluconeogenesis because the conversion of alanine to glucose is enhanced by promoting alanine uptake by the liver (Goldstein *et al.*, 1992, 1993). Glucocorticosteroids may thus regulate gluconeogenesis by stimulating supplies of hepatic gluconeogenic precursors and maintaining hepatic glycogen availability in conjunction with catecholamines, glucagon and insulin (Fujiwara *et al.*, 1996).

In rats white adipose tissue (WAT) is more sensitive than brown adipose tissue (BAT) to glucocorticosteroids. In adrenalectomized rats, doses of corticosterone above the daily mean level in blood increase BAT lipid stores and elevate WAT stores even more so (Strack *et al.*, 1995b). Furthermore, corticosterone decreases UCP (uncoupling protein–a BAT protein involved in thermogenesis) and the binding characteristics of GDP to BAT mitochondria (B_{max} and dissociation constant, K_d). Thus, corticosterone seems to depress thermogenesis but promotes storage of lipid (Strack *et al.*, 1995b). In birds corticosterone treatment increases plasma levels of glucose as well as triglyceride, fatty acids, glycerol, protein and uric acid levels (Davidson *et al.*, 1983). Furthermore, corticosterone administration results in atrophy of the flight muscles, enhanced activity of muscle lipoprotein lipase and a large increase in subcutaneous fat depots suggesting that protein is metabolized and fat synthesized (Davidson *et al.*, 1983; Wingfield and Silverin, 1986; Gray *et al.*, 1990). King penguins, *Aptenodytes patagonica*, can tolerate 4–5 months fasting in the parental phase of the breeding cycle and also during molt. Corticosterone levels remain low as fat depots are slowly mobilized but as they near depletion circulating corticosterone levels suddenly rise, paralleled by an increase in protein utilization (Le Ninan *et al.*, 1988). The pectoralis muscles (used to power flight) in birds may be an important protein store as a source for gluconeogenesis and other nutrients such as amino acids (Kendall *et al.*, 1973; Jones and Ward, 1976). This reserve may consist of soluble proteins (separate from the contractile components) that can be mobilized preferentially by glucocorticosteroids. Captive house sparrows, *Passer domesticus*, treated with corticosterone lose body weight and mass of the pectoralis muscles. Fractionation of these muscle proteins shows that the soluble fraction is mobilized while the contractile components remain intact. In this way, mobility would not be impaired at least in the short-term (Honey, 1990). In the longer term chronic elevation of glucocorticosteroids may deplete contractile components of muscle as well. It should also be noted that corticosterone increases muscle lipoprotein lipase activity which would maintain or elevate delivery of fatty acids for oxidation (Gray *et al.*, 1990).

1.2.2.3 'Take it' or 'leave it' strategies

Facultative behaviors associated with LPFs vary depending upon the species observed and context. Some seek shelter (take it strategy) whereas others may abandon their territory or home range (leave it strategy). For example, experimental restriction of food to simulate one type of LPF increases locomotor activity in birds (Ketterson and King, 1977; Freeman *et al.*, 1980; Stuebe and Ketterson, 1982; Astheimer *et al.*, 1992), and rats (File and Day, 1972), but reduces activity in fish (Robinson and Pitcher,

1989) and humans (Grande, 1964). These two strategies may overlap in some circumstances. For example, individuals may forage beyond their normal home range but still return to their refuge at night–i.e. movements over relatively short distances of a few hundred meters. In other species poor local environmental conditions may lead to spectacular facultative migrations (better known as irruptions) over thousands of kilometers (Wingfield and Ramenofsky, 1997). In the white-crowned sparrow, perch hopping activity is a measure of facultative movements associated with an ELHS. Corticosterone treatment decreases activity if food is available, but if food is removed then perch hopping activity and 'escape-behavior' is increased dramatically compared to controls. These behaviors are more consistent with movements away (irruptive migration) from the source of the LPF (Astheimer *et al.*, 1992). CRF may have additional action here because evidence suggests that it stimulates locomotor activity (Sutton *et al.*, 1982; Moore *et al.*, 1984; Veldhuis and de Wied, 1984), and depresses exploratory behavior (Berridge and Dunn, 1989), all consistent with the 'leave it' strategy outlined above.

In species in which irruptive migration is not possible, locating a refuge and quiescence is an appropriate strategy. This may be the major ELHS in vertebrate taxa such as reptiles and amphibians, but is also likely to occur widely in mammals, birds and fish. Hormonal mechanisms under-lying the 'take it' strategy (to ride-out the LPF) are largely unexplored but some provocative studies suggest possible lines of investigation. Western fence lizards, *Sceloporus occidentalis*, treated with human interleukin-1β show a decrease in daily activity within 2 h (Dunlap and Church, 1996). This effect on activity is very similar to that of lizards infected with malaria, *Plasmodium mexicanum*. These authors raise the hypothesis that interleukin-1β may reduce activity in pathogen-induced alterations of behavior as well as those activated by other forms of stress, and paralleled by elevated corticosterone levels (Dunlap and Schall, 1995). ACTH may also activate behavior consistent with seeking a refuge in an ELHS. This peptide has been shown to affect excessive stretching and yawning, and slowed extinction of avoidance learning (Bertolini and Gessa, 1981; de Wied and Jolles, 1982).

1.2.2.4 *Promote night restfulness*

An effect of glucocorticosteroids on metabolic rate and oxygen consumption might be expected given the well-known actions on metabolism cited above. However, the experimental evidence is rather contradictory. In great tits, *Parus major*, and black-headed gulls, *Larus ridibundus*, corticosterone treatment increases oxygen consumption (Hissa and Palokangas, 1970; Palokangas and Hissa, 1971), decreases nocturnal energy expenditure in domestic fowl (Mitchell *et al.*, 1986), but has no effect in the pigeon, *Columba livia* (Hissa *et al.*, 1980). More recently, sub-cutaneous implants of corticosterone in white-crowned sparrows, and Pine Siskins, *Spinus pinus*, result in uniformly low oxygen consumption throughout the observation period at night, compared with episodic increases in oxygen consumption in controls (Buttemer *et al.*, 1991). An overall energy savings of about 20% is obtained overnight. Further investigations will clarify the actions of glucocorticosteroids in regulating metabolic rate, particularly in relation to whether a species may seek a refuge or emigrate.

1.2.2.5 Recovery and return to the normal life history stage

Individuals return to an appropriate life history stage for that time of year once an LPF passes and stimuli for an ELHS decline. That is, if the perturbation is prolonged, then the LHS that follows may not be the one which was originally interrupted by the LPF (J.D. Jacobs, 1996). A period of recovery follows during which energy reserves are replenished, etc. The role glucocorticosteroids play in recovery from an emergency requiring activation of the immune system has been discussed in detail (e.g. Munck *et al.*, 1984) but other aspects remain equivocal. Corticosterone treatment of male song sparrows increases re-feeding after a fast (Astheimer *et al.*, 1992) suggesting that glucocorticosteroids may actually facilitate recovery from acute stress. On the other hand, glucocorticosteroids appear to increase the time required for recovery of blood and muscle metabolites and acid–base status in rainbow trout, *Oncorhynchus mykiss*, subjected to exhaustive exercise (Eros and Milligan, 1996). This impediment to recovery may seem contradictory, but the post-exercise rise in cortisol may be involved with clearing increased blood lactate levels and may actually potentiate full recovery. In the desert iguana, *Dipsosaurus dorsalis*, five minutes of exhaustive exercise results in a rapid rise of circulating glucagon (within 5 min) whereas corticosterone took longer to rise (about 45 min). Glucagon appeared to be more involved in lactate metabolism during recovery because inhibition of corticosterone by metyrapone has no effect on lactate clearance (Scholnick *et al.*, 1997). The existing data are intriguing, but much more investigation is needed to clarify the endocrine basis of recovery following an ELHS.

1.2.2.6 Overview

Numerous experiments point to the highly adaptive effects of glucocorticosteroids (and several peptide hormones associated with the HPA axis) on the facultative physiological and behavioral process in response to LPFs. A crucial point here is that these effects are rapid (minutes to hours) and trigger the ELHS that is designed to avoid stress, particularly the deleterious effects of more chronic exposure to high circulating levels of glucocorticosteroids. The ELHS can be triggered at any time of year and in response to a broad spectrum of LPFs in the physical as well as social environment (Wingfield, 1994; Wingfield *et al.*, 1998). Although much more work needs to be done to determine the interactions of glucocorticosteroids with other hormones, particularly central peptides, we are now in a position to ask some more fundamental questions concerning what conditions constitute an LPF, how rapidly an individual responds and if there are any common themes and underlying mechanisms that provide a unifying concept of an ELHS. These questions will be addressed next.

1.3   A theoretical framework to unify concepts of the emergency life history stage in response to diverse perturbations of the environment

The question of whether a common physiological pathway exists by which diverse labile perturbation factors in the physical, social and internal environments are transduced into secretions of the HPA axis remains obscure. The following scheme is postulated that may provide a unifying framework to explain how extremely diverse LPFs trigger an ELHS. There may be many common characteristics of the ELHS regardless of the population expressing it, and the LHS from which it was activated (Wingfield and Ramenofsky, 1997; Wingfield *et al.*, 1998). The model has simple heuristic value to begin identifying possible common themes underlying these phenomena. It is based on an energetic theme where **E** represents the energy available to an individual in its environment, as well as that required to survive day to day and pursue it's activities as demanded by the progression of normal LHSs. It is important to note that this framework has no assumptions or adjustments for specialized nutrient requirements, vitamins, etc., although these could be modeled separately. The reasoning is as follows:

E_G = Energy to be gained from food in the environment
E_E = Existence energy (i.e. maintenance level = resting metabolic rate)
E_I = Energy required to obtain food, process and assimilate it under ideal conditions
E_O = Additional energy required to obtain food under non-ideal conditions

In the theoretical example given in Figure 1.1a, broken lines represent E_G, E_I and E_E over time (such as the annual cycle of LHSs). In reality of

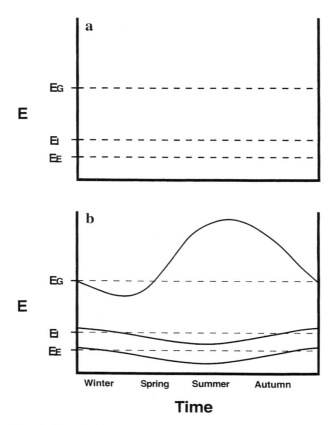

Figure 1.1 A simple theoretical framework to model how energy available in the environment and energy required by an individual to live may interact. E = overall energy levels (with no adjustments made for specific nutritional requirements); E_E = existence energy; E_I = energy required to obtain food and process it under ideal conditions. In the top panel (a) these energy levels are constant with time (for purposes of simplicity). In the lower panel (b), an example of how these may vary (superimposed on panel (a)) with seasons is given. In most temperate zones E_E and E_I will be greater in winter than summer for simple energetic reasons. Also, E_G tends to be greater in spring and summer because these are the primary production seasons. See text for further details.

course, they will vary as a function of predictable changes in the environment (Figure 1.1b). However, here the energy lines are held constant for simplicity. Normally, $E_G - (E_I + E_E) > 0$ and thus the individual remains in an appropriate LHS. However, environmental conditions are rarely ideal and the energy required to obtain food is usually greater than E_I. The line E_O represents the additional energy required for an individual to locate, obtain and process food that is represented by line **E$_G$** (Figure 1.2). As long as **E$_O$** remains below **E$_G$** (**E$_G$** − (**E$_I$** + **E$_E$** + **E$_O$**) > 0), then positive energy balance is maintained and the individual can continue in the appropriate LHS for that time of year. If an LPF occurs that increases **E$_O$** further, then the additional energy

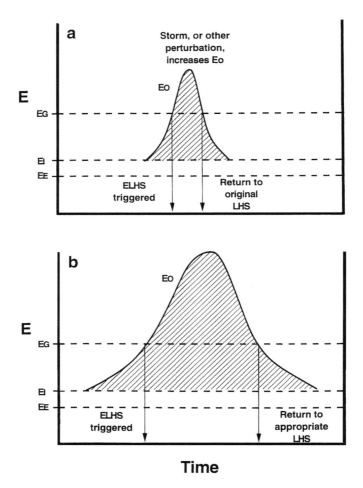

Figure 1.2 Using Figure 1.1a as a framework, we can introduce the line **E$_O$** as the extra energy required to obtain food and process it under less than ideal conditions. The area under this line is shaded for emphasis. If labile perturbation factors (LPF) occur, then **E$_O$** may exceed **E$_G$** and an emergency life history stage (ELHS) is activated (indicated by the arrow). As the LPF subsides, **E$_O$** decreases and when it falls below **E$_G$** the individual can return to a normal LHS (indicated by the right-hand arrow). Variation in the intensity and duration of LPFs can result in **E$_O$** profiles of different periods (upper and lower panels–a and b). See text for details.

required to obtain food may increase such that $E_G - (E_I + E_O + E_E) < 0$. In this case the individual should trigger an ELHS. Note that once the perturbation passes and $E_G - (E_I + E_O + E_E) > 0$ once again, then the individual can return to a LHS appropriate for that time (Figure 1.2.). On the other hand, if an alternate habitat is discovered that allows positive energy balance, then the individual may settle there and resume its normal LHS.

The intensity and duration of the LPF can vary resulting in a corresponding short period that the ELHS is expressed (Figure 1.2a) or a longer period (Figure 1.2b). In the latter case, the original LHS may be inappropriate and the next LHS, or most appropriate one, may be assumed. This exemplifies the flexibility an organism must have to deal with a capricious environment. The individual is able to adjust LHSs to maximize survival and ultimately lifetime reproductive success in response to both predictable and unpredictable environmental events. It is also possible to construct a similar framework but varying E_G rather than E_O. Here the assumption is that food resources may fluctuate without necessarily resulting in an increase in E_O above E_I. Additionally, an LPF may result in a decline of E_G. The result, however, is the same as illustrated in Figure 1.3. When E_G drops below E_I then the individual is in negative energy balance and an ELHS is activated. Both scenarios, or a combination of these (i.e. an increase in E_O or a decrease in E_G), probably occur regularly under natural conditions, but the basic premise that negative energy balance triggers the ELHS remains the same.

1.3.1 Negative energy balance, glucocorticosteroid secretion, and activation of the ELHS

An important question now is: how is negative energy balance perceived? Immediately one thinks of nutritional requirements. As energy reserves are tapped to meet the falling levels of energy intake, then negative energy balance is the peripheral trigger that provides an internal signal to the HPA axis resulting in release of glucocorticosteroids. However, this mechanism may require several hours, especially in larger vertebrates in which negative energy balance may take some time to manifest itself. It may be a function of how much food is already in the gastrointestinal tract, and how long it takes to digest the intestinal contents so that flow of new nutrients ceases. Nevertheless, this may be one important way in which negative energy balance is perceived resulting in activation of corticosterone secretion. It is also possible that detection of the LPF via sensory perception may provide a rapid way to respond to diverse unpredictable events. Typical examples are the 'fight-or-flight' responses mediated within seconds or less by catecholamines (Axelrod and Reisine,

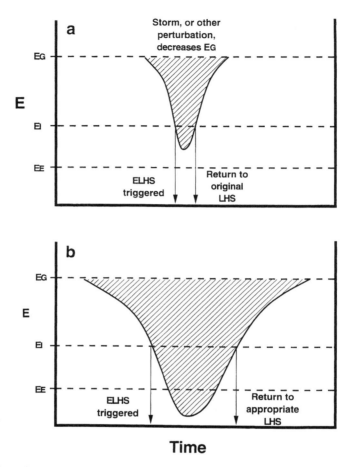

Figure 1.3 Using Figures 1.1 and 1.2 as frameworks, it is possible to model the effects of LPFs of varying intensity and duration on E_G (panels a and b). In these cases E_G declines during an LPF and when it drops below E_I, an ELHS is activated (left-hand arrows in both panels). As the LPF passes E_G increases again and when it exceeds E_I (right-hand arrows in both panels), the individual may return to an appropriate LHS. See text for details.

1984). These reactions to very rapid LPFs such as predators, attack by a dominant conspecific, etc. are usually over within seconds and do not necessarily result in an ELHS. If predator attacks persist, then the effects could become cumulative and trigger an ELHS but, by and large, they are not chronic. Such responses are usually mediated by behavioral and other sensory modalities. However, there is no reason per se why such modalities may not also be used to perceive other types of LPFs. For example, sudden severe storms often trigger facultative behaviors such as seeking a refuge, suggesting that some birds may react to LPFs before going into negative energy balance. In other words the 'fight or flight' response may overlap with an ELHS in some cases. Additional evidence for possible sensory perception of LPFs comes from the domestic fowl. Just showing individuals food after a fast was sufficient to reduce corticosterone levels even though they did not actually get to eat the food (Harvey *et al.*, 1983). Also in mammals there is extensive evidence that psychological variables modulate stress physiology such as 'lack of control' over an LPF or exposure and unpredictability (e.g. Sapolsky, 1992a,b). This emphasizes a fundamental issue in relation to responses to LPFs and perhaps stress in general–how is the negative stimulus perceived? Purely nutritional, non-sensory mechanisms such as negative energy balance in relation to internal levels of glucose, etc., may not be always appropriate mechanisms to activate the ELHS. Sensory mechanisms whereby an organism is in some way able to assess negative environmental stimuli associated with an LPF and react immediately, whether it be by release of catecholamines, glucocorticosteroids or other hormones, may be much more adaptive for most LPFs. More critical research needs to be done here using appropriate animal models and relevant stimuli mimicking natural LPFs.

1.3.2   How is negative energy balance transduced into corticosterone secretion and how quickly does it affect release?

A critical question is how quickly an LPF can trigger an ELHS. This will, of course, depend to a great extent on the severity and intensity of the LPF. Experimental evidence suggests that, in white-crowned sparrows, food withdrawal results in a decrease in blood glucose and an increase in free fatty acid levels for up to 22 h of fasting. Plasma levels of corticosterone rose within at least 2 h of fasting (Richardson, 1996). In rats, food deprivation overnight results in a delay in diel changes in ACTH and corticosterone of about 3 h compared to controls, and a decreased responsivity of ACTH release to stress in the morning (Akana *et al.*, 1994). Overnight fasts also reduce pituitary concentrations of ACTH suggesting increased release during the fast (Hanson *et al.*, 1994). These effects may be exacerbated by a decrease in corticosteroid-binding globulins in blood because food restriction in rats resulted in a decrease in the bound component of circulating corticosterone even though absolute (total) levels in plasma did not change (Sabatino *et al.*, 1991; Nelson *et al.*, 1995). Although there is still much work to be done at this level of analysis, the experimental evidence thus far suggests that time courses of glucocorticosteroid secretion in response to metabolic challenge are within credible limits for the frameworks proposed above. Of particular interest is whether an LPF triggers an increase in glucocorticosteroid secretion via purely metabolic signals in the internal environment, or whether an individual's perception of the LPF is more important. Combinations of these two extremes are also possible, especially in relation to body condition.

1.3.3 What mediates the different effects of corticosterone at different circulating concentrations?

The next question concerns what changes in levels of glucocorticosteroids mean in the contexts of different energy levels over time (Figures 1.1–1.3). That is, different levels of glucocorticosteroids are hypothesized to trigger different things. How do we formalize these concepts? To illustrate this point we propose three levels of secretion, and thus action, of glucocorticosteroids (Wingfield *et al.*, 1997, 1998). In Figure 1.4, level A is a hypothetical baseline of glucocorticosteroid secretion that is required to maintain feedback signals for ACTH release, Na^+/K^+ ATPase, and glucose transporters in many cells (e.g. Chester-Jones *et al.*, 1972; Hadley, 1996). Note that many vertebrates die soon after adrenalectomy, unless given glucose and salt solutions to replace lost ability to regulate glucose and salt balance (Chester-Jones *et al.*, 1972). It is possible that this low level of secretion may be more or less continuous (constitutive) from adrenal cortex cells. Superimposed on level A is the regulated periodic secretion of glucocorticosteroids as stimulated by changes in ACTH release on a daily/seasonal basis. These actions of glucocorticosteroids include homeostatic regulation of glucose, salt balance, activation of daily locomotor activity and a myriad of permissive actions, especially on the sympathetic nervous system (e.g. Chester-Jones *et al.*, 1972; Hadley, 1996). Level B, then, represents changes in glucocorticosteroid titers as directed by predictable environmental fluctuations such as night and day, high tide–low tide, the seasons, etc. These are important for the LHS expressed at any time in the life cycle. Level C represents the regulated but facultative rises of glucocorticosteroid secretion above level B. These surges are transitory, stimulated by LPFs, and trigger the ELHS. Glucocorticosteroid titers remain above level B until the LPF passes or an alternate habitat is located. Note, however, that if glucocorticosteroid concentrations remain above level B for too long then serious debility typical of chronic stress can result. In Figure 1.4 we have also indicated how energy levels may correspond to levels of glucocorticosteroid secretion. Level A corresponds to the existence energy (**E**ᴇ) in our theoretical framework. Daily/seasonal fluctuations in glucocorticosteroid secretion (Level B) during the

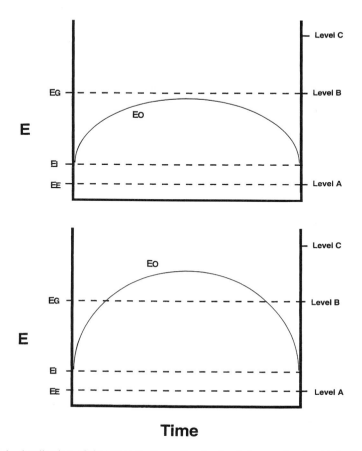

Time

Figure 1.4   Application of the concept of secretion levels of glucocorticosteroids to the energy level framework. Here energy levels are modeled as in Figures 1.1 and 1.2. However, on the right-hand vertical axis, levels of corticosterone secretion are superimposed. Level A refers to the absolute baseline levels of glucocorticosteroids required to maintain life (i.e. corresponding to E_E); B refers to the normal daily or seasonal changes in glucocorticosteroids in relation to the predictable life cycle (i.e. corresponding to $E_E + E_I + E_O$ as long as it remains below E_G). Once E_O exceeds E_G then a different level of glucocorticosteroid secretion is triggered (level C) and the ELHS is activated.

predictable LHSs cover the E_I and E_O levels of energy required as long as they remain below E_G. During an LPF, if $E_E + E_I + E_O$ exceeds E_G (as in Figures 1.2 and 1.3), then glucocorticosteroid secretion increases further, above level B toward level C (Figure 1.4, lower panel). It is this transition in glucocorticosteroid titer in blood that we postulate activates the ELHS. It is possible that excursions of circulating concentrations of glucocorticosteroids to level C may have additional functions, but nonetheless this concept of change in level of secretion can provide a focus for designing future experiments to explore this overall framework further. The HPA is physiologically regulated by glucocorticosteroid feedback under most conditions throughout the 24-h day (and probably seasons as well), but how these feedback signals are over-ridden when secretion increases above level B has been of interest to endocrinologists for some time. Another interesting question is: when hyperactivity occurs (i.e. above level B to C), is it because of increased drive to CRF/AVP neurons from chronic/intermittent stimuli or because of altered feedback efficacy of glucocorticosteroids (e.g. Dallman *et al.*, 1994)?

1.3.4   How quickly does corticosterone act to trigger an ELHS?

Control of secretion of glucocorticosteroids is not the only issue because the levels of secretion postulated in Figure 1.4 suggest different biological actions for glucocorticosteroids at different concentrations. How do target cells differentiate among these levels and respond appropriately? Glucocorticosteroids act through classic intracellular receptors that bind to the genome and regulate gene expression. Two types of intracellular receptors have been identified for glucocorticosteroids in mammals (see McEwen *et al.*, 1988 for review). The type I receptor has a high affinity for corticosteroids and may regulate day-to-day actions of this hormone. This receptor may thus be saturated at intermediate and low levels of hormone, i.e. at levels A and B (Figure 1.4). A second receptor, type II, has a lower affinity for corticosteroids and requires higher concentrations of steroid to become saturated. It is tempting to suggest that type II receptors may mediate the effects of corticosteroids at level C (Figure 1.4). There may, however, be some exceptions to this rule. Prairie voles (*Microtus ochrogaster*) have extremely high plasma levels of glucocorticosteroids. Evidence suggests that their tissues have reduced sensitivity to these high levels, although this is poorly understood at present (Taymans *et al.*, 1997).

Genomic actions of steroid hormones require at least 30 min, usually hours, for the responses to become apparent. More recently it has been shown that some actions of glucocorticosteroids occur within minutes–a time frame inconsistent with classical genomic actions. In rough-skinned newts, *Taricha granulosa*, injections of corticosterone inhibit courtship behavior in males within minutes (Moore and Miller, 1984; Orchinik *et al.*, 1991). Furthermore, non-invasive administration of corticosterone to male white-crowned sparrows results in an increase in plasma levels of corticosterone within 5–10 min and heightens perch hopping activity within 15 min (Breuner *et al.*, 1998). These data point to the presence of a non-genomic receptor that may be able to mediate glucocorticosteroid effects much more rapidly. Evidence for a membrane receptor for corticosterone has been presented for newts (Orchinik *et al.*, 1991). If such membrane receptors for steroid hormones prove to be more widespread, then it is possible that they may play an additional role in mediating the ELHS in response to LPFs. A combination of membrane and genomic actions of glucocorticosteroids may mediate different effects at levels A, B and C.

There is evidence in mammals for activation of different types of corticosteroid receptors in different physiological states. In rats, changes in feedback sensitivity appear to be paralleled by changes in the type of receptor that is activated. In the morning when sensitivity to feedback is greatest, type I receptors may predominate, whereas later in the day when sensitivity to feedback decreases, type II receptors may be more important (Bradbury *et al.*, 1994). Moreover, occupation of type I receptors may potentiate actions of type II receptors as they then become occupied. In adrenalectomized female rats, high doses of corticosterone proved to be catabolic as expected. However, in adrenalectomized rats with lesions of the ventromedial hypothalamus, all doses of corticosterone resulted in weight gain. Thus, damage to the basomedial hypothalamus appears to influence the response to corticosterone at both ends of a dose-response curve. Occupation of both type I and II receptors appear to be involved (King *et al.*, 1993). It has also been demonstrated that the basal daily peak of corticosterone coincides with the point when stress responsiveness is lowest; and, stress responsiveness is highest when basal daily level of corticosterone is lowest (Dallman *et al.*, 1993).

In general these phenomena are entirely consistent with the hypotheses and frameworks relating to responses to natural LPFs. Different levels of glucocorticosteroid secretion mediate different effects and at high doses may be equivalent to level C (Figure 1.4) and trigger the ELHS. It is hoped that the framework developed in Figures 1.1–1.4 will have heuristic value in designing experiments to explore the mechanisms underlying the responses of organisms to unpredictable events (LPFs) and how the ELHS is orchestrated.

1.4   Examples of what happens when $E_O + E_I + E_E > E_G$ in free-living animals

Given the theoretical framework outlined above, it is important to turn to the field and determine whether organisms under natural conditions show elevated circulating levels of glucocorticosteroids when challenged by LPFs, and then whether the ELHS is triggered. There are now numerous studies indicating that individuals responding to unpredictable events in the environment, such as direct LPFs, show elevated levels of glucocorticosteroids in blood, consistent with development of an ELHS (see Wingfield, 1994; Wingfield *et al.*, 1998 for reviews). Endocrine and neuroendocrine evidence to date supports the theoretical framework– allowing further, more critical, experiments to be designed in order to determine whether common basic mechanisms may be involved, despite great diversity of LPFs, habitats, and stages in the life cycle when an ELHS may be activated. Next we wish to describe several scenarios in the field when an ELHS was triggered, and how the theoretical framework may provide a unifying base to explain potential mechanisms. In the space available it is not possible to review all of the evidence, but we will choose examples from widely different habitats and LHSs.

1.4.1   Breeding seasons

Reproduction entails additional energetic costs over and above E_E and E_I (Figure 1.5). These costs are represented by the line E_Y that includes the added energy required to produce young and raise them to independence. In many ways it has parallels to E_O in Figures 1.2–1.4, but E_Y is always part of the predictable life cycle. Natural selection has favored the cost of E_Y to remain below E_G. However, as E_Y increases, susceptibility to storms and other LPFs that result in an increase in E_O becomes greater (Figure 1.5, upper panel). The outcome is the same if we model this as a decrease in E_G (Figure 1.5, lower panel). For example, in male white-crowned sparrows baseline corticosterone levels increase normally during the nesting season (within level B of Figure 1.5; Wingfield *et al.*, 1997) and decline thereafter (toward level A of Figure 1.5; Wingfield *et al.*, 1997). However, in May 1980, a severe and prolonged storm resulted in abandonment of their nests and territories. Circulating levels of corticosterone were greatly elevated (level C of Figure 1.5) at this time compared with males sampled in a year with no storm (Wingfield and Farner, 1978; Wingfield *et al.*, 1983). Later in the season, after the severe storm had passed and birds were re-nesting, plasma levels of corticosterone had returned to normal for that time of year (i.e. within level B of Figure 1.5). During the storm, subcutaneous fat depots were virtually depleted, but returned to normal after the storm had passed and when re-nesting was initiated. Thus corticosterone levels were high when an ELHS had been triggered. It should also be noted that during the storm of 1980, male white-crowned sparrows had normal levels of luteinizing hormone and testosterone, thus supporting the hypothesis that corticosterone may be acting directly to suppress expression of reproductive behavior rather

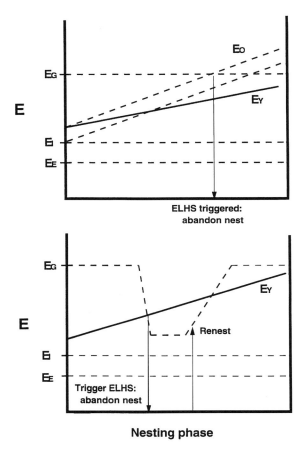

Figure 1.5 Energy framework in relation to breeding seasons of birds. As the nesting phase of reproduction progresses then the line E_Y represents the increasing additional energy required to incubate eggs and feed young to independence. Natural selection on this reproductive effort has favored the slope of E_Y to remain below E_G thus maximizing reproductive success. However, if an LPF should occur then E_O increases energy requirements such that it may exceed E_G (upper broken line for E_O) resulting in an ELHS (indicated by the arrow in the upper panel). For animals not breeding, E_O would take longer to trigger an ELHS because the line starts from E_I, not E_Y (see lower broken line for E_O). Alternatively, E_G may decrease and an ELHS (including abandonment of the nest) will occur when it drops below E_Y (left-hand arrow of lower panel). Note that as the LPF passes and E_G increases again, re-nesting will occur.

than indirectly through decreased secretion of sex steroids. Further research is needed to determine the mechanisms and locus of corticosterone action in this regard. Note in Figure 1.5 that re-nesting occurs when E_G returns to normal or when E_O drops to a sufficiently low level.

1.4.2   Modeling LPF intensity–a different approach
applicable to all seasons

Instead of modeling changes in energy levels with time (such as an annual cycle, etc.), it is also possible to model storm intensity at any point in time. Figure 1.6 illustrates the normal lines E_E, E_I and E_G, while the X axis depicts increasing storm (or other LPF) intensity. As E_O increases with LPF intensity, it crosses E_G, glucocorticosteroid secretion increases

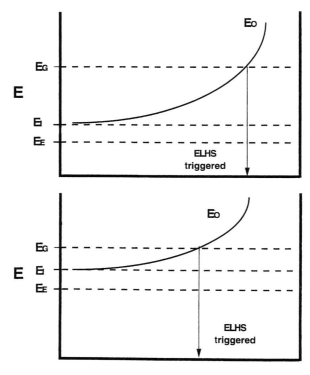

Labile Perturbation Factors
(snow, wind speed, rain, temperature,
predator pressure, human disturbance etc.)

Figure 1.6   Modeling the energy framework in relation to intensity of the labile perturbation factor (LPF). The vertical axis is as in Figures 1.1–1.5, but the horizontal axis now represents intensity and duration of LPFs such as snowfall, rain, wind speed, temperature, predator pressure, human disturbance, etc. As intensity (or duration) of the LPF increases then E_O increases and triggers an emergency life history stage (ELHS) when it crosses E_G (upper panel). If local conditions are more energetically demanding (e.g. winter conditions) then E_E is higher (lower panel) and the LPF will trigger an ELHS at lower intensity (or duration).

above level B and an ELHS is triggered. An alternative way to describe this would be when **EG** decreases as a function of LPF intensity (not shown). Note also that the same intensity of LPF can trigger an ELHS at varying times depending upon local conditions at the time. For example, if ambient temperature were lower then **EE** would be higher, **EI** the same, but **Eo** would increase at the same rate resulting in an earlier activation of the ELHS (Figure 1.6, lower panel). Many other local environmental variables could modeled in this way. There are numerous examples from free-living vertebrates–we present four types in the non-breeding and breeding seasons.

1.4.2.1 Snow and ground-feeding birds
Dark-eyed juncos, *Junco hyemalis*, have significantly higher plasma levels of corticosterone during a snow storm than before or after (Rogers *et al.*, 1993). This elevation is accompanied by abandonment of home range. Similarly in European blackbirds, *Turdus merula*, in southern Germany, severe cold and snow results in first-year birds of both sexes migrating south leaving adults behind. Young European blackbirds of both sexes have significantly higher plasma levels of corticosterone just prior to their departure than in the non-migratory adults (Schwabl *et al.*, 1985). These data are consistent with a role for elevated corticosterone secretion triggering an ELHS in response to an LPF. As snow and/or ice covered resources of ground-feeding birds, then **Eo** expended in digging for food would soon exceed **EG** resulting in an increase in corticosterone. Severe weather in the non-breeding season is also accompanied by elevated circulating corticosterone in Harris' sparrows, *Zonotrichia querula* (Rohwer and Wingfield, 1981). In contrast, these sparrows did not leave the area but became inactive to 'ride-out' the storm (i.e. a 'take it' strategy).

1.4.2.2 Oceanic weather and marine birds
By contrast, an example in a totally different habitat, the open ocean, illustrates how the framework provides a potential common pathway for triggering an ELHS in response to LPFs. In the southern oceans a guild of seabirds has evolved that are almost entirely pelagic; they usually return to land only to breed. The common diving petrel, *Pelecanoides urinatrix*, may be an exception because, under very severe weather conditions, it may retreat to oceanic islands to wait out the storm. Normally these diving petrels feed on krill swarms within 30 m of the ocean surface and withstand high winds and mountainous seas, as do many seabirds in this region. In June 1991 a severe storm occurred including high winds, low temperatures, snow, and near zero visibility. These conditions tend to reduce feeding efficiency on the open ocean (Veit *et al.*, 1991), and can be interpreted either as an increase in **Eo** or a

decrease in E_G (Figure 1.6). Body masses of birds during the storm are lower than those of birds captured during calm weather and they have significantly higher levels of corticosterone (Smith *et al.*, 1994). During the storm large numbers of diving petrels were flying toward Annekov Island–an island known to be a breeding locality and where burrows could provide shelter. These responses to an LPF are remarkably similar to those of the ground-feeding passerines described above.

1.4.2.3   Prolonged human disturbance
Recent investigations demonstrate that human disturbance may also elicit the ELHS in natural populations. Human disturbance associated with building development, agriculture, harvesting natural resources, etc. is an unpredictable event to wildlife and qualifies as an LPF. Wasser *et al.* (1997) have measured fecal levels of glucocorticosteroids as an indication of circulating levels extended over time. Additionally, non-invasive collection of droppings is a way of obtaining useful endocrine information from threatened or endangered species for which capture and handling may not be appropriate. The presence of logging roads near nests of Northern spotted owls (*Strix occidentalis*), and disruptive logging practices such as felling trees over large areas (clear cutting), are correlated with elevated glucocorticosteroid levels in feces, at least in males. Although these data do not yet indicate a causal relation, they suggest that triggering an ELHS may be one mechanism by which human disturbance reduces populations of wildlife.

1.4.2.4   Intraspecific competition
It has long been known that social disruption caused by immigration of conspecifics is often unpredictable (i.e. qualifying as an LPF) and has profound effects on the endocrine system. There can be long-term changes in glucocorticosteroid levels depending upon an individual's social status (e.g. Sapolsky, 1987; Schwabl, 1995; Creel *et al.*, 1996). Most of these studies have determined that the endocrine profiles of individuals in stable dominance hierarchies, and endocrine differences between high and low ranking animals, may remain stable for a considerable period. Responses of the HPA axis to short-term perturbations in a dominance hierarchy trigger release of cortisol in a free-living population of olive baboons, *Papio anubis* (Alberts *et al.*, 1992; Sapolsky, 1992a,b). During these periods aggression increases dramatically as well. Whether or not these increased levels of cortisol resulting from unpredictable social interactions may also push an individual into an ELHS is an intriguing possibility. On the other hand, moving from one troop to another is extremely difficult and living alone is impossible. In these cases, the possibility of chronic stress in subordinates, especially during poor

trophic conditions, is likely (Sapolsky, 1987, 1992a,b)—an unusual event in free-living populations.

In tree lizards (*Urosaurus ornatus*), both a territorial morph and a non-territorial morph show increases in plasma corticosterone following male–male encounters, but the territorial morph appears to show less of a decline in testosterone levels as a result (Knapp and Moore, 1996). Physical restraint (experimental application of an LPF that mimics a predation attempt, see below) results in an increase in corticosterone in both morphs and a negative correlation with testosterone levels in the non-territorial lizards (Knapp and Moore, 1997). Furthermore, implants of corticosterone induce a decline in testosterone in both morphs but more robustly in the non-territorial morph (Knapp and Moore, 1997). These data clearly suggest not only differential sensitivity to corticosterone in the two morphs, but also an effect of social status on responses to an LPF.

These examples from different taxa and breeding status in widely varying habitats can be modeled by the energy framework in Figure 1.6. Although more experimental work is required, the data thus far are consistent with a common pathway by which adrenococortical function is triggered and the ELHS activated.

1.5 Modulation of the adrenocortical responses to LPFs–possible ecological bases of endocrine phenomena

Adrenocortical responses to LPFs vary considerably from species to species, among populations within a species, with gender, season and individual, or even in some cases variation between laboratories using different techniques (e.g. in reptiles: Gregory *et al.*, 1996; Moore *et al.*, 1991; birds: Wingfield, 1994; mammals: Walker, 1994). There is little doubt that changes in HPA axis responses (i.e. changing sensitivity) of individuals to LPFs are occurring (Sapolsky, 1987; Schwabl, 1995; Walker, 1994; Wingfield, 1994; Wingfield *et al.*, 1998). One intriguing question is whether such variation has ecological and physiological bases, or is this physiological 'noise'? Controlled field investigations are critical here because data collected from free-living organisms are much less likely to represent 'noise'. However, before exploring possible ecological bases it is necessary to discuss the evidence for modulation of HPA responses to stress. There are roughly four main types of modulation as follows (see also Figure 1.7 for examples):

(a) Variation among species living in different habitats (e.g. Wingfield *et al.*, 1992; O'Reilly, 1995; Silverin *et al.*, 1997). Comparisons of

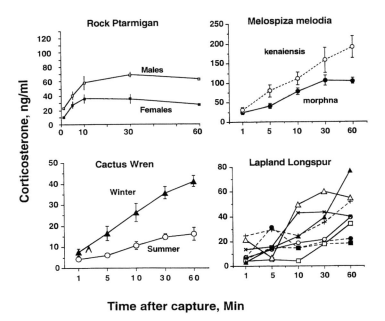

Time after capture, Min

Figure 1.7 Examples of modulation of the hypothalamo–pituitary–adrenal axis (HPA). There are clear gender differences in breeding rock ptarmigan (*Lagopus mutus*), and locality differences in two sub-species of song sparrow (*Melospiza melodia morphna* at mid-latitudes, Seattle, Washington State and *M.m. kenaiensis* at higher latitudes, Cordova, Alaska). In the cactus wren (*Campylorhynchus brunneicapillus*), there is a decrease in sensitivity of the HPA to an LPF in summer. In Lapland longspurs (*Calcarius lapponicus*) there is extreme individual variation within a population at the same stage in breeding. Data compiled from Wingfield *et al.*, 1992, 1994b, 1995b).

closely related species decreases the likelihood of phylogenetic differences (see upper right hand panel of Figure 1.7). This could include seasonal variation or with time of day, sexual dimorphism (upper left hand panel of Figure 1.7), or during development within a population, e.g. breeding season and non-breeding seasons. See also lower left hand panel of Figure 1.7.

(b) Individual variation within a population and season. For example, adrenocortical sensitivity to acute stress may vary as a function of social status, body condition, infection, and other factors, see lower right hand panel of Figure 1.7).

(c) Variation in physiological and behavioral responses to elevated levels of glucocorticosteroids (Sapolsky, 1992a,b). Changes in receptor numbers and distribution, as well as intracellular enzymes that have the potential to convert glucocorticosteroids to inactive

11-keto forms could be involved. For example, 11β-hydroxyster-oid-dehydrogenase converts cortisol to an inactive form of cortisone, or corticosterone to 11-dehydrocorticosterone. Regulation of this enzyme within target cells is an additional mechanism by which the action of glucocorticosteroids may be modulated (Funder *et al.*, 1988; Seckl and Brown, 1994).

(d) Recent evidence suggests that there is variation in the ability to turn off the adrenocortical response to LPFs and thus prevent further increases in secretion of glucocorticosteroids (e.g. Whittier *et al.*, 1987; Sapolsky, 1992a,b; Dufty and Belthoff, 1997). This may give some individuals an advantage in resisting the effects of an LPF.

Given these types of examples, it appears that as the sensitivity of the HPA axis to LPFs decreases there is an increasing resistance potential, perhaps to LPFs in general. This is represented on the vertical axis of Figure 1.8. Variation in this resistance potential may be a function of

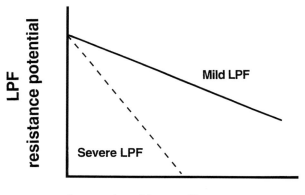

Length of breeding season

Figure 1.8   The relationship of changing sensitivity of the hypothalamic–pituitary–adrenal axis to labile perturbation factors (LPFs). As the life history stage (LHS) or other component of the life cycle changes (e.g. in this case length of the breeding season), then the resistance potential to LPFs also changes. In this example, if the length of the breeding season is short then the number of attempts at reproducing will be few and thus reduced sensitivity to LPFs might maximize the chances of reproductive success in relation to an unpredictable environment. As the length of the breeding season increases (and hence the number of potential attempts at reproducing increases) then greater sensitivity to LPFs should be retained so as to maximize the potential of breeding when environmental conditions are most conducive to success. Thus, this scheme predicts that adrenocortical responses to acute stress would be reduced in a population that has a short breeding season versus a population with a long breeding season. Note that severity of the LPF may have an effect. The most severe LPFs would likely result in reproductive failure and activation of an emergency life history stage (ELHS) regardless of length of the breeding season. Hence this line (broken) is steeper than for a mild LPF. See text for further examples.

many ecological factors such as, for example, length of the breeding season (Figure 1.8). Note that the change in resistance potential may be much more rapid with severe LPFs so that there is no resistance at all in many cases (broken line in Figure 1.8). At this point all individuals should respond with an increase in glucocorticosteroid secretion and activate an ELHS. With milder LPFs, resistance potentials may be more effective over a wider range of ecological variation (solid line of Figure 1.8). But how can we establish what these ecological factors may be so that we can then generate hypotheses designed to investigate mechanisms by which such modulation occurs? To do this it is critical that an experimental LPF be applied in a comparable manner across all species, populations and individuals so that possible ecological bases can be tested in a controlled manner. A standardized stress protocol has been devised so that such broad comparisons can be made. Capture, handling and restraint elicit marked increases in circulating glucocorticosteroids in virtually all species from teleost fish to mammals (Holmes and Phillips, 1976; Harvey *et al.*, 1984; Greenberg and Wingfield, 1987). Because adrenocortical responses to capture are likely to be comparable across all species, then a 'capture stress' protocol is an effective way of assessing sensitivity of the HPA axis to acute stress in general (see Schwabl, 1995; Wingfield, 1994 for details). Similarly, Sapolsky (1982, 1987) used the stress of darting olive baboons with an anesthetic to follow changes in plasma levels of cortisol because all individuals were treated the same way. At first it may appear more logical to use other techniques that more closely resemble potential LPFs, such as low or high temperature, food restriction, etc., but responses of individuals to these stimuli vary as a function of season and body condition and many other factors (Wingfield, 1994). The capture stress protocol appears highly artificial, but it is a reasonable assumption and all individuals regard the procedure as a potential 'predation attempt' by the investigator. Virtually all animals struggle, show elevated respiration rates and may give distress vocalizations when they are captured and handled. We feel that this approach provides a repeatable and uniform acute stress that is a meaningful measure of responsiveness of the HPA axis. The technique has the advantage that it can be compared across individuals, populations, seasons, etc. to provide insight into possible ecological bases of population and individual variation (Wingfield, 1994).

The capture stress protocol entails collecting approximately 30 μl of whole blood from an appropriate vein (e.g. wing vein for birds, orbital sinus for small mammals, reptiles, caudal vein for many species of fish) as soon as possible after capture (usually within 2 min). Samples collected within 2 min after capture approximate closely the baseline concentrations of glucocorticosteroids just prior to capture. Further samples are then collected at, for example, 5, 10, 30 and 60 min following capture. Between sample collections, individuals can be restrained in cloth bags closed by a draw string for restraint (or similar device appropriate for the species investigated). Plasma levels of glucocorticosteroids in these samples is an indication of the degree and time course of the response to capture, handling and restraint (e.g. Wingfield, 1994). Because heightened adrenocortical secretion occurs following an extremely wide spectrum of stresses (acute and chronic), we feel that the subsequent rise of plasma glucocorticosteroid levels during the capture stress protocol is a useful indication of the sensitivity of the HPA axis to acute stress. With such an experimental tool in hand it is possible to test hypotheses in the field and laboratory, on free-living populations at specific seasons, etc., or in captive animals subjected to controlled conditions.

This protocol also allows us to investigate the pattern of glucocorticosteroid secretion during the early responses to an LPF. For example, there may be variations in the rate of increase of glucocorticosteroids, the maximum level obtained, and also in the degree to which secretion is turned off quickly resulting in a decline of glucocorticosteroid levels. This has been observed in baboons (e.g. Sapolsky, 1992b), Western screech owls, *Otus kennicottii*, (Dufty and Belthoff, 1997) and in the red-sided garter snakes, *Thamnophis sirtalis parietalis*, where there is a significant decline in corticosterone after 1 h of confinement (Whittier *et al.*, 1987). Much less well understood is how responsiveness to elevated glucocorticosteroid concentrations may change. This is a very important possibility that can be approached in the field with experimental implants of glucocorticosteroids or the peptides that regulate glucocorticosteroid secretion. Changes in receptor types, numbers and distribution will also likely prove to be important. Some examples of what these variations in responses of the HPA axis to LPFs are discussed next.

1.5.1 Variation in sensitivity of the HPA axis among populations, and within populations across seasons

In Figure 1.8, it is suggested that as the length of the breeding season increases (horizontal axis) then the LPF resistance potential (i.e. sensitivity of the HPA axis to LPFs) should be lower. For example, spring weather at high latitudes (such as the Arctic) is often very severe, but the breeding season is so short that only one reproductive attempt is possible and any delay could reduce reproductive success. If inclement spring weather in the Arctic induced an increase in adrenocortical response, then an ELHS would be triggered that would in turn disrupt breeding. Therefore, sensitivity of the HPA axis to LPFs should be reduced. This would allow individuals to initiate breeding despite potentially stressful conditions. It is possible that such resistance to LPFs early in the breeding season might increase the potential for debilitation or even mortality, but the 'pay-off' is maximum reproductive success. Many other ecological factors could be modeled in the horizontal axis of Figure 1.8, but here we will discuss three: seasonal changes in relation to length of breeding seasons (especially in severe environments), breeding strategy (such as expression of parental care), and facultative responses to local conditions.

1.5.1.1   Length of the breeding season and severe environments
In the Alaskan Arctic, sensitivity of the HPA axis to the capture stress protocol in breeding snow buntings, *Plectrophenax nivalis*, sampled at Barrow, Alaska (71°N), female redpolls, *Carduelis flammea*, and Lapland longspurs, *Calcarius lapponicus*, sampled at Barrow and Toolik Lake (68°N), Alaska, are generally lower than those of passerine species sampled in temperate zone regions (Dawson and Howe, 1983; Wingfield et al., 1992, 1994a,b). Furthermore, two breeding populations of semi-palmated sandpiper, *Calidris pusilla*, studied at a location in the low arctic (near Nome, Alaska) and another in the high arctic (Barrow/ Prudhoe Bay, Alaska) show that maximum circulating levels of corticosterone are lower at the most northerly sites with most severe weather (O'Reilly, 1995). These data are consistent with the hypothesis of increased LPF resistance potential in severe environments. This hypothesis is further bolstered by the findings of Wingfield et al. (1992), that birds breeding in another extreme environment, the Sonoran Desert of Arizona, have lower responsiveness of circulating levels of corticosterone to capture stress than in the non-breeding season (winter). Species breeding in more benign riparian habitat nearby show no such modulation. Those breeding in the Sonoran Desert have by far the greatest reproductive success during the ephemeral monsoons of July and August. In contrast, those species breeding in riparian habitat with permanent shade and water have opportunity for good reproductive success over a much longer period of the year. Hence, there should be selection for mechanisms to modulate the adrenocortical responses to acute stress in desert birds (i.e. increase LPF resistance potential), but not in species that inhabit riparian zones nearby.

It should be noted, however, that not all species breeding in extreme environments suppress the sensitivity of the HPA to LPFs. Some species sampled at intermediate latitudes show a different pattern. Preliminary data from white-crowned sparrows sampled at Fairbanks, Alaska (64°N) suggest that breeding females have much lower levels of corticosterone following capture, handling and restraint than males (Wingfield et al., 1982). However, further studies reveal that early in the breeding season, males actually increase their sensitivity to the capture stress protocol, possibly as a result of reduced sensitivity to glucocorticosteroid feedback (Astheimer *et al.*, 1994). Comparisons between two taxa of male song sparrow further complicate the issue. Males in a northern sub-species (*Melospiza melodia kenaiensis*) sampled from a breeding population on the Copper River Delta near Cordova, Alaska (61°N) in May 1992, show a slightly more pronounced increase in plasma levels of corticosterone following capture, handling and restraint than do males in a population of song sparrows (*M.m. morphna*) breeding in western Washington State (48°N) (Wingfield *et al.*, 1995b). Similar results are found when comparing northern and southern populations of bush warblers, *Cettia diphone*, in Japan (Wingfield *et al.*, 1995a). Although some species breeding in extreme environments show reduced sensitivity to capture stress (LPF resistance potential) compared with those in more temperate climates, others do not. We should be careful, however, to temper these conclusions until information on the distribution and number of corticosterone receptors in the central nervous system becomes available. Nonetheless, reduced sensitivity of the HPA system to the capture stress protocol may not be a general phenomenon in arctic breeding birds–other ecological factors may apply.

Variation in the magnitude of adrenocortical responses to stress (both seasonal and across populations) raises a number of questions concerning the underlying causes. Firstly, there appears to be a phylogenetic component to species differences in maximum corticosterone level attained during the capture stress protocol (Wingfield *et al.*, 1995b). The mean maximum corticosterone level in charadriiformes is significantly higher than in both passeriformes and galliformes. Whether this has functional significance and/or is simply phylogenetic remains to be determined. Secondly, although galliformes and charadriiformes tend to be larger than the passeriformes, there is no relationship of body mass with either maximum corticosterone level or the ratio of maximum to minimum levels during the capture stress protocol. Even though the charadriiformes had higher maximum corticosterone levels than the other orders, there is no trend within groups, and this phylogenetic component does not appear to be biasing the relationship with body mass (Wingfield *et al.*, 1995b). Thirdly, species with a greater life expectancy should have more potential attempts at breeding than those with lower life expectancy. Thus, longer lived species should retain sensitivity to acute stress while short-lived species should be resistant. The galliformes and two charadriiformes have greater longevity than other charadriiformes and the passeriformes, but there is no relationship with either maximum corticosterone level or the ratio of maximum to minimum corticosterone levels. Again, there are also no trends within groups and it is unlikely that the phylogenetic relationship is biasing the results (Wingfield *et al.*, 1995b).

1.5.1.2 Breeding strategy, parental care

Sexual dimorphism in profiles of corticosterone plasma levels following capture, handling and restraint, suggest that expression of parental care by each sex and species may be related to the modulation of adreno-cortical responses to acute stress (see the upper left hand panel of Figure 1.7; Wingfield *et al.*, 1995b). Arctic-breeding birds showing less parental care have higher maximum corticosterone levels generated by the capture stress protocol and the ratio of maximum/minimum corticosterone level tends to be higher than in birds which express more parental care (Wingfield *et al.*, 1995b). Moreover, in shorebirds breeding in northern Alaska in which each sex displays varying degrees of parental care, the sex showing most parental behavior always had lower maximal levels of corticosterone after 30 min of the capture stress protocol. Interestingly, a species in which males and females provide equal amounts of parental care had similar maximal levels of corticosterone in the same experimental procedure (O'Reilly, 1995). In the latter study, phylogenetic problems were minimized since the species are closely related. Thus, it is possible that expression of parental behavior is an ecological base for increased LPF resistance potential. This modulation may be more evident if the species also breeds in extreme environments.

1.5.1.3 Facultative variation within a population
in relation to local conditions

We have emphasized repeatedly that modulation of the adrenocortical responses to stress applies to acute perturbations–over minutes to hours. If the perturbation turns out to be more persistent, i.e. extend duration to several days, then abandonment of the nest (i.e. trigger an emergency life history stage) may become advantageous after all and the LPF resistance potential should be overcome. Only if the perturbation is transient is it likely that modulation of the HPA axis would be favored. Recent field evidence from arctic Alaska suggests that modulation of the HPA axis may be far more labile than we previously thought. A prolonged snow storm (four days) at Toolik Lake, Alaska, in June 1990 was resisted by breeding Lapland longspurs for at least three days. Females remained on nests under snow. By the end of the third day, conditions were still severe and the Lapland longspurs started to abandon nests and territories. A number of these birds were captured after they ceased breeding and were wandering over the tundra. The rate of increase in corticosterone levels in response to capture stress was greatly increased over rates before the storm (Astheimer *et al.*, 1995). These data suggest that longspurs actually up-regulated their responsiveness to acute stress within a few days during the prolonged and severe snow storm. Clearly, modulation of the adrenocortical response to capture stress (LPF resistance potential) can occur in both directions and possibly serves to adjust responsiveness to perturbations of the environment thereby maximizing reproductive success in the long term.

1.5.2   Individual variation within a population and season

Comparisons of individual profiles of corticosterone levels in blood during the capture stress protocol reveal marked variation (e.g. Figure 1.7, lower right hand panel) in addition to that seen at the population level. This may occur in either sex, involve variation in initial level of corticosterone, as well as the rate of increase, maximal level generated during the 60 min protocol, and whether levels decline quickly after an initial increase (Wingfield, 1994). The example in the lower right hand panel of Figure 1.7 is for Lapland longspurs sampled at Barrow Alaska. Some birds (e.g. profile with solid squares) show no adrenocortical response to the capture stress protocol, whereas others (e.g. profile with solid triangles) show an order of magnitude increase in circulating corticosterone levels. This type of individual variation within a population, gender and LHS has been observed in several other species and may represent characteristic individual LPF resistance potentials (see Wingfield et al., 1994a,b). What basis, if any, is there for this pronounced variation?

1.5.2.1   Variation due to social status

It has long been known that subordinate animals in a social hierarchy either have higher baseline levels of glucocorticosteroids circulating in blood or have a greater adrenocortical response to other stresses (e.g. Sapolsky, 1982, 1987; Axelrod and Reisine, 1984). Thus, we can predict that for a population exposed to any given LPF, the subordinates would be more susceptible to that LPF and trigger an ELHS stage before dominants in that population. In Figure 1.9 we have applied this hypothesis to the theoretical framework. In the top panel (Figure 1.9a) we have E_E, E_I and E_G as usual with time (e.g. season, day, etc.) on the horizontal axis. When an LPF is applied E_O increases but the line will be generally lower for dominants than for subordinates. Dominant individuals in the population have greater access to food and shelter and thus would be less energetically challenged than subordinates and hence the different lines for E_O. Note that in this case, the top dominants should not trigger an ELHS whereas at least three subordinates have such a high E_O profile that it triggers an ELHS (indicated by the left-hand

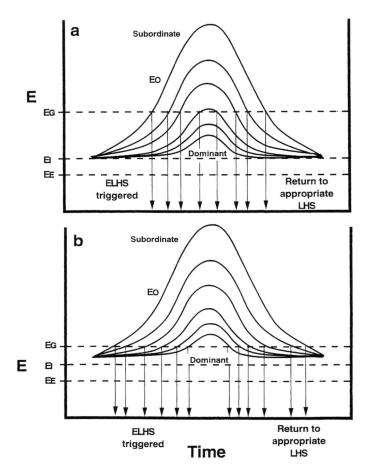

Figure 1.9 Social status and individual variation in **Eo** of a population subjected to the same labile perturbation factor (LPF). The lines **Ee**, **Ei** and **Eg** are as in earlier figures (Figures 1.1–1.6). However, the line **Eo** (increase in energy required to find food and process it) increases as a function of social status in a population. The smallest **Eo** lines (i.e. low amplitude) represent the increased energy in the face of an LPF for dominant individuals who have priority of access to food resources and shelter. **Eo** increases in intensity as status decreases and the most subordinate animals with lowest priority of access to food and shelter should trigger an ELHS earlier, and for longer periods than dominants (arrows on left-hand side of upper panel–a). They should also return to a normal LHS later than dominants (right-hand arrows of Figure 1.9a). Note that in the upper panel some top dominants may not have to trigger an ELHS at all and should remain in their normal LHS. In the lower panel (b), **Eg** has been decreased as another way of modeling the effects of social status. In this scenario **Eo** exceeds **Eg** in all cases and all individuals should trigger an ELHS. However, the time taken for this to occur is longer in dominants (left-hand arrows of Figure 1.9b), and they return to a normal LHS much more quickly as LPF and **Eo** subside (right-hand arrows of Figure 1.9b). These models indicate that dominant individuals have a distinct advantage in dealing with LPFs.

arrows in Figure 1.9a). As the LPF subsides and **Eo** declines, then these subordinates may rejoin the group, if they survive (right-hand arrows of Figure 1.9a).

We can also model this slightly differently by showing that if there is a decline in **EG** (e.g. as during winter), and/or an increase in **EE**, then an LPF will increase **Eo** such that all individuals of the population will eventually trigger an ELHS, but the time taken to do this will vary as a function of social status. Subordinates will always have **Eo** exceed **EG** before dominants (left-hand arrows of Figure 1.9b). As the LPF subsides then individuals will resume the normal LHS with dominants recovering before subordinates (right-hand arrows of Figure 1.9b). Here again, the theoretical framework makes specific predictions concerning when glucocorticosteroids rise and trigger an ELHS in relation to individual social status. Is there evidence for this in the wild?

In the olive baboon, subordinate animals tend to have higher baseline cortisol levels than dominants, but responsiveness to acute stress (darting and anesthesia) is muted in subordinates (Sapolsky, 1982, 1987, 1995). The mechanism of cortisol release is disrupted in subordinate males, and dominants are more sensitive to feedback (Sapolsky, 1995). Social subordinance or social isolation results in hypercortisolism or feedback resistance (Sapolsky *et al.*, 1997). In a drought year in East Africa, food resources became scarce as a result (e.g. a form of LPF), and subordinate animals had reduced levels of testosterone compared with other years suggesting a stressed state (Sapolsky, 1987). In the European blackbird, first-year males and females are subordinate to adults in wintering populations in southern Germany. In a year when temperatures were low and snowfall high many first birds left the wintering range and flew south whereas those that stayed were mostly adults. Plasma of corticosterone in first-year birds that left were higher (in both sexes) than those of adults that stayed (Schwabl *et al.*, 1985). In winter flocks of white-throated sparrows, dominant birds had lower profiles of corticosterone following the capture stress protocol than did subordinates (Schwabl, 1995). The evidence, although limited at present, thus supports the hypotheses and predictions generated from the model. Note, however, in free-living Cape hunting dogs, *Lycaon pictus*, of Africa, fecal glucocorticosteroid levels indicate that the reverse may be true (Creel *et al.*, 1996).

There is additional evidence that individuals react differently to similar LPFs. Even among dominant baboons, some individuals appear more able to deal with stress than others (styles of dominance–Sapolsky, 1992a,b). A subset of subordinate males tends to fare better than other subordinates and tends to move into more dominant positions later in life. These males had higher adrenocortical sensitivity to stress as well as higher baseline levels of cortisol. These data suggest that factors other

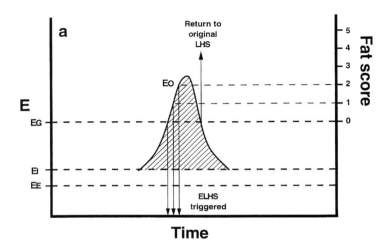

Figure 1.10a and b Variation in activation of an emergency life history stage (ELHS) in relation to body condition measured in this case as fat score (this scale on the upper right-hand vertical axis is the average of an arbitrary score for fat depots both subcutaneous and intraperitoneal, as follows: 0 = no fat and thus no reserves, to 5 = bulging fat depots; see Wingfield and Farner, 1978). The lines E_E, E_I and E_G are as in Figures 1.1–1.6. In response to a labile perturbation factor (LPF), E_O increases (line with shading underneath) and when it crosses E_G an emergency life history stage (ELHS) should be triggered. However, if fat can be mobilized quickly as an energy source then the LPF resistance potential will also be increased.

Figure 1.10a E_O exceeds lines representing those individuals with low fat scores (poorer body condition) and they will thus activate an ELHS (downward arrows on the left-hand side of the upper panel). Those with larger fat scores (better body condition) will have LPF resistance potential sufficiently great so that E_O does not trigger an ELHS and they can remain in their normal LHS. However, when the LPF subsides and E_O decreases, those individuals in poor body condition should not return to a normal LHS until E_G is greater than E_O and they can then replenish reserves (upward pointing arrow on the right-hand side of Figure 1.10a).

than dominance status alone may also play a role (Virgin and Sapolsky, 1997). Stable hierarchies also tend to allow greater resistance to additional stress than unstable hierarchies (Sapolsky, 1992a,b). Some differences in resistance to stress among individuals may be related to experience during development. Early environmental events have a profound influence on development of the HPA response to stressful stimuli. Rats exposed to short periods of handling neonatally show decreased responsiveness to stress when adult. On the other hand, maternal separation, physical trauma, endotoxin, etc. when young can increase HPA responses to stress in the adult. These effects persist throughout adult life and include increases in hypothalamic levels of mRNA for CRF and AVP. Changes in feedback sensitivity and

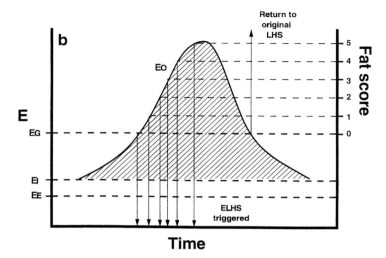

Figure 1.10b An LPF of greater intensity and duration is depicted. In this scenario **Eo** increases to such an extent that even individuals in best body condition should trigger an ELHS, although those with the highest fat scores will take longer to do so (downward arrows on left-hand side of Figure). Because fat score will be depleted once **Eo** exceeds **EG**, return to a normal LHS should not occur until **Eo** drops below **EG** and all individuals can replenish reserves (upward arrow on right-hand side of Figure).

glucocorticosteroid receptor expression also occur (e.g. Francis *et al.*, 1996; Meaney *et al.*, 1996).

1.5.2.2   Variation with body condition

Although this hypothesis is not necessarily mutually exclusive from variation due to social status it may, nonetheless, be important in some populations. It is suggested that if an individual is able to increase its LPF resistance potential by mobilizing fat stores (and possibly other sources such as glycogen and protein), then it can delay triggering an ELHS and perhaps remain in a normal LHS. This idea is modeled in Figure 1.10. In the upper panel (Figure 1.10a), **EE**, **EI** and **EG** are as normal and **Eo** (line shaded underneath) represents the increase in energy required to locate food and process it during an LPF. As in earlier figures, when **Eo** surpasses **EG** then an ELHS is activated. However, if fat depots can be utilized quickly then this can raise the line that **Eo** must exceed. This is indicated in the scale on the upper right-hand vertical axis as fat score (a measure of increasing fat depot from 0 (no fat) to 5 (bulging fat depots)). In the scenario in Figure 1.10a, the LPF is sufficiently strong to increase **Eo** above the fat score lines for individuals with 0–2 fat scores and these individuals should trigger an ELHS (downward arrows on the left-hand side of Figure 1.10a). Those individuals with greater fat (scores 3–5) should not trigger an ELHS and continue in their normal LHS. In the lower panel (Figure 1.10b) a much stronger LPF is modeled with a much greater increase in **Eo**. In this scenario **Eo** exceeds all fat scores and all individuals should trigger an ELHS although the time when they do this will be delayed in individuals in best condition (downward pointing arrows on the left-hand side of Figure 1.10b). Note that return to the normal LHS after the LPF passes and **Eo** subsides may not be proportional to body condition because individuals may mobilize their fat stores at different rates. In any event they will be lower than when the ELHS was triggered. Hence, we postulate that most individuals should resume their normal LHS at about the same time when **Eo** drops below **EG** (upward pointing arrows on right-hand side of both Figures 1.10a and 1.10b).

It is also possible to model the effects of body condition by changing **EG** as a function of an LPF (Figure 1.11). As **EG** decreases and crosses **EI** (i.e. the sum of **EE** + **EI**) then an ELHS should be triggered. However, if fat stores can be mobilized as in Figure 1.10, then LPF resistance potential is increased. In the case of Figure 1.11a, fat score (scaled on the lower right-hand vertical axis) can depress the line needed for **EG** to cross. In this case, the LPF reduced **EG** to an extent that individuals with fat scores of 1 or 0 should activate an ELHS (arrows on the left-hand side of Figure 1.11a). Individuals with fat scores of 2–5 have sufficient LPF resistance potential to remain in their normal LHS. In the case of a more intense and longer duration LPF, **EG** is depressed much further (Figure 1.11b). In this case **EG** drops below all the fat score lines and all individuals should trigger an EHLS (arrows on the left-hand side of Figure 1.11b). Note that return to the normal LHS after the LPF subsides and **EG** increases again may not be proportional to starting fat scores (body condition) for the same reasons as in Figure 1.10. Since fat scores will be depleted (albeit to varying degrees), return to the normal LHS may only occur as **EG** exceeds **EE** (arrows on right-hand side of Figures 1.11a, 1.11b).

Since most vertebrates accumulate stored energy in some form, or multiple forms, for future contingencies (e.g. Stephens, 1991), then the scenarios in Figures 1.10 and 1.11 are entirely possible, indeed probable. What is the evidence that body condition does indeed contribute to LPF resistance potential? In common diving petrels studied at large in the southern oceans there is individual variation in the adrenocortical responses to capture stress. At least some of this variation may result from differences in body condition. During calm conditions there is a significant negative relationship between maximum corticosterone level and ratio of body mass to the cube of wing cord. These data suggest that

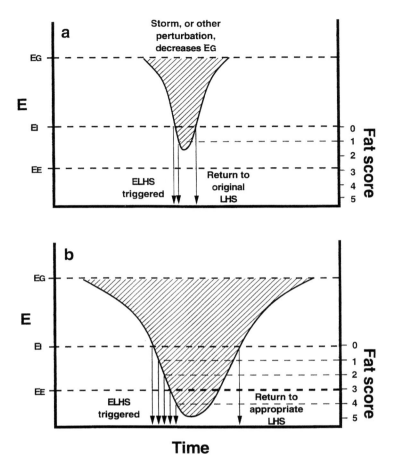

Figure 1.11 Variation in activation of an emergency life history stage (ELHS) in relation to body condition (fat score, see Figure 1.10). The lines **E**ᴇ, **E**ɪ and **E**ɢ are as in Figures 1.1–1.6. Here we model the decrease of **E**ɢ in response to a labile perturbation factor (LPF), the line with shading above. If fat can be mobilized quickly as an energy source then the LPF resistance potential will also be increased. In the upper panel (Figure 1.11a), **E**ɢ drops below **E**ɪ and a line representing a fat score of 1 (i.e. those individuals with poorer body condition), thus activating an ELHS (downward arrows on the left-hand side of the upper panel). Those with larger fat scores (better body condition), will have LPF resistance potential sufficiently great so that the decline in **E**ɢ does not trigger an ELHS and they can remain in their normal LHS. However, when the LPF subsides and **E**ɢ increases, those individuals in poor body condition should not return to a normal LHS until **E**ɢ is greater than **E**ᴇ + **E**ɪ, and they can then replenish reserves (downward pointing arrow on the right-hand side of Figure 1.11a). In the lower panel (Figure 1.11b), an LPF of greater intensity and duration is depicted resulting in a larger decrease of **E**ɢ In this case even individuals in best body condition should trigger an ELHS, although those with the highest fat scores will take longer to do so (downward arrows on left-hand side of Figure 1.11b). Because fat score will be depleted once **E**ɢ drops below **E**ᴇ + **E**ɪ, then return to a normal LHS should not occur until **E**ɢ increases again and all individuals can replenish reserves (upward arrow on right-hand side of Figure 1.11b).

birds in better body condition may be more resistant to acute stress. However, birds captured during the storm showed no such relationship, suggesting either that their body condition had already deteriorated (body mass was lower), or that responsiveness to acute stress may be regulated rapidly (Smith *et al.*, 1994). More recent studies show similar relationships with body condition in some, but not all species (Wingfield *et al.*, 1994a,b, 1995a). Free-living red-eared slider turtles, *Trachemys scripta elegans*, show a rapid increase in corticosterone levels (within 10 min) after capture handling and restraint. There were no differences between the sexes, nor was there any correlation of initial plasma corticosterone levels with energetic condition (Cash *et al.*, 1997).

It should be noted here that the ELHS should be initiated before the individual becomes severely stressed, or energy stores (e.g. fat) become so depleted that none is left to fuel emigration (see also Cherel *et al.*, 1988). Although fat and other components contributing to body condition may provide LPF resistance potential, some must be held in reserve for fueling the ELHS should it be triggered in the strategy where the individual may 'take-it' at first and then leave if conditions do not improve. Observations of white-throated-sparrows in New York State show that fat stores are maintained at high levels at all times. Even on nights when temperature drops to near $-30°C$, i.e. the coldest night of winter at this location, there is no significant change in body mass throughout the afternoon or overnight. However, fat score may increase during the afternoon to a maximum at dusk, and to the lowest value the next morning. Nevertheless, fat stores are still nearly 85% of those measured the previous day despite enduring the coldest night of the winter. Clearly these birds retain far more fat than they need for overnight survival (Wingfield and Ramenofsky, 1997). This fat may be used when ELHS is triggered to provide fuel for a flight south. Apparent 'excess' fat stores may represent an additional 'insurance' reserve against LPFs.

1.5.2.3   Disease as a source of variation in adrenocortical responses to LPFs

Western fence lizards, *Sceloporus occidentalis*, infected with the malarial parasite *Plasmodium mexicanum*, have baseline levels of corticosterone identical to uninfected individuals, but their responsiveness to capture and handling is greater (Dunlap and Schall, 1995). Baseline levels of testosterone and glucose are lower in infected males, and they have lower testis mass, dull nuptial coloration, give fewer courtship displays and are less aggressive, resulting in loss of territories. In females, reduced fat stores lead to lower fecundity in the following breeding season (Dunlap and Schall, 1995). Experimental implants of corticosterone that maintain high circulating levels similar to those measured during the capture stress protocol result in a decrease in testis mass, plasma levels of testosterone and fat score, but increase blood glucose concentrations in otherwise healthy male fence lizards. These data suggest that several deleterious morphological, physiological and behavioral changes reduce overall fitness owing to increased adrenocortical responsiveness to LPFs resulting from a natural cause such as malarial infection. Similarly in the marine turtle, *Chelonia mydas*, those individuals with fibropapillomas had higher stress levels of corticosterone than healthy individuals (Aguirre *et al.*, 1995).

1.5.2.4 Variation in physiological and behavioral responses to elevated levels of glucocorticosteroids

Regardless of whether there is modulation of sensitivity of the HPA axis to acute stress at the population or individual level, it is possible that physiological and behavioral responses to elevated circulating levels of corticosterone may be regulated independently. There is little evidence for this as yet, possibly because the appropriate studies have not been performed on free-living species. We can expect exciting new advances in this area in the near future, but in the interim it is important to remember that such modulation may occur at the intracellular target level either through regulation of receptor number and types (e.g. McEwen *et al.*, 1988; Dallman *et al.*, 1994), or through expression of enzymes that metabolize glucocorticosteroids to inactive forms before they have a chance to interact with a receptor (Funder *et al.*, 1988; Seckl and Brown, 1994). Other mechanisms are also possible, especially in relation to corticosteroid-binding proteins in blood. In the dark-eyed junco, implants of testosterone into young birds increased plasma levels of corticosterone but not the acute response of corticosterone levels to capture and handling. Thus, increased plasma levels of corticosterone were not a result of increased sensitivity to stress. The ability of the plasma to bind corticosterone (corticosterone-binding proteins) were elevated 2- to 3-fold in testosterone-treated birds (Klukowski *et al.*, 1997).

1.6 Conclusions

One of the fascinating aspects of biology is how organisms deal with a changing environment. In most cases the environment fluctuates on a predictable scale (night and day, high tide, low tide, seasons) and organisms can adjust their morphology, physiology and behavior in anticipation of these changes. However, the environment can be capricious and individuals must deal with unpredictable perturbations. We have long known that neuroendocrine and endocrine systems regulate the developmental, daily and seasonal changes, but the mechanisms involved have, by necessity, been determined under highly controlled laboratory conditions with animal subjects often selected for genetic uniformity to reduce individual variation. This has led to an enormous literature on how hormones work and how they orchestrate adaptive changes. Investigations on whether these mechanisms apply to individuals under natural conditions is much less well known because field studies have always been thought to be fraught with problems of individual variation and uncontrollable conditions. However, in many ways these variations are the most interesting and it is important to ask whether there are underlying ecological factors that explain them. Now that we have such an enormous base of laboratory experimentation that provides mechanisms, we can go into the field and ask questions as to which are most important under certain conditions, or how they interact with other processes. This, in turn, develops new questions that can be approached by further field experiments in close conjunction with laboratory investigation. This concept of 'environmental endocrinology' provides an experimental way in which to explore possible ecological bases of endocrine phenomena in general, including the behavioral ecology of stress and the hormone mechanisms that underlie it.

The responses of the HPA axis to stress are considered deleterious because chronic high levels of glucocorticosteroids result in physiological and morphological deterioration. Here we argue that the actions of glucocorticosteroids in response to acute stress or perturbations of the environment (LPFs) may be highly advantageous, although they do have the potential to be stressful. The ELHS, a facultative physiological and behavioral response to LPFs, is highly adaptive in re-directing an individual away from non-essential activities such as reproduction, migration, or defending a territory and promotes survival. This allows an individual to endure the effects of an LPF in the best possible condition so that an appropriate LHS can be resumed as soon as the LPF subsides. If an LPF occurs during the reproductive season, then breeding is interrupted–an apparently deleterious event because reproductive success is decreased. However, the individual will survive the LPF in good body condition and can begin breeding again immediately after the LPF passes. In the longterm this may result in higher reproductive success than trying to maintain breeding in the face of an LPF and suffering deteriorating body condition (see Wingfield, 1988; Wingfield *et al.*, 1998). Animals that are responding to LPFs in this manner under many different environmental conditions have circulating levels of glucocorticosteroids above the normal seasonal changes in baseline levels (i.e. above level B to level C, Wingfield *et al.*, 1997, 1998). A combination of field and laboratory experiments indicates that glucocorticosteroids, and peptides of the HPA axis, are involved in the regulation of many of these behaviors and physiological responses. Transient increases in glucocorti-costeroid secretion to level C may thus play a major role in orchestrating the ELHS. Furthermore, it is important to note that these rapid responses to increased glucocorticosteroid levels may be highly adaptive in *avoiding* the deleterious effects of chronic, severe stress. We are fully aware that under certain circumstances severe chronic stress may occur in the field, but mass mortality is a common result. The ELHS reduces this possibility and clearly may enhance lifetime fitness.

The adaptive features of the ELHS notwithstanding, there are periods in an organism's life cycle when it is possible that the ELHS might not be the most advantageous response to an LPF. For example, for populations breeding in severe environments where only one reproductive attempt is likely, it may be an advantage to be resistant to LPFs that would normally trigger an ELHS. There may be 'costs' associated with this resistance (e.g. decreased body condition, even mortality), but the long-term gain is greater reproductive success. In support of this hypothesis, there is considerable evidence that animals can modulate their adrenocortical responsiveness to acute stress (LPFs). The capture stress protocol is an experimental approach that can be applied in laboratory and field and has proven to be a useful method of determining the responsiveness of the HPA axis to acute stress (including LPFs). This has relevance to how responsive the HPA axis may be to a wide spectrum of LPFs including inclement weather. The capture stress protocol and LPFs such as severe weather conditions have the potential to increase circulating levels of corticosterone above the predictable daily or seasonal norm (i.e. level B) to a higher range of circulating levels often equated with stress (level C). We do understand that many LPFs and the capture stress protocol cannot be equated ideally, but we can, nonetheless, use the profile of corticosterone levels during the experimental protocol to analyze the dynamics of the HPA axis response which then allows us to explore possible ecological bases for variation across populations. Field endocrine analyses of this sort provide critical insight into WHY there is such variation. These data may then point the way to laboratory experiments designed to reveal mechanisms.

The analysis presented here combines a theoretical framework with a comparative field approach that generates testable hypotheses. The framework allows us to bring the great diversity of LPFs into a perspective that suggests a common underlying suite of mechanisms. Much work remains to be done and it is hoped that the framework will have at least heuristic value in pointing the way to more relevant schemes. The comparative field approach has also allowed us to pinpoint possible key ecological relationships that will allow us test the framework further, particularly the incorporation of cell and molecular mechanisms.

Acknowledgements

Many of the investigations on stress in free-living animals cited herein, and the theoretical modeling were supported by a series of grants from the Office of Polar Programs and the Integrative Biology and Neuroscience Program, National Science Foundation; a Shannon Award from the National Institutes of Health; a Benjamin Meaker Fellowship from the University of Bristol, U.K.; and a John Simon Guggenheim Fellowship to J.C.W.

References

Aguirre, A.A., Balazs, G.H., Sparker, T.R. and Gross, T.S. (1995) Adrenal and hematological responses to stress in juvenile green turtles (*Chelonia mydas*) with and without fibropapillomas. *Physiological Zoology*, **68** 831-854.

Akana, S.F., Strack, A.M., Hanson, E.S. and Dallman, M.F. (1994) Regulation of activity in the hypothalamic-pituitary-adrenal axis is integral to a larger hypothalamic system that determines caloric flow. *Endocrinology*, **135** 1125-1134.

Alberts, S.C., Sapolsky, R.M. and Altmann, J. (1992) Behavioral endocrine and immunological correlates of immigration by an aggressive male into a natural primate group. *Hormones and Behavior*, **26** 167-178.

Astheimer, L.B., Buttemer, W.A. and Wingfield, J.C. (1992) Interactions of corticosterone with feeding, activity, and metabolism in passerine birds. *Ornis Scandinavica*, **23** 355-365.

Astheimer, L.B., Buttemer, W.A. and Wingfield, J.C. (1994) Gender and seasonal differences in the adrenocortical response to ACTH challenge in an arctic passerine, *Zonotrichia leucophrys gambelii*. *General and Comparative Endocrinology*, **94** 33-43.

Astheimer, L.B., Buttemer, W.A. and Wingfield, J.C. (1995) Seasonal and acute changes in adrenocortical responsiveness in an arctic-breeding bird. *Hormones and Behavior*, **29** 442-457.

Axelrod, J. and Reisine, T.D. (1984) Stress hormones: their interaction and regulation. *Science*, **224** 452-459.

Barna, I., Koenig, J.I. and Péczely, P. (1998) Characteristics of the proopiomelanocortin system in the outdoor-bred domestic gander. *General and Comparative Endocrinology*, **109** 44-52.

Berridge, C.W. and Dunn, A.J. (1989) CRF and restraint-stress decrease exploratory behavior in hypophysectomized mice. *Pharmacology and Biochemistry of Behavior*, **34** 517-519.

Bertolini, A. and Gessa, G.L. (1981) Behavioral effects of ACTH and MSH peptides. *Journal of Endocrinological Investigation*, **4** 241-251.

Bohus, B. and De Kloet, E.R. (1981) Adrenal steroids and extinction behavior: antagonism by progesterone, deoxycorticosterone and dexa-methasone of a specific effect of corticosterone. *Life Sciences*, **28** 433-440.

Bradbury, M.J., Akana, S.F. and Dallman, M.F. (1994) Roles of type I and II corticosteroid receptors in regulation of basal activity in the hypothalamo-pituitary-adrenal axis during the diurnal trough and the peak: evidence for a non additive effect of combined receptor occupation. *Endocrinology*, **134** 1286-1296.

Breuner, C.W., Greenberg, A.L. and Wingfield, J.C. (1998) Non-invasive corticosterone treatment rapidly increases activity in Gambel's White-crowned Sparrows (*Zonotrichia leucophrys gambelii*). *General and Comparative Endocrinology*, **111** 386-394.

Buttemer, W.A., Astheimer, L.B. and Wingfield, J.C. (1991) The effect of corticosterone on standard metabolic rates of small passerines. *Journal of Comparative Physiology B*, **161** 427-431.

Carsia, R.V. (1990) Hormonal control of avian adrenocortical function: cellular and molecular aspects, in *Progress in Comparative Endocrinology* (eds. A. Epple, C.G. Scanes and M.H. Stetson), Wiley-Liss, New York, pp. 439-444.

Cash, W.B., Holberton, R.L. and Knight, S.S. (1997) Corticosterone secretion in response to capture and handling in free-living red-eared slider turtles. *General and Comparative Endocrinology*, **108** 427-433.

Cherel, Y., Robin, J.P., Walch, O., Karmann, H., Netchatalio, P. and le Maho, Y. (1988) Fasting in the king penguin. 1. Hormonal and metabolic changes during breeding. *American Journal of Physiology*, **23** R170-R177.

Chester-Jones, I., Bellamy, D., Chan, D.K.O., Follett, B.K., Henderson, I.W., Phillips, J.G. and Snart, R.S. (1972) Biological actions of steroid hormones in nonmammalian vertebrates, in *Steroids in Nonmammalian Vertebrates* (ed. D.R. Idler), Academic Press, New York, pp. 414-480.

Creel, S., Creel, N.M. and Monfort, S.L. (1996) Social stress and costs of dominance. *Nature*, **379** 212.

Dallman, M.F., Strack, A.M., Akana, S.F., Bradbury, M.J., Hanson, E.S., Scribner, K.A. and Smith, M. (1993) Feast and famine: critical role of glucocorticosteroids with insulin in daily energy flow. *Frontiers in Neuroendocrinology*, **14** 303-347.

Dallman, M.F., Akana, S.F., Levin, N., Walker, C.D., Bradbury, M.J., Suemaru, S. and Scribner, K.S. (1994) Corticosteroids and the control of function in the hypothalamo-pituitary-adrenal (HPA) axis. *Annals of the New York Academy of Sciences*, **746** 22-31.

Dallman, M.F., Akana, S.F., Strack, A.M., Hanson, E.S. and Sebastian, R.J. (1995) The neural network that regulates energy balance is responsive to glucocorticosteroids and insulin and also regulates HPA axis responsivity at a site proximal to CRF neurons. *Annals of the New York Academy of Sciences*, **771** 730-742.

Davidson, T.F., Rea, J. and Rowell, J.G. (1983) Effects of dietary corticosterone on the growth and metabolism of immature *Gallus domesticus*. *General and Comparative Endocrinology*, **50** 463-468.

Dawson, A. and Howe, P.D. (1983) Plasma corticosterone in wild starlings (*Sturnus vulgaris*) immediately following capture and in relation to body weight during the annual cycle. *General and Comparative Endocrinology*, **51** 303-308.

DeNardo, D.F. and Licht, P. (1993) Effects of corticosterone on social behavior of male lizards. *Hormones and Behavior*, **27** 184-199.

DeNardo, D.F. and Sinervo, B. (1994a) Effects of corticosterone on activity and home range size of free-living male lizards. *Hormones and Behavior*, **28** 53-62.

DeNardo, D.F. and Sinervo, B. (1994b) Effects of steroid hormone interaction on activity and home range size of free-living male lizards. *Hormones and Behavior*, **28** 273-287.

Denver, R.J. (1997) Proximate mechanisms of phenotypic plasticity in amphibian metamorphosis. *American Zoologist*, **37** 172-184.

Denver, R.J. (1998) Hormonal correlates of environmentally induced metamorphosis in the western spadefoot toad, *Scaphiopus hammondii*. *General and Comparative Endocrinology*, **110** 326-336.

Deviche, P. (1983) Interactions between adrenal function and reproduction in male birds, in *Avian Endocrinology: Environmental and Ecological Perspectives* (eds. S. Mikami, S. Ishii and M. Wada), Jap. Sci. Soc. Press and Springer-Verlag, pp. 243-245.

Deviche, P. and Delius, J.D. (1981) Short-term modulation of domestic pigeon (*Columbia livia* L.) behaviour induced by intraventricular administration of ACTH. *Zeitschrift für Tierpsychologie*, **55** 335-342.

de Wied, D. and Jolles, J. (1982) Neuropeptides derived from proopio-melanocortin: behavioral, physiological and neurochemical effects. *Physiological Reviews*, **62** 976-1059.

Dufty, A.M. Jr. and Belthoff, J.R. (1997) Corticosterone and the stress response in young Western screech owls: effects of captivity, gender, and activity period. *Physiological Zoology*, **70** 143-149.

Dunlap, K.D. and Church, D.R. (1996) Interleukin-1β reduces daily activity level in male lizards, *Sceloporus occidentalis. Brain Behavior and Immunology*, **10** 68-73.

Dunlap, K.D. and Schall, J.J. (1995) Hormonal alterations and reproductive inhibition in male fence lizards (*Sceloporus occidentalis*) infected with the malarial parasite (*Plasmodium mexicanum*). *Physiological Zoology*, **68** 608-621.

Eros, S.K. and Milligan, C.L. (1996) The effect of cortisol on recovery from exhaustive exercise in rainbow trout (*Oncorhynchus mykiss*): potential mechanisms of action. *Physiological Zoology*, **69** 1196-1214.

File, S.E. and Day, S. (1972) Effects of time of day and food deprivation on exploratory behavior in the rat. *Animal Behaviour*, **20** 758-762.

Francis, D., Diorio, J., LaPlante, P., Weaver, S., Seckl, J.R. and Meaney, M.J. (1996) The role of early environmental events in regulating neuroendocrine development. Moms, pups, stress and glucocorticoid receptors. *Annals of the New York Academy of Sciences*, **794** 136-152.

Freeman, B.M., Manning, A.C. and Flack, I.H. (1980) Short-term stressor effects of food withdrawal on the immature fowl. *Comparative Biochemistry and Physiology*, **67A** 569-571.

Fujiwara, T., Cherrington, A.D., Neal, D.N. and McGuiness, O.P. (1996) Role of cortisol in the metabolic response to stress hormone infusion in the conscious dog. *Metabolism*, **45** 571-578.

Funder, J.W., Pearce, P.T., Smith, R. and Smith, A.I. (1988) Mineralocorticoid action: target tissue specificity is enzyme, not receptor, mediated. *Science*, **242** 583-585.

Goldstein, R.E., Reed, G.W., Wasserman, D.H., Williams, P.E., Brooks Lacy, D., Buckspan, R., Abumrad, N.N. and Cherrington, A.D. (1992) The effects of acute elevations in plasma cortisol levels on alanine metabolism in the conscious dog. *Metabolism*, **41** 1295-1303.

Goldstein, R.E., Wasserman, D.H., McGuinness, O.P., Brooks Lacy, D., Cherrington, A.D. and Abumrad, N.N. (1993) Effects of chronic elevation in plasma cortisol on hepatic carbohydrate metabolism. *American Journal of Physiology*, **264** E119-E127.

Grande, F. (1964) Man under caloric deficiency, in *Handbook of Physiology, Sec. 4.* (eds. D.B. Dill, E.F. Adolph and C.G. Wilbur), American Physiology Society, Washington, D.C., pp. 911-937.

Gray, J.M., Yarian, D. and Ramenofsky, M. (1990) Corticosterone, foraging behavior, and metabolism in dark-eyed juncos, *Junco hyemalis. General and Comparative Endocrinology*, **79** 375-384.

Gregory, L.F., Gross, T.S., Bolten, A.B., Bjorndal, K.A. and Guillette, L.J. (1996) Plasma corticosterone concentrations associated with acute captivity stress in wild loggerhead sea turtles (*Caretta caretta*). *General and Comparative Endocrinology*, **104** 312-320.

Greenberg, N. and Wingfield, J.C. (1987) Stress and reproduction: reciprocal relationships, in *Reproductive Endocrinology of Fishes, Amphibians and Reptiles* (eds. D.O. Norris and, R.E. Jones), Wiley, New York, pp. 389-426.

Hadley, M.E. (1996) *Endocrinology,* fourth edition. Prentice Hall, Upper Saddle River, New Jersey, pp. 518.

Hanson, E.S., Bradbury, M.J., Akana, S.F., Scribner, K.S., Strack, A.M. and Dallman, M.F. (1994) The diurnal rhythm in adrenocorticotropin responses to restraint in adrenalecto-mized rats is determined by caloric intake. *Endocrinology*, **134** 2214-2220.

Harvey, S., Klandorf, H. and Pinchasov, Y. (1983) Visual and metabolic stimuli cause adrenocortical suppression in fasted chickens during refeeding. *Neuroendocrinology*, **37** 59-63.

Harvey, S., Phillips, J.G., Rees, A. and Hall, T.R. (1984) Stress and adrenal function. *Journal of Experimental Zoology*, **232** 633-645.

Hayes, T.B. (1997) Steroids as potential modulators of thyroid hormone activity in anuran metamorphosis. *American Zoologist*, **37** 185-194.

Hissa, R. and Palokangas, R. (1970) Thermoregulation in the titmouse (*Parus major* L.). *Comparative Biochemistry and Physiology*, **33** 941-953.

Hissa, R., George, J.C. and Saarela, S. (1980) Dose-related effects of nor-adrenaline and corticosterone on temperature regulation in the pigeon. *Comparative Biochemistry and Physiology*, **65C** 25-32.

Holmes, W.N. and Phillips, J.G. (1976) The adrenal cortex of birds, in *General, Comparative and Clinical Endocrinology of the Adrenal Cortex* (eds. I. Chester-Jones and, I.W. Henderson), Academic Press, New York, pp. 293-420.

Honey, P.K. (1990) Avian flight muscle *Pectoralis major* as a reserve of proteins and amino acids. M.S. Thesis, University of Washington.

Idler, D.R. (1972) *Steroids in Non-Mammalian Vertebrates*. Academic Press, New York,

Iuvone, P.M. and van Hartesveldt, C. (1977) Diurnal locomotor activity in rats: Effects of hippocampal ablation and adrenalectomy. *Behavioral Biology*, **19** 228-237.

Jacobs, J.D. (1996) Regulation of Life History Strategies Within Individuals in Predictable and Unpredictable Environments. Ph.D. Thesis, University of Washington.

Jacobs, L.F. (1996) The economy of winter: phenotypic plasticity in behavior and brain structure. *Biological Bulletin*, **191** 92-100.

Jones, P.J. and Ward, P. (1976) The level of reserve protein as the proximate factor controlling the timing of breeding and clutch size in the red-billed quelea, *Quelea quelea. Ibis*, **118** 547-574.

Kendall, M.D., Ward, P. and Bacchus, S. (1973) A protein reserve in the *pectoralis major* flight muscle of *Quelea quelea. Ibis*, **115** 600-601.

Ketterson, E.D. and King, J.R. (1977) Metabolic and behavioral responses to fasting in the white-crowned sparrow (*Zonotrichia leucophrys gambelii*). *Physiological Zoology*, **50** 115-129.

King, B.M., Zansler, C.A., Tatford, A.C., Neville, K.L., Sam, H., Kass, J.M. and Dallman, M.F. (1993) Level of corticosterone replacement determines body weight gain in adrenalectomized rats with VMH lesions. *Physiology and Behavior*, **54** 1187-1190.

Klukowski, L.A., Cawthorn, J.M., Ketterson, E.D. and Nolan, Jr., V. (1997) Effects of experimentally elevated testosterone on plasma corticosterone and corticosteroid-binding globulin in dark-eyed juncos (*Junco hyemalis*). *General and Comparative Endocrinology*, **108** 141-151.

Knapp, R. and Moore, M.C. (1996) Male morphs in tree lizards, *Urosaurus ornatus*, have different delayed hormonal responses to aggressive encounters. *Animal Behaviour*, **52** 1045-1055.

Knapp, R. and Moore, M.C. (1997) Male morphs in tree lizards have different testosterone responses to elevated levels of corticosterone. *General and Comparative Endocrinology*, **107** 273-279.

Lance, V.A. (1994) Life in the slow lane: hormones, stress, and the immune system in reptiles, in *Perspectives in Comparative Endocrinology* (eds. K.G. Davey, R.E. Peter and S.S. Tobe), National Research Council of Canada, Ottawa, pp. 529-534.

Le Ninan, F., Cherel, Y., Sardet, C. and Le Maho, Y. (1988) Plasma hormone levels in relation to lipid and protein metabolism during prolonged fasting in king penguin chicks. *General and Comparative Endocrinology*, **71** 331-337.

Maney, D.L. and Wingfield, J.C. (1998) Neuroendocrine suppression of female courtship in a wild passerine: corticotropin-releasing factor and endogenous opioids. *Journal of Neuroendocrinology*, **10** 593-599.

Meaney, M.J., Diorio, J., Francis, D., Widdowson, J., LaPlante, P., Caldji, C., Sharma, S., Seckl, J.R. and Plotsky, P.M. (1996) Early environmental regulation of forebrain glucocorticoid receptor gene expression: implications for adrenocortical responses to stress. *Developmental Neuroscience*, **18** 49-72.

McEwen, B., Brinton, R.E. and Sapolsky, R.M. (1988) Glucocorticoid receptors and behavior: implications for the stress response. *Advances in Experimental Medicine and Biology*, **245** 35-45.

McMahon, M., Gerich, J. and Rizza, R. (1988) Effects of glucocorticoids on carbohydrate metabolism. *Diabetes/Metabolism Reviews*, **4** 17-30.

Micco, D.J., Meyer, J.S. and McEwen, B.S. (1980) Effects of corticosterone replacement on the temporal patterning of activity and sleep in adrenalectomized rats. *Brain Research*, **200** 206-212.

Mitchell, M.A., MacLeod, M.G. and Raza, A. (1986) The effects of ACTH and dexamethasone upon plasma thyroid hormone levels and heat production in the domestic fowl. *Comparative Biochemistry and Physiology*, **85A** 207-215.

Moore, F.L. and Miller, L.J. (1984) Stress-induced inhibition of sexual behavior: corticosterone inhibits courtship behaviors of a male amphibian (*Taricha granulosa*). *Hormones and Behavior*, **18** 400-410.

Moore, F.L., Roberts, J. and Bevers, J. (1984) Corticotropin-releasing factor (CRF) stimulates locomotor activity in intact and hypophysectomized newts (Amphibia). *Journal of Experimental Zoology*, **231** 331-333.

Moore, M.C., Thompson, C.W. and Marler, C.A. (1991) Reciprocal changes in corticosterone and testosterone levels following acute and chronic handling stress in the tree lizard, *Urosaurus ornatus*. *General and Comparative Endocrinology*, **81** 217-226.

Moyer, J.A. and Leshner, A.I. (1976) Pituitary-adrenal effects on avoidance-of-attack in mice: separation of the effects of ACTH and Corticosterone. *Physiology of Behavior*, **17** 297-301.

Munck, A., Guyre, P. and Holbrook, N. (1984) Physiological functions of glucocorticosteroids in stress and their relation to pharmacological actions. *Endocrine Reviews*, **5** 25-44.

Nelson, J.F., Karelus, K., Bergman, M.D. and Felicio, L.S. (1995) Neuroendocrine involvement in aging: evidence from studies of reproductive aging and caloric restriction. *Neurobiology of Aging*, **16** 849-850.

Norris, D.O. (1997) *Vertebrate Endocrinology*. Third, Edition, Academic Press, New York.

O'Reilly, K.M. (1995) Ecological Bases of Endocrine Phenomena. Ph.D. Thesis, University of Washington.

Orchinik, M., Murray, T.F. and Moore, F.L. (1991) A corticosteroid receptor in neuronal membranes. *Science*, **252** 1848-1851.

Palokangas, R. and Hissa, R. (1971) Thermoregulation in young black-headed gulls (*Larus ridibundus* L.). *Comparative Biochemistry and Physiology*, **38A** 743-750.

Pickering, A.D. and Fryer, J.N. (1994) Hormones and stress: a comparative approach, in *Perspectives in Comparative Endocrinology* (eds. K.G. Davey, R.E. Peter and S.S. Tobe), National Research Council of Canada, Ottawa, pp. 517-519.

Richardson, R.D. (1996) Central Regulation of Food Intake in the White-crowned Sparrow. Ph.D. Thesis, University of Washington.

Robinson, C.J. and Pitcher, T.J. (1989) The influence of hunger and ration level on shoal density, polarization and swimming speed of herring, *Clupea harengus* L. *Journal of Fish Biology*, **34** 631-633.

Rogers, C.M., Ramenofsky, M., Ketterson, E.D., Nolan, Jr., V. and Wingfield, J.C. (1993) Plasma corticosterone, adrenal mass, winter weather, and season in non-breeding populations of dark-eyed juncos (*Junco hyemalis hyemalis*). *Auk*, **110** 279-285.

Rohwer, S. and Wingfield, J.C. (1981) A field study of social dominance; plasma levels of luteinizing hormone and steroid hormones in wintering Harris' sparrows. *Zeitschrift für Tierpsychologie*, **47** 173-183.

Sabatino, F., Masoro, E.J., McMahan, C.A. and Kuhn, R.W. (1991) Assessment of the role of the glucocorticoid system in aging and in the action of food restriction. *Journal of Gerontology (Biological Sciences)*, **46** B171-B179.

Sapolsky, R.M. (1982) The endocrine stress response and social status in the wild baboon. *Hormones and Behavior*, **16** 279-292.

Sapolsky, R.M. (1987) Stress, social status, and reproductive physiology in free-living baboons, in *Psychobiology of Reproductive Behavior: an Evolutionary Perspective* (ed. D. Crews), Prentice-Hall, Englewood Cliffs, New Jersey, pp. 291-322.

Sapolsky, R.M. (1992a) Cortisol concentrations and the social significance of rank instability among wild baboons. *Psychoneuroendocrinology*, **17** 701-709.

Sapolsky, R.M. (1992b) Neuroendocrinology of the stress response, in *Behavioral Endocrinology* (eds. J.B. Becker, S.M. Breedlove and D. Crews), MIT Press, Cambridge, Mass, pp. 287-324.

Sapolsky, R.M. (1995) Social subordinance as a marker of hypercortisolism. Some unexpected subtleties. *Annals of the New York Academy of Sciences*, **771** 626-639.

Sapolsky, R.M. (1996) Why stress is bad for your brain. *Science*, **273** 749-750.

Sapolsky, R.M., Alberts, S.C. and Altmann, J. (1997) Hypercortisolism associated with social subordinance or social isolation among wild baboons. *Archives of General Psychiatry*, **54** 1137-1143.

Scholnick, D.A., Weinstein, R.B. and Gleeson, T.T. (1997) The influence of corticosterone and glucagon on metabolic recovery from exhaustive exercise in the desert iguana *Dipsosaurus dorsalis. General and Comparative Endocrinology*, **106** 147-154.

Schwabl, H. (1995) Individual variation of the acute adrenocortical response to stress in the white-throated sparrow. *Zoology*, **99** 113-120.

Schwabl, H., Wingfield, J.C. and Farner, D.S. (1985) Influence of winter on behavior and endocrine state in European blackbirds (*Turdus merula*). *Zeitschrift für Tierpsychologie*, **68** 244-252.

Seckl, J.R. and Brown, R.W. (1994) 11-beta-hydroxysteroid dehydrogenase: on several roads to hypertension. *Journal of Hypertension*, **12** 105-112.

Silverin, B. (1986) Corticosterone binding proteins and behavioral effects of high plasma levels of corticosterone during the breeding period in the pied flycatcher. *General and Comparative Endocrinology*, **64** 67-74.

Silverin, B., Arvidson, B. and Wingfield, J.C. (1997) The adrenocortical responses to stress in breeding willow warblers, *Phylloscopus trochilus,* in Sweden: effects of latitude and gender. *Functional Ecology*, **11** 376-384.

Smith, G.T., Wingfield, J.C. and Veit, R.R. (1994) Adrenocortical response to stress in the common diving-petrel, *Pelecanoides urinatrix. Physiological Zoology*, **67** 526-537.

Stephens, D.W. (1991) Change, regularity, and value in the evolution of animal learning. *Behavioral Ecology*, **2** 77-79.

Stuebe, M.M. and Ketterson, E.D. (1982) A study of fasting in tree sparrows (*Spizella arborea*) and dark-eyed juncos (*Junco hyemalis*): ecological implications. *Auk*, **99** 299-308.

Strack, A.M., Sebastian, R.J., Schwartz, M.W. and Dallman, M.F. (1995a) Glucocorticosteroids and insulin: reciprocal signals for energy balance. *American Journal of Physiology*, **268** R142-R149.

Strack, A.M., Bradbury, M.J. and Dallman, M.F. (1995b) Corticosterone decreases nonshivering thermogenesis and increases lipid storage in brown adipose tissue. *American Journal of Physiology*, **268** R183-R191.

Sumpter, J.P., Pottinger, T.G., Rand-Weaver, M. and Campbell, P.M. (1994) The wide-ranging effects of stress on fish. in *Perspectives in Comparative Endocrinology* (eds. K.G. Davey, R.E. Peter and S.S. Tobe), National Research Council of Canada, Ottawa, pp. 535-538.

Sutton, R.E., Koob, G.F., Le Moal, M., Rivier, J. and Vale, W. (1982) Corticotrophin-releasing factor produces behavioral activation in rats. *Nature*, **297** 331-333.

Taymans, S.E., DeVries, A.C., DeVries, M.B., Nelson, R.J., Friedman, C., Castro, M., Detera-Wadleigh, S., Carter, C.S. and Chrousos, G.P. (1997) The hypothalamic-pituitary-adrenal axis of prairie voles (*Microtus ochrogaster*): evidence for target tissue glucocorticoid resistance. *General and Comparative Endocrinology*, **106** 48-61.

Tempel, D.L. and Leibowitz, S.F. (1989) PVN steroid implants: Effects on feeding patterns and macronutrient selection. *Brain Research Bulletin*, **23** 553-560.

Tyrrell, C.L. and Cree, A. (1998) Relationships between corticosterone concentration and season, time of day and confinement in a wild reptile (Tuatara, *Sphenodon punctatus*). *General and Comparative Endocrinology*, **110** 97-108.

Veit, R.R., Kareiva, P.M., Doak, D.F., Engh, A., Heppell, S.F., Hollon, M., Jordan, C.E., Morgan, R.A., Morris, W.F., Nevitt, G.A. and Smith, G.T. (1991) Foraging interactions between pelagic seabirds and Antarctic krill at South Georgia during winter 1991. *Antarctic Journal of the U. S. A.*, **28** 183-185.

Veldhuis, H.D. and de Wied, D. (1984) Differential behavioral actions of corticotropin-releasing factor (CRF). *Pharmacology and Biochemistry of Behavior*, **21** 707-713.

Veldhuis, H.D., De Kloet, E.R., Van Zoest, I. and Bohus, B. (1982) Adrenalectomy reduces exploratory activity in the rat: a specific role of corticosterone. *Hormones and Behavior*, **16** 191-198.

Vergoni, A.V., Poggioli, R. and Bertolini, A. (1986) Corticotropin inhibits food intake in rats. *Neuropeptides*, **7** 153-158.

Virgin, C.E. Jr. and Sapolsky, R.M. (1997) Styles of male social behavior and their endocrine correlates among low ranking baboons. *American Journal of Primatology*, **42** 25-39.

Walker, C.-D. (1994) Regulation of adrenocortical activity in rats during development and under situations of chronic stress: the interplay between circadian inputs, stress activation, and corticosteroid feedback, in *Perspectives in Comparative Endocrinology* (eds. K.G. Davey, R.E. Peter and, S.S. Tobe), National Research Council of Canada, Ottawa, pp. 548-551.

Wasser, S.K., Bevis, K., King, G. and Hanson, E. (1997) Non-invasive physiological measures of disturbance in the Northern spotted owl. *Conservation Biology*, **11** 1019-1022.

West-Eberhard, M.J. (1989) Phenotypic plasticity and the origin of diversity. *Annual Review of Ecology and Systematics*, **20** 249-278.

Whittier, J.M., Mason, R.T. and Crews, D. (1987) Plasma steroid hormone levels of female red-sided garter snakes, *Thamnophis sirtalis parietalis*: relationship to mating and gestation. *General and Comparative Endocrinology*, **67** 33-43.

Wingfield, J.C. (1988) Changes in reproductive function of free-living birds in direct response to environmental perturbations, in *Processing of Environmental Information in Vertebrates* (ed. M.H. Stetson), Springer-Verlag, New York, pp. 121-148.

Wingfield, J.C. (1994) Modulation of the adrenocortical response to stress in birds, in *Perspectives in Comparative Endocrinology* (eds. K.G. Davey, R.E. Peter and, S.S. Tobe) National Research Council Canada, Ottawa, pp. 520-528.

Wingfield, J.C. and Farner, D.S. (1978) The endocrinology of a naturally breeding population of the white-crowned sparrow (*Zonotrichia leucophrys pugetensis*). *Physiological Zoology*, **51** 188-205.

Wingfield, J.C. and Ramenofsky, M. (1997) Corticosterone and facultative dispersal in response to unpredictable events. *Ardea*, **85** 155-166.

Wingfield, J.C. and Silverin, B. (1986) Effects of corticosterone on territorial behavior of free-living song sparrows, *Melospiza melodia*. *Hormones and Behavior*, **20** 405-417.

Wingfield, J.C., Smith, J.P. and Farner, D.S. (1982) Endocrine responses of white-crowned sparrows to environmental stress. *Condor*, **84** 399-409.

Wingfield, J.C., Moore, M.C. and Farner, D.S. (1983) Endocrine responses to inclement weather in naturally breeding populations of white-crowned sparrows. *Auk*, **100** 56-62.

Wingfield, J.C., Vleck, C.M. and Moore, M.C. (1992) Seasonal changes in the adrenocortical response to stress in birds of the Sonoran Desert. *Journal of Experimental Zoology*, **264** 419-428.

Wingfield, J.C., Deviche, P., Sharbaugh, S., Astheimer, L.B., Holberton, R., Suydam, R. and Hunt, K. (1994a) Seasonal changes of the adrenocortical responses to stress in redpolls, *Acanthis flammea,* in Alaska. *Journal of Experimental Zoology*, **270** 372-380.

Wingfield, J.C., Suydam, R. and Hunt, K. (1994b) Adrenocortical responses to stress in snow buntings and Lapland longspurs at Barrow, Alaska. *Comparative Biochemistry and Physiology*, **108** 299-306.

Wingfield, J.C., Kubokawa, K., Ishida, K., Ishii, S. and Wada, M. (1995a) The adrenocortical response to stress in male bush warblers, *Cettia diphone:* a comparison of breeding populations in Honshu and Hokkaido, Japan. *Zoological Science*, **12** 615-621.

Wingfield, J.C., O'Reilly, K.M. and Astheimer, L.B. (1995b) Ecological bases of the modulation of adrenocortical responses to stress in Arctic birds. *American Zoologist*, **35** 285-294.

Wingfield, J.C., Breuner, C. and Jacobs, J. (1997) Corticosterone and behavioral responses to unpredictable events, in *Perspectives in Avian Endocrinology* (eds. S. Harvey and R.J. Etches) Journal of Endocrinology Ltd., Bristol, pp. 267-278.

Wingfield, J.C., Breuner, C., Jacobs, J., Lynn, S., Ramenofsky, M. and Richardson, R. (1998) Ecological bases of hormone-behavior interactions: The emergency life history stage. *American Zoologist*, **38** 191-206.

Yon, L., Contesse, V., Leboulenger, F., Feuilloley, M., Esneu, M., Kodjo, M. and Lesouhaitier, O. (1994) New concepts concerning the regulation of corticosteroid secretion in amphibians, in *Perspectives in Comparative Endocrinology* (eds. K.G. Davey, R.E. Peter and S.S. Tobe), National Research Council of Canada, Ottawa, pp. 539-547.

2 Respiratory and cardiovascular systems during stress

Steve F. Perry and Kathleen M. Gilmour

2.1 Introduction

The cardiovascular and respiratory systems of animals are integrated in an efficient and co-ordinated manner to sustain the fluctuating energetic requirements of metabolising tissues. Although often reviewed separately in the literature, the inter-dependence of the cardiovascular and respiratory systems in physiological homeostasis cannot be overstated. Thus, in this chapter we will address the involvement of both systems in the physiological responses of animals to stress.

The nature or definition of stress is arguably one of the most ambiguous and controversial concepts in integrative animal biology (Pickering, 1981). Although there is a general belief that stress is obligately associated with an elevation of circulating stress hormones (in particular corticosteroids), this traditional view has recently been challenged (Pollard, 1995). In this chapter, we have opted to interpret the concept of stress in the broadest sense. Thus, we consider stress to be a situation elicited by one or more stressors in which physiological function is compromised or in which the ability to meet energetic requirements is challenged. Ensuing adjustments to the cardiovascular and respiratory systems ensure that the detrimental effects of stressors are minimised or that energetic requirements continue to be met. In certain instances, the physiological adjustments to stressors are linked to changes in circulating stress hormone concentrations (see Randall and Perry, 1992; Thomas and Perry, 1992; Gamperl et al., 1994c), yet frequently they occur in the absence of changing hormone levels.

To varying degrees, all animals experience stressors, both natural and artificial. Certain groups of animals encounter stressors more frequently than others and thus may have evolved mechanisms for coping with stress. This chapter will focus on such animals and in particular will emphasise aquatic organisms that inhabit fluctuating and often harsh environments. Three underlying themes will prevail: (i) the nature of adaptive versus maladaptive responses to stress, (ii) inter-specific differences in the ability to tolerate stressors, and (iii) the relative involvement of the so-called stress hormones in mediating cardiovascular and respiratory responses to stressors.

Animals routinely might encounter numerous different types of stressors. However, the following discussion will focus predominantly on natural environmental stressors to illustrate basic principles of cardiovascular and respiratory control during stress. Two specific themes will be addressed in detail: exercise and oxygen availability. We have opted to focus on these particular topics because they have been studied extensively in both invertebrates and vertebrates, and because they are among the most common stressors facing animals in their natural habitat.

2.2   Exercise

In all animals, exercise requires an increase in O_2 delivery to exercising muscle and a roughly equivalent increase in the removal of metabolically produced CO_2 (aerobic exercise) or anaerobic end-products (anaerobic exercise). Adjustments to the cardiovascular system ensure that exercising tissues are supplied with adequate blood flow and also are essential to increase the rate of respiratory gas transfer at the gas exchange organ. Adjustments to the respiratory system are aimed at matching gas transfer and blood-gas transport to the increased metabolic demands imposed by exercise.

2.2.1   Types of exercise

Several categories of exercise exist, depending on the intensity and/or the duration of activity. Sustainable exercise can be maintained indefinitely and is powered exclusively by aerobic metabolism. In fish, this type of exercise is termed 'cruising' and is defined as exercise that can be maintained for periods exceeding 200 min (Beamish, 1978). In mammals, exercise generally can be sustained aerobically at O_2 consumption rates (Vo_2) less than 50–60% Vo_2Max. At greater intensities, exercise is fuelled both by aerobic and anaerobic metabolism. In mammals, the switch from strictly aerobic exercise to combined anaerobic–aerobic exercise is termed the 'lactate threshold'. Although this threshold varies among species, a conservative estimate is approximately 65–75% of Vo_2Max (Mazzeo and Marshall, 1989; Podolin et al., 1991). This type of exercise is analogous to prolonged swimming in fish (2–200 min duration). During prolonged swimming, the importance of anaerobic metabolism varies according to swimming speeds and exercise duration (Driedzic and Hochachka, 1978). A third type of exercise, intense burst activity, relies almost exclusively on anaerobic metabolism within the glycolytic 'white' muscle, is often terminated by fatigue, and is performed in brief bouts (e.g. < 20 s duration in fish).

2.2.2   Stress hormones during exercise

The potential involvement of stress hormones in cardiovascular and respiratory control during exercise is clearly dependent on the type of exercise being performed (Tables 2.1 and 2.2). Generally, the acute stress hormones, adrenaline and noradrenaline, are unlikely to contribute significantly during sustained aerobic activity (Table 2.1). In a few fish species, however, plasma catecholamine levels do increase during sustained swimming to levels that could potentially impact on cardiovascular and respiratory systems. In mammals, plasma catecholamine concentrations are not usually substantially elevated until the intensity of exercise exceeds about 60–65% Vo_2Max (Mazzeo and Marshall, 1989; Mazzeo, 1991; Podolin et al., 1991). Indeed, physiologically relevant levels may not be achieved until the intensity of exercise reaches about 80% Vo_2Max. In mammals, there is generally an excellent correlation between the lactate and catecholamine release thresholds during exercise (Mazzeo and Marshall, 1989; Podolin et al., 1991). Unlike in many lower vertebrates, noradrenaline is the predominant circulating catecholamine in mammals and its increase during moderate exercise is usually attributed to neuronal 'spillover' rather than to adrenal secretion. With few exceptions, exhaustive exercise is associated with pronounced increases in circulating levels of catecholamines. In mammals, a sudden increase in the ratio of plasma [adrenaline]/[noradrenaline] signals an abrupt release of catecholamines (predominantly adrenaline) from the adrenal gland. In lower vertebrates, exhaustive exercise is usually associated with large increases in both catecholamine hormones, although in most species that have been examined adrenaline tends to predominate. Amongst fish, the elasmobranchs tend to be an exception because equivalent quantities of adrenaline and noradrenaline are released into the blood during exhaustive exercise; this may reflect the relatively greater levels of noradrenaline stored in the chromaffin tissue within the axillary bodies (see Table 1 in Reid et al., 1998). Recently, Egginton (1997) demonstrated that three species of Antarctic fish did not exhibit a humoral adrenergic stress response during exhaustive exercise (Table 2.1). While it is possible that this insensitivity reflects their extremely cold and stenothermal environment, it is more likely a consequence of their sluggish lifestyle. In support of this idea, Milligan and Wood (1987) demonstrated stable levels of plasma catecholamines during exhaustive exercise in a temperate sedentary species, the starry flounder, Platichthys stellatus.

The classical studies of Nakano and Tomlinson (1967) and Opdyke et al. (1982) demonstrated that exercise elicited by physical disturbance of fish (tail grabbing) could elicit increases in circulating catecholamine

Table 2.1 Levels of plasma catecholamines (nmol l^{-1}) during exercise in selected animals. The data are presented as means $\pm$ 1 standard error of the mean except in cases where values were estimated from graphs

	Rest		Exercise		Reference
	[adrenaline]	[noradrenaline]	[adrenaline]	[noradrenaline]	
FISH					
Sustained aerobic swimming					
Gadus morhua	4	2.5	5	4	Axelsson and Nilsson, 1986
Oncorhynchus mykiss	0.2 ± 0.1	0.4 ± 0.1	0.5 ± 0.2	0.5 ± 0.3	Gallaugher et al., 1992
Oncorhynchus mykiss	1.4 ± 0.5	10.2 ± 2.4	0.3 ± 0.7	2.5 ± 2.0	Butler et al., 1986
Oncorhynchus mykiss	1.8 ± 0.2	3.9 ± 0.8	2.1 ± 0.2	5.9 ± 0.9	Hughes et al., 1988
Oncorhynchus mykiss	1.2 ± 0.1	1.3 ± 0.1	1.3 ± 0.1	1.1 ± 0.1	Ristori and Laurent, 1985
Scyliorhinus canicula	5.9 ± 1.2	14.0 ± 4.6	19.3 ± 6.8	32.5 ± 11.9	Butler et al., 1986
Labrus mixtus	4	2	11	9	Axelsson et al., 1987
Pollachius pollachius	6	2	28	13	Axelsson et al., 1987
Swimming at U_{crit}					
Gadus morhua	4	3	30	50	Butler et al., 1989
Oncorhynchus mykiss	0.2 ± 0.1	0.4 ± 0.1	11.6 ± 5.4	2.4 ± 0.7	Gallaugher et al., 1992
Oncorhynchus mykiss	1.4 ± 0.5	10.2 ± 2.4	14.4 ± 3.3	22.8 ± 6.1	Butler et al., 1986
Burst swimming until exhaustion, chasing until exhaustion or physical disturbance					
Oncorhynchus mykiss	1	1	37	28	Primmett et al., 1986
Oncorhynchus mykiss	1.4 ± 0.5	10.2 ± 2.4	212 ± 89	85 ± 46	Butler et al., 1986
Oncorhynchus mykiss	3	2	275	40	Perry et al., 1996
Oncorhynchus mykiss	30 ± 5	30 ± 3	358 ± 102	445 ± 160	Van Dijk and Wood, 1988
Oncorhynchus mykiss	2.2 ± 1.6	2.7 ± 1.8	29.7 ± 10.3	36.4 ± 8.4	Milligan and Wood, 1987
Oncorhynchus mykiss	1.2 ± 0.1	1.3 ± 0.1	7.9 ± 1.7	4.5 ± 2.0	Ristori and Laurent, 1985
Oncorhynchus mykiss	2.6	3.3	179.0	49.5	Tang and Boutilier, 1988
Oncorhynchus mykiss	15	2	210	27	Wood et al., 1990
Platichthys stellatus	19.1 ± 6.5	22.5 ± 6.4	NC	NC	Milligan and Wood, 1987
Notothenia coriiceps	0.6 ± 0.1	NR	0.4 ± 0.1	NR	Egginton, 1997

Table 2.1 (Continued).

	Rest		Exercise		Reference
	[adrenaline]	[noradrenaline]	[adrenaline]	[noradrenaline]	
Notothenia Rossii	0.5±0.1	NR	0.6±0.1	NR	Egginton, 1997
Chaenocephalus aceratus	0.4±0.2	NR	0.2±0.1	NR	Egginton, 1997
Scyliorhinus canicula	5.9±1.2	14.0±4.6	96.3±28	90.5±38	Butler et al., 1986
AMPHIBIANS					
Physical disturbance					
Bufo marinus	2.2±0.4	0.3±0.1	36.5±3.2	2.7±0.5	Tufts et al., 1987
Bufo marinus (Vo_2Max)	13.1±2.9	2.1±0.6	71.8±12.0	9.8±3.0	Withers et al., 1988a
REPTILES					
Exhaustive exercise					
Dipsosaurus dorsalis	10.4±4.4	16.0±4.7	116.3±40.4	109.3±16.0	Gleeson et al., 1993
MAMMALS					
Moderate/strenuous exercise					
Capra aegagrus (5.6 km h^{-1})	1.0±0.1	4.3±0.4	2.7±0.5	10.8±2.4	Warner and Mitchell, 1991
Rattus norvegicus (15 m min^{-1})	10.9±3.3	NR	19.1±4.9	NR	McDermott et al., 1987
Homo sapiens (50% Vo_2Max)	0.6	4.7	1.6	5.9	Mazzeo, 1991
Homo sapiens (50% Vo_2Max)	0.2±0.01	1.5±0.05	0.4±0.06	4.6±0.8	Brenner et al., 1997
Homo sapiens (80% Vo_2Max)	0.6	4.7	5.5	17.7	Mazzeo, 1991
Homo sapiens (85% H_F Max)	0.1±0.02	0.7±0.06	0.3±0.04	3.6±0.3	Kinugawa et al., 1996
Exhaustive exercise					
Homo sapiens	0.3±0.1	3.0±0.3	3.0±0.8	21.9±4.3	Young et al., 1992
Homo sapiens (Vo_2Max)	0.7	NR	7.4±1.4	54.1±13.8	Podolin et al., 1991
H. sapiens (Vo_2Max; cycling)	NR	NR	8.2±3.4	39.2±5.3	Mazzeo and Marshall, 1989
H. sapiens (Vo_2Max; running)	NR	NR	14.3±2.1	39.4±3.3	Mazzeo and Marshall, 1989

U_{crit}, critical swimming velocity; NC, no change; NR, not reported; Vo_2Max, maximal oxygen consumption during exercise; H_F, cardiac frequency.

levels. On the basis of these studies, it was generally accepted that catecholamine hormones could play a potential role in the physiological responses of fish to heavy exercise. In recent years, however, there has been considerable debate concerning the physiological relevance of elevated catecholamine levels in lower vertebrates during exhaustive exercise. The origin of this debate stems from the protocol generally used to elicit exhaustion. In studies of fish, the current standard protocol is to chase and prod animals within a small tank until they are exhausted. In studies of amphibians, the standard protocol is to repeatedly flip animals onto their backs to force a righting reflex. Clearly, such procedures must elicit a stress component that is independent of pure exercise. However, as discussed in detail by Wood (1991a), examples of such types of stressful or violent exercise are probably commonplace in the natural environments of lower vertebrates. For example, fish might experience exhaustive exercise in their natural habitat to avoid capture by a predator. Thus, while standard protocols to elicit exhaustive exercise in fish in the laboratory surely include a stress component, they are nevertheless physiologically relevant.

The impact of exercise on the circulating levels of the so-called chronic stress hormones, the corticosteroids (Table 2.2) differs markedly from the effects of exercise on the catecholamine hormones. An intriguing observation reported for several species, including fish and mammals, is that prolonged light (fish) or moderate (mammals) exercise may cause a decline in the circulating levels of cortisol (Davies and Few, 1973; Few, 1974; Boesgaard et al., 1993). Whether this reflects increased clearance of cortisol in the face of elevated cardiac output (see below) or a true reduction in the secretion of cortisol has not been ascertained. Unlike the catecholamine response to exercise, cortisol levels are elevated in fish both during sustained moderate exercise (> 1 BL s^{-1}) and during exhaustive 'violent' exercise. In mammals, cortisol levels are elevated at exercise levels exceeding $\sim 65\%$ of V_{O_2}Max.

2.2.3   Potential interactions between catecholamines and corticosteroids

The simultaneous elevation of corticosteroids and catecholamines or prior elevation of corticosteroids may have important consequences on the responses to exercise. In mammals, cortisol is known to increase the synthesis of phenylethanolamine-N-methyltransferase (PNMT), the enzyme responsible for the methylation of noradrenaline to form adrenaline (Evinger et al., 1992; Betito et al., 1993). This stimulatory effect of corticosteroids on PNMT appears to be absent in lower vertebrates (Jönsson et al., 1983; Reid et al., 1996). Thus, in mammals, prior elevation of cortisol levels during moderate exercise might serve to

Table 2.2 Levels of plasma cortisol or [a]corticosterone ($nmol\,l^{-1}$) during exercise in selected animals. The data are presented as means ± 1 standard error of the mean except in cases where values were estimated from graphs

	Rest	Exercise	Reference
FISH			
Sustained swimming			
Salmo salar; $0.5\,BL\,s^{-1}$ 1 h	25.4 ± 5.5	76.7 ± 5.2	Boesgaard *et al.*, 1993
Salmo salar; $0.5\,BL\,s^{-1}$ 4–24 h	25.4 ± 5.5	~13	Boesgaard *et al.*, 1993
Salmo salar parr; $50\,cm\,s^{-1}$—8 h	136.9	958	Virtanen and Forsman, 1987
Salmo salar smolt; $50\,cm\,s^{-1}$—8 h	520	2,191	Virtanen and Forsman, 1987
Oncorhynchus mykiss; $1\,BL\,s^{-1}$ 2 h	209.2 ± 24.9	353.8 ± 24.9	Zelnik and Goldspink, 1981
Oncorhynchus mykiss; $2.6\,BL\,s^{-1}$ 2 h	198.2 ± 20.8	696.6 ± 42.2	Zelnik and Goldspink, 1981
Oncorhynchus mykiss; $5\,BL\,s^{-1}$ 2 h	190.3 ± 33.6	893.8 ± 47.6	Zelnik and Goldspink, 1981
Chasing until exhaustion			
Oncorhynchus mykiss	11.6 ± 6.3	415.0 ± 37.5	Perry *et al.*, 1996
Oncorhynchus mykiss	78.0 ± 39.2	~329	Milligan and Wood, 1987
Oncorhynchus mykiss	~205	~465	Pagnotta *et al.*, 1994
Platichthys stellatus	277.9 ± 98.3	NC	Milligan and Wood, 1987
REPTILES			
Exhaustive exercise			
[a]*Dipsosaurus dorsalis*	40.8	131.2	Gleeson *et al.*, 1993
BIRDS			
Moderate exercise			
[a]*Anas platyrhynchos* $1.1\,km\,h^{-1}$—30 min	11.5	28.9	Rees *et al.*, 1985
[a]*Anas platyrhynchos* $1.1\,km\,h^{-1}$—60 min	11.5	20.2	Rees *et al.*, 1985

MAMMALS

Light – moderate exercise

Homo sapiens; 50% V_{O_2}Max	~300	~375	Brenner *et al.*, 1997
Homo sapiens; < 50% V_{O_2}Max	260	158	Davies and Few, 1973
Homo sapiens; 6.4 km h^{-1}—1 h	375.1 ± 73.9	197.2 ± 57.5	Few, 1974

Heavy exercise

Homo sapiens; 65–90% V_{O_2}Max	NR	+192.2	Davies and Few, 1973
Homo sapiens; 65–80% V_{O_2}Max—1 h	205.4 ± 54.7	539.4 ± 84.9	Few, 1974

BL, body lengths; NC, no change; NR, not reported; V_{O_2}Max, maximal oxygen consumption during exercise.

enhance the secretion of adrenaline during more intense exercise. Similarly, elevated plasma catecholamines may influence cortisol secretion. In mammals and birds, catecholamines stimulate cortisol secretion (Mokuda et al., 1992; Mazzocchi et al., 1998). In lower vertebrates, the paracrine influences of catecholamines on corticosteroid release are poorly understood (Mazzocchi et al., 1998) although in fish, catecholamines may inhibit cortisol secretion (Gfell et al., 1997). In addition to possible paracrine interactions, corticosteroids are known to influence synthesis and distribution of hormone receptors including β-adrenoreceptors (Hadcock and Malbon, 1988; Reid and Perry, 1991; Reid et al., 1992; Perry and Reid, 1993) and muscarinic receptors (Scherrer et al., 1997). Consequently, cardiovascular and respiratory responses to heavy or exhaustive exercise are likely to be modified by prior elevation of plasma corticosteroid levels. Finally, the hormonal response to acute exercise may be influenced by prior chronic exercise. For example, Perry et al. (1996) demonstrated that repetitive daily chasing of rainbow trout was associated with a blunting of the catecholamine secretory response during subsequent bouts of exercise. This likely reflected a decreased responsiveness of the chromaffin cells to cholinergic stimuli (Reid et al., 1994). These effects cannot be attributed to chronically elevated levels of cortisol because chronic treatment of trout with cortisol enhances the responsiveness of chromaffin cells to cholinergic stimuli (Reid et al., 1996).

2.2.4 Cardiovascular responses to exercise

Numerous comprehensive reviews focusing exclusively on, or highlighting aspects of, cardiovascular control during exercise, have been written (Jones and Randall, 1978; Taylor, 1982; Randall, 1982; Wood and Perry, 1985; Butler, 1991; Gleeson, 1991; Turner, 1991; Bushnell and Jones, 1992; Farrell, 1993, 1996; Olson, 1998). With a few exceptions, there are several universal cardiovascular responses to exercise in animals including an elevation of cardiac output ($\dot{V}b$), redistribution of blood flow, changes in blood pressure and peripheral vascular resistance, and adjustments to coronary blood flow.

2.2.4.1 Elevation of $\dot{V}b$

In the invertebrate decapod crustaceans, increases in $\dot{V}b$ are accomplished by simultaneous elevations of cardiac frequency (H_f) and stroke volume (H_{sv}) (Wood and Randall, 1981b; Hamilton and Houlihan, 1992). In lower vertebrates, the contributions of H_f and H_{sv} adjustments to the increases in $\dot{V}b$ during exercise are highly variable amongst the species that have been examined (e.g. see Figure 1 in Gleeson, 1991). Although there is a general belief that adjustments to $\dot{V}b$ during exercise in fish predominantly reflect increases in H_{sv}, this conclusion does not appear to be supported by the results of the relatively few species that have been examined (see also Olson, 1998). As in other lower vertebrates, the increases in $\dot{V}b$ in fish during exercise reflect variable contributions of elevated H_f and H_{sv} (Kiceniuk and Jones, 1977; Piiper *et al.*, 1977; Smith, 1978; Axelsson and Nilsson, 1986; Axelsson *et al.*, 1987, 1994; Butler *et al.*, 1989; Kolok *et al.*, 1993; Davison *et al.*, 1997). Elasmobranchs, however, appear to rely mostly on increases in H_{sv} (Piiper *et al.*, 1977). In birds, increases to H_{sv} and H_f contribute to elevated $\dot{V}b$ although the changes in H_f appear to be more important (Butler, 1991). In mammals, increases in $\dot{V}b$ during exercise are caused largely by increases in H_f.

At least three mechanisms contribute to the increases in $\dot{V}b$ during exercise: (i) a stimulation of cardiac β-adrenoreceptors via sympathetic nerves or circulating catecholamines, (ii) a reduction of parasympathetic cholinergic tonus, and (iii) an increase in venous return. The relative involvement of cardiac sympathetic nerves versus circulating catecholamines in the control of $\dot{V}b$ varies according to species and exercise intensity. During sustained exercise (light to moderate activity), the increases in $\dot{V}b$ largely reflect decreased parasympathetic activity coupled with increased sympathetic activity. Exceptions to this generalisation, however, can be found within several groups of fish. In particular, the hearts of elasmobranchs are devoid of adrenergic neural innervation (Nilsson, 1984, 1997) and thus rely exclusively on a reduction in cholinergic tonus and increases in circulating catecholamines for cardiac control during exercise. This may explain the substantial increase in plasma catecholamine levels in the dogfish (*Scyliorhinus canicula*) during spontaneous sustained swimming (Butler *et al.*, 1986). Within the agnathans, the hearts of hagfish lack any neuronal innervation (Nilsson, 1984). Thus, any change to $\dot{V}b$ in exercising hagfish would arise from altered venous return, blood-borne hormones or catecholamines secreted from the chromaffin cells located in the heart itself (Axelsson *et al.*, 1990; Forster *et al.*, 1992; Bernier and Perry, 1998b). Amongst the teleosts, there has been considerable debate concerning the possible role of circulating catecholamines in cardiovascular control during sustained swimming. For example, there is a prevailing view that the levels achieved in the plasma are insufficient to evoke cardiovascular responses. This view stems from studies that have compared *in vivo* levels of circulating catecholamines to those levels required to elicit significant responses *in vitro* or in *in situ* preparations (Butler *et al.*, 1986; Xu and Olson, 1993). In general, the levels of catecholamines achieved *in vivo* during sustained swimming are much lower than the levels required to elicit responses *in vitro* or *in situ*. Clearly, however, such comparisons are inappropriate and do not take into account the synergistic effects of other hormones such as the corticosteroids (see above) and the progressive deterioration of *in vitro* and *in situ* preparations. Recently, several studies (Gamperl *et al.*, 1994a; Bernier and Perry, 1998a) have demonstrated that significant cardiovascular responses could be triggered in rainbow trout at circulating levels of adrenaline between 10 and $20 \, \text{nmol} \, \text{l}^{-1}$ (see also Perry and Bernier, 1998). Such levels are achieved in several teleost species during sustained aerobic swimming and while swimming at critical velocity (U_{crit}; Table 2.1). Further support for a role of circulating catecholamines in cardiovascular control during sustained swimming was provided by Butler *et al.* (1989). In that study, prevention of catecholamine release by denervating the spinal nerves of Atlantic cod caused a significant reduction in U_{crit} that was re-established by infusion of denervated fish with a physiological dosage of catecholamines.

During heavy or exhaustive exercise, increases in plasma levels of catecholamines are likely to impact on $\dot{V}b$ except in sluggish species that do not display any appreciable increase in plasma catecholamine levels (Table 2.1). Interestingly, the Antarctic species that lack a humoral adrenergic response during intense exercise (Egginton, 1997) appear to exhibit an unusually high cardiac cholinergic tonus and thus rely predominantly on a reduction of this tonus to increase $\dot{V}b$ during intense exercise (Axelsson *et al.*, 1992; Davison *et al.*, 1997).

A well-documented response to an increase in plasma catecholamine levels is down-regulation of β-adrenoreceptors (Hausdorff *et al.*, 1990). For example, in rainbow trout, chronically elevated plasma catecholamine levels were shown to reduce the number of erythrocyte plasma membrane β-adrenoreceptors (Gilmour *et al.*, 1994). Thus, there is a potential for circulating catecholamines to attenuate the adrenergically mediated cardiovascular responses during exercise. This possibility has received little attention, although Gamperl *et al.* (1994d) demonstrated that in rainbow trout, the number of cardiac β_2-adrenoreceptors was unaffected by an elevation of plasma catecholamine levels.

An increase in $\dot{V}b$ during exercise, coupled with an elevation of blood viscosity owing to increases in haematocrit (see below), clearly will increase the work performed by the heart. However, increases in viscosity owing to polycythaemia may be partially offset by elevated levels of the stress hormones, catecholamines and cortisol. For example, it was recently demonstrated that both adrenaline and cortisol are able to effectively lower viscosity of rainbow trout blood *in vitro* (Sorensen and Weber, 1995).

2.2.4.2   *Redistribution of blood flow*
The mechanisms underlying the redistribution of blood flow during exercise are well understood in mammals and only poorly understood in

the lower vertebrates. In mammals, increased flow to exercising skeletal muscle commences with anticipatory sympathetic cholinergic vasodilatation of arterioles. This is followed by widespread sympathetic adrenergic vasoconstriction of arterioles within most vascular beds, a response mediated by α-adrenoreceptors. Because the brain and heart lack α-receptors, blood flow to these tissues is unaffected by the generalised increase in sympathetic activity. In exercising muscle, the tendency for sympathetic vasoconstriction is counteracted by profound metabolic vasodilatation leading to active hyperaemia. Consequently, blood flow is redistributed to areas experiencing increased metabolism while directed away from tissues exhibiting lower levels of metabolic activity. It is unlikely that circulating catecholamines play a role in the redistribution of blood flow during exercise in mammals.

Only a few studies have examined blood flow redistribution during exercise in fish (Stevens, 1968; Randall and Daxboeck, 1982; Neumann *et al.*, 1983; Axelsson and Fritsche, 1991; Kolok *et al.*, 1993; Thorarensen *et al.*, 1993). During sustained aerobic swimming, there is a massive increase in the proportion of $\dot{V}b$ directed to red muscle and a corresponding decrease in blood flow to white muscle (Randall and Daxboeck, 1982; Kolok *et al.*, 1993). During exhaustive exercise, there are pronounced increases in blood flow to both red and white muscle (Neumann *et al.*, 1983). It is likely that increased blood flow to exercising tissues, as in mammals, reflects active hyperaemia under the control of local metabolites (CO_2, H^+, K^+). This presumably overrides generalised sympathetic vasoconstriction (see below). During exercise in fish, there is a shunting of blood away from the gut (Axelsson and Fritsche, 1991; Kolok *et al.*, 1993). The mechanisms, although not totally understood, likely involve α-adrenergic vasoconstriction (Axelsson and Fritsche, 1991).

2.2.4.3   Changes in blood pressure and peripheral vascular resistance
Despite a 2- to 3-fold increase in $\dot{V}b$ during heavy exercise in mammals, mean systemic blood pressure generally remains constant or increases only slightly (Smith and Kampine, 1990). This presumably reflects the vasodilatation of skeletal muscle vasculature and the associated reduction in total peripheral vascular resistance. As a result of the decreased systemic vascular resistance, diastolic pressure is reduced markedly during heavy exercise. Thus, mean blood pressure is maintained by a concomitant increase in systolic blood pressure. In mammals, therefore, heavy exercise is associated with large increases in pulse pressure.

In fish, exercise is associated with pronounced increases in systemic blood pressure that vary with the intensity of exercise (Bushnell and Jones, 1992; Farrell, 1993; Olson, 1998). The increases in blood pressure can be attributed to the large increases in $\dot{V}b$. In most fish, the blood pressure increases are often lower than otherwise expected because of concurrent decreases in systemic vascular resistance (Bushnell and Jones, 1992; Farrell, 1993; Olson, 1998). With few exceptions (e.g. *Anguilla australis* (Hipkins *et al.*, 1986) and *Pagothenia borchgrevinki* (Axelsson *et al.*, 1994; Davison *et al.*, 1997)), the decreases in systemic vascular resistance during exercise reflect the opposing effects of metabolic vasodilatation and α-adrenergic vasoconstriction (Smith, 1978; Axelsson and Nilsson, 1986). The latter effect is mediated by sympathetic nerves and/or circulating catecholamines. An increase in ventral aortic pressure is likely to contribute to lamellar recruitment and thus an enhancement of gas transfer during exercise (see below).

2.2.4.4   Changes in coronary blood flow

The relative importance of the coronary circulation to cardiac function varies widely amongst the vertebrates. In amphibians and reptiles, the coronary circulation is relatively unimportant because the spongy nature of the myocardium allows the metabolic requirements of the heart to be met by the oxygen contained within the returning venous blood. Within fish, coronary vessels are found in all elasmobranchs and some active teleosts (Axelsson, 1995). The importance of the coronary circulation in fish varies according to the relative mass of the compact myocardium (Davie and Farrell, 1991). In fish, coronary blood flow accounts for approximately 1% of cardiac output (Axelsson and Farrell, 1993; Gamperl *et al.*, 1994b) whereas in birds and mammals, coronary flow is approximately 5% of $\dot{V}b$.

Although apparently unimportant during normoxia at rest (Gamperl *et al.*, 1994a), Farrell and Steffensen (1987) demonstrated the importance of the coronary circulation during exercise in fish. In that study, ligation of the coronary artery caused a 36% reduction in U_{crit} in Chinook salmon (*Oncorhynchus tshawytscha*). It is unknown whether coronary blood flow increases during exercise in fish. The coronary resistance in fish is controlled by constrictory α-adrenoreceptors, dilatory β-adrenoreceptors and probably local metabolites (Farrell, 1987; Axelsson and Farrell, 1993; Gamperl *et al.*, 1994b; Axelsson, 1995). Because the α-constrictory response dominates over the β-dilatory response, increases in circulating catecholamines during exercise might tend to increase coronary resistance. It is likely, however, that coronary flow increases during exercise owing, at least in part, to the increased work performed by the heart (Farrell, 1987) and metabolic vasodilatation.

In mammals, coronary blood flow increases during exercise in relation to the increase in cardiac work. Numerous metabolic factors have been implicated including increased P_{CO_2}, lowered pH and in particular, local hypoxia. It is possible that the dilatory influence of hypoxia reflects both a direct effect on the coronary vasculature as well as an indirect effect mediated by the vasodilator, adenosine (Smith and Kampine, 1990).

2.2.5   *Respiratory responses to exercise*

The respiratory responses to exercise in both vertebrates and invertebrates have been the subject of numerous detailed reviews (e.g. Jones and Randall, 1978; Randall, 1982; Taylor, 1982; Whipp and Ward, 1982; Wood and Perry, 1985; Gleeson and Bennett, 1985; Butler, 1986, 1991; Wasserman *et al.*, 1986; Gleeson, 1991; Turner, 1991; Wood, 1991a; Wasserman, 1994; Saunders and Fedde, 1994; Mateika and Duffin, 1995). In response to exercise, the convective, diffusive, and blood gas transport properties of the gas exchange system are altered to match respiratory gas transfer to the metabolic requirements of the exercising tissues.

2.2.5.1   *Ventilation*

An apparently universal response to exercise among both the vertebrates and invertebrates examined to date is an increase in ventilation (e.g. invertebrates: McMahon *et al.*, 1979; Wood and Randall, 1981b; fish: Piiper *et al.*, 1977; Kiceniuk and Jones, 1977; Wood and Munger, 1994; amphibians: McDonald *et al.*, 1980; Withers *et al.*, 1988b; reptiles: Mitchell *et al.*, 1981; Gleeson and Bennett, 1985; Hopkins *et al.*, 1995; birds: Butler *et al.*, 1977; Kiley *et al.*, 1985; Fedde *et al.*, 1989; mammals: Whipp *et al.*, 1982; Kuhlmann *et al.*, 1985; Evans and Rose, 1988b; Warner and Mitchell, 1991; Butler *et al.*, 1993). Hyperventilation occurs immediately with the onset of exercise and serves to increase the delivery of O_2 to the gas exchange surface to meet the demand for elevated O_2 uptake; indeed, ventilation volume increases are often in proportion to those in O_2 uptake (e.g. Piiper *et al.*, 1977; Kiceniuk and Jones, 1977; Butler, 1991; Butler *et al.*, 1993). Although the increase in ventilation will decrease the residence time of the respiratory medium at the gas exchange surface, the percentage of O_2 removed from the water or air (utilisation) generally does not decrease and may increase during sustainable exercise (Jones and Randall, 1978; Butler, 1991), presumably because of elevated O_2 diffusive conductance across the gas exchange surface (see below).

Hyperventilation may be achieved through increases in ventilation frequency and/or ventilatory stroke volume. The relative contributions of these two parameters to the elevated ventilation volume vary with both species and the level of exercise. In horses, for example, large increases in breathing frequency are the major contributor to elevated pulmonary ventilation during walking and trotting, but at higher speeds (cantering and galloping), frequency ceases to increase and substantial changes in tidal volume are observed (Butler *et al.*, 1993). The constraint on frequency increases at higher speeds is probably a reflection of the fact that limb movements and ventilation are mechanically coupled in cantering and galloping horses (Butler *et al.*, 1993). Breathing frequency and stride frequency are linked during strenuous exercise in a variety of mammals, and in such cases the forces generated during locomotion may assist to a small extent in the work of breathing (Baudinette, 1991; Ainsworth *et al.*, 1997). Similarly, a constant ratio of wing beats to breaths is observed in many species of birds during flight (Saunders and Fedde, 1994), and the respiratory and wing-beat cycles may be phasically co-ordinated in some species so as to achieve a net assistance (or at least minimal interference) to respiration from flight-induced forces (Boggs *et al.*, 1997). The relative contributions of frequency and tidal volume changes to increased pulmonary ventilation during exercise in birds appear to be quite species specific (Butler, 1991; Saunders and Fedde, 1994); such species specific variation also appears to occur among reptiles (Shelton *et al.*, 1986; Hopkins *et al.*, 1995).

In contrast to the relatively small contributions of locomotory muscles to breathing in air-breathers, fish swimming at speeds at or above 50–80 cm s^{-1} may transfer all of the work of breathing from the respiratory to the swimming musculature by switching from rhythmic breathing movements to ram ventilation (Roberts and Rowell, 1988). By means of this strategy, the energetic cost of breathing can be kept constant and independent of the level of exercise, a considerable advantage given that the cost of breathing at rest is probably 10% of the resting oxygen consumption (versus 1–2% in air-breathers) owing to the relatively low capacitance of water for O_2 together with the relatively high density and viscosity of this respiratory medium (Jones and Randall, 1978). At lower swimming speeds, gill ventilation volume increases are accomplished in an energetically efficient manner through small increases in breathing frequency and large changes in stroke volume (Piiper *et al.*, 1977; Jones and Randall, 1978). An alternative ventilatory strategy to support activity that is available to a few bimodally breathing fish species is an increase in the extraction of O_2 from air relative to water during exercise; in two species of air-breathing fish, the frequency of surfacing to breathe was found to increase with the intensity of exercise (Farmer and Jackson, 1998).

The mechanisms through which ventilation is increased at the onset of exercise and matched to the O_2 demand during exercise are not yet fully understood. The rapidity (0–15 s) with which ventilation increases in response to the onset of exercise argues for neurally based control mechanisms (see reviews by Whipp and Ward, 1982; Shelton *et al.*, 1986; Wasserman *et al.*, 1986; Turner, 1991; Mateika and Duffin, 1995). Two such mechanisms have been proposed: (i) feedback reflexes, consisting of neural signals from mechanical or chemical nerve receptors in the active muscle mass which act upon the central cardiorespiratory control centres and, (ii) feedforward control mechanisms, in which a centrally generated command signal is produced to drive both locomotion and the cardiorespiratory responses required to maintain it. In addition, cardio-pulmonary coupling mechanisms have been proposed, involving the direct activation of ventilation by cardiac, pulmonary vascular and/or peripheral vascular factors (Whipp and Ward, 1982; Wasserman et al., 1986; Mateika and Duffin, 1995; Haouzi et al., 1996). Experimental evidence supporting roles for each of these control mechanisms has been obtained, but the relative importance of each and the exact pathways involved remain uncertain (Wasserman et al., 1986; Turner, 1991; Mateika and Duffin, 1995). As exercise proceeds, cardiorespiratory variables change more slowly until a new steady-state condition is reached. Both neural and humoral mechanisms may be involved in controlling this stage of the ventilatory response to exercise (Wasserman et al., 1986; Turner, 1991; Mateika and Duffin, 1995). The neural mechanisms responsible for the stimulation of ventilation at the onset of exercise will also operate to control ventilation as exercise is sustained. For example, muscle mechanoreceptors may be important in matching respiratory frequency and locomotory gait in mammals (Turner, 1991), while flow- or velocity-sensitive mechanoreceptors may initiate the transition from rhythmic breathing movements to ram ventilation in fish (Shelton et al., 1986). Additionally, however, blood-borne chemical factors produced by the active muscle could now play a role in controlling ventilation, although it is noteworthy that respiratory adjustments to sustainable exercise occur in the absence of marked changes in arterial blood pH (pHa), Po_2 (Pao_2) or Pco_2 ($Paco_2$), and there is little evidence for the existence of venous chemoreceptors (Turner, 1991). Increases in arterial temperature in birds and mammals also have been suggested to contribute to the elevated ventilation during sustained exercise (Butler et al., 1993; Saunders and Fedde, 1994; Mateika and Duffin, 1995).

With respect to exercise above the lactate threshold and exhaustive exercise, decreased arterial pH as well as elevated levels of circulating stress hormones may provide additional mechanisms through which ventilation could be controlled. At these intensities, exercise results in significant increases in muscle and blood lactate concentrations concomitant with a metabolic acidosis in the arterial blood that is usually attributed to protons generated in association with lactate production (Gleeson, 1996). This metabolic acidosis will, in air-breathers, drive a hyperventilatory response through arterial (carotid body) and central chemoreceptor mechanisms, and causes a lowering of $Paco_2$ (Wasserman et al., 1986). Blood lactate accumulations are often lower in teleost fish than in terrestrial vertebrates owing to intracellular retention of lactate in the white muscle (Gleeson, 1996), but two additional factors can contribute to the acidosis observed following exhaustive exercise in teleost fish. Protons extruded from red blood cells (RBCs), a consequence of the action of elevated circulating catecholamines on the β-adrenergically mediated Na^+/H^+ antiporter of the RBC membrane (see below), add to the metabolic acidosis (Wood, 1991a; Tufts and Perry, 1998). Furthermore, the post-exhaustive exercise acidosis in teleost fish has a respiratory component. The basis of this respiratory acidosis remains somewhat controversial (Wood, 1991a; Tufts and Perry, 1998), but it is likely that arterial P_{CO_2} is elevated by CO_2 produced from the titration of extracellular HCO_3^- with protons extruded from white muscle and erythrocytes, and by a β-adrenergically mediated relative inhibition of HCO_3^- flux through the red blood cells (Wood, 1994). Together, these metabolic and respiratory components produce a pronounced depression of arterial pH which probably serves to stimulate ventilation after exercise (Wood and Munger, 1994), i.e. at a time when the fish is motionless, circumventing proprioceptive stimulation of ventilation, and the arterial O_2 content is close to normal, such that hyperventilation cannot be elicited through the primary O_2-keyed ventilatory drive (Wood and Perry, 1985; Perry and Wood, 1989; Wood, 1991a). Interestingly, the elevated cortisol levels observed following exhaustive exercise appear to increase the time required for recovery of the extracellular acid–base status (Pagnotta et al., 1994; Eros and Milligan, 1996), and may therefore indirectly contribute to the post-exercise hyperventilation.

The potential involvement of circulating catecholamines in stimulating ventilation directly has been examined in mammals and fish. In mammals exercising above the lactate threshold, elevated levels of circulating catecholamines could act as a humoral stimulus for ventilation (Mateika and Duffin, 1995). Experimental results, however, tend not to support a major role for catecholamines in stimulating ventilation during exercise. For example, infusion of adrenaline into exercising humans did not increase ventilation significantly (Gaesser et al., 1994), while intra-arterial infusion of noradrenaline in exercising goats was found to have an inhibitory effect on ventilation (Pizarro et al., 1992). Ventilatory responses to exercise were also unaffected by β-adrenergic blockade in goats (Warner and Mitchell, 1991) and humans (Wasserman et al., 1986). Similarly, hypoventilatory or no effects on ventilation following the administration of physiological doses of catecholamines have been documented in a number of studies on fish (Perry et al., 1992), suggesting that the role of catecholamines in stimulating ventilation following exhaustive exercise is limited to the indirect effects mediated through arterial P_{CO_2} and pH in teleost fish. Experiments designed to assess the contribution of circulating catecholamines to the control of ventilation in fish have focused largely on hypoxia or hypercapnia and will be discussed below.

2.2.5.2 Diffusive conductance at the gas exchange surface

In general, percentage utilisation of O_2 from air or water does not decrease during exercise (Jones and Randall, 1978; Wasserman et al., 1986; Butler, 1991), even though ventilation is greatly elevated and hence residence time of the respiratory medium at the gas exchange surface must be decreased. For example, the residence time of water flowing over the gills of fish may be reduced from 250 ms at rest to 35 ms during intense exercise (Randall and Daxboeck, 1984). Reductions in venous Po_2 (Pvo_2) and a consequent increase in the partial pressure gradient for O_2 diffusion may increase the overall transfer of O_2 across the gas exchange surface (Wood and Perry, 1985; Longworth et al., 1989), but to account for the maintenance of O_2 utilisation in the face of decreased residence time, O_2 diffusive conductance across the gas exchange surface must be enhanced during exercise. In species such as the dogfish, where increases in O_2 diffusive conductance with exercise are insufficient to balance the increases in ventilation, O_2 utilisation decreases during exercise (Piiper et al., 1977).

Elevated ventilation in fish may increase the gill O_2 diffusive conductance by reducing unstirred or boundary layers next to the gill lamellae (Randall and Daxboeck, 1984); diffusion of O_2 across the interlamellar water is predicted to contribute significantly to limitations on diffusive O_2 transfer between the respiratory medium and blood because the diffusion of O_2 in water is orders of magnitude slower than in air (Piiper et al., 1986; Swenson, 1990). Crustaceans face an additional limitation in this respect, in that the gills are covered with a thin layer of chitin and chitin is even less permeable to O_2 than the underlying gill tissue (Taylor, 1982). The changes in blood flow associated with exercise in fish may increase the functional surface area of the gill by lamellar recruitment and a more even distribution of blood flow within the lamellae (Farrell et al., 1979; Randall and Daxboeck, 1984; Wood and Perry, 1985), reduce the blood-to-water diffusion distance through a thinning of the respiratory epithelium (i.e. pillar cell flanges, epithelium and interstitial space) to accommodate the increased vascular volume (Farrell et al., 1980), and increase the effective epithelial permeability (Davie and Daxboeck, 1982). Changes in blood flow together with elevated ventilation may also reduce ventilation-perfusion inequalities in the gills, thereby improving the efficiency of gas transfer across the gill (Jones and Randall, 1978). Further increases in the gill O_2 diffusive conductance may be achieved through the mobilisation of catecholamines into the circulation in response to exhaustive exercise (Randall and Perry,

1992); catecholamines are thought to increase the permeability of the respiratory epithelium (Isaia et al., 1978a,b; Perry et al., 1985) and will increase the functional surface area of the gill by lamellar recruitment through β-adrenoreceptor-mediated dilation of afferent lamellar arterioles (Booth, 1979; Holbert et al., 1979). In contrast to the beneficial effects of catecholamines, elevated cortisol levels in response to exercise could potentially decrease the gill O_2 diffusive conductance since the treatment of rainbow trout with cortisol for 10 days caused an increase in the blood-to-water diffusion distance (Bindon et al., 1994a) and a concomitant impairment of respiratory gas transfer (Bindon et al., 1994b) that were associated with a cortisol-induced proliferation of the ion-transporting chloride cells of the gill epithelium. While the enhanced diffusive conductance of the gill for O_2 is adaptive for the maintenance of O_2 uptake during exercise, it is accompanied by increased water and ionic fluxes across the gills (Wood, 1988; Gonzalez and McDonald, 1992; Postlethwaite and McDonald, 1995), which may contribute to the metabolic cost of exercise and recovery from exercise (Wood, 1991a).

In air-breathers, O_2 diffusion in the respiratory medium is not thought to be a significant limitation in gas exchange, as is the case for water-breathers (Swenson, 1990). Increases in O_2 diffusive conductance with exercise have been reported for birds, and have been attributed to increases in the functional surface area of the lung resulting from capillary dilation and/or recruitment and reductions in ventilation-perfusion inequalities (Kiley et al., 1985; Powell, 1994). Similar effects would be expected to increase lung O_2 diffusive conductance during exercise in other air-breathers (Truchot et al., 1980). However, ventilation-perfusion heterogeneities in both reptiles (Hopkins et al., 1995) and mammals (Hopkins et al., 1994) have been found to increase with exercise and together with diffusion limitations may represent significant limitations during maximal exercise (Powell, 1994). It is noteworthy that, in mammals with very high aerobic exercise capacities, such as the dog and horse, estimates of lung O_2 diffusing capacity based on morphometric measurements tend to be higher than in less 'athletic' species of similar size (Longworth et al., 1989), while the O_2 diffusing capacity of the avian lung is much higher than that of the mammalian lung owing to thinner blood-to-gas diffusion barriers and increased functional surface areas, structural adaptations which are probably important in meeting the high O_2 demands of flight (Saunders and Fedde, 1994).

2.2.5.3 Blood gas transport

In mammals or reptiles exercising above the lactate threshold, arterial pH is reduced (Gleeson and Bennett, 1985; Wasserman, 1994), while exhaustive exercise in fish is characterised by a marked depression of pHa coupled with a significant increase in Pa_{CO_2} (Wood, 1991a).

However, except at these intense levels of exercise, Pa_{O_2}, Pa_{CO_2} and pHa during exercise do not in general differ markedly from their resting values in birds (e.g. Butler *et al.*, 1977; Kiley *et al.*, 1985; Fedde *et al.*, 1989), mammals (e.g. Kuhlmann *et al.*, 1985; Taylor *et al.*, 1987; Jones *et al.*, 1989; Warner and Mitchell, 1990; Butler *et al.*, 1993; Stringer *et al.*, 1994), reptiles (e.g. Gleeson and Bennett, 1985), or fish (e.g. Piiper *et al.*, 1977; Kiceniuk and Jones, 1977; Thomas *et al.*, 1987; Gallaugher *et al.*, 1992; Korsmeyer *et al.*, 1997); note that exercise in decapod crustaceans results in changes in haemolymph gas transport that are qualitatively similar to the changes in blood gas transport observed in vertebrates (McMahon *et al.*, 1979; Wood and Randall, 1981a; Taylor, 1982). Haemoglobin-oxygen (Hb-O_2) saturation in arterial blood remains close to the resting level during sustainable exercise, while arterial O_2 content (Ca_{O_2}) tends to be maintained or even increased. Increases in the arterial haemoglobin concentration may contribute to the maintenance or elevation of Ca_{O_2} (e.g. Kuhlmann *et al.*, 1985; Thomas *et al.*, 1987; Taylor *et al.*, 1987; Evans and Rose, 1988a; Jones *et al.*, 1989; Butler *et al.*, 1993) and can be achieved through erythrocyte recruitment from the spleen (Yamamoto *et al.*, 1980; Evans and Rose, 1988a; Gallaugher *et al.*, 1992; Laub *et al.*, 1993). Contraction of the spleen in most vertebrates is under adrenergic nervous control, although an unusual cholinergic control mechanism has been documented in the red-blooded Antarctic fish *Pagothenia borch-grevinki* (Nilsson *et al.*, 1996).

Whereas Ca_{O_2} is maintained or increased during sustainable exercise, mixed venous O_2 content (Cv_{O_2}) is typically significantly reduced, such that the arterial-venous O_2 content difference (ΔC_{O_2}) is enhanced. For example, ΔC_{O_2} increased by 80% during flight in pigeons (Butler *et al.*, 1977), 111% during trotting in horses (Butler *et al.*, 1993), and 63% during swimming at a moderate speed in rainbow trout (Kiceniuk and Jones, 1977). The lower Cv_{O_2} during exercise reflects increased O_2 extraction from the blood. Sustainable exercise commonly results in decreases in venous Po_2 and pH (pHv) together with an increase in venous Pco_2 (Pv_{CO_2}) (e.g. mammals: Kuhlmann *et al.*, 1985; Taylor *et al.*, 1987; Evans and Rose, 1988a; Jones *et al.*, 1989; Butler *et al.*, 1993; Stringer *et al.*, 1994; birds: Butler *et al.*, 1977; Kiley *et al.*, 1985; amphibians: Withers *et al.*, 1988b; fish: Kiceniuk and Jones, 1977; Korsmeyer *et al.*, 1997); the net effect of these changes is a reduction in venous Hb-O_2 saturation, thereby increasing O_2 extraction from the blood. In addition to the direct effect of the lower Pv_{O_2} on venous Hb-O_2 saturation, the lower pHv and/or elevated Pv_{CO_2} (in fish the specific effect of CO_2 is small or absent) may elicit a right shift of the O_2 equilibrium curve through the Bohr effect, with the resultant decrease in Hb-O_2 binding affinity augmenting O_2 unloading (Jensen, 1991).

Exercise at intensities above the lactate threshold in mammals may result in significant changes in arterial blood gases and pH, as well as elevated plasma lactate concentrations. A significant decline in Pao_2 together with an arterial acidosis have been reported for horses and steer exercising at Vo_2Max (Evans and Rose, 1988a; Jones et al., 1989; Butler et al., 1993). Although these changes would be expected to reduce Hb-O_2 saturation, the concomitant large increases in the arterial haemoglobin concentration were sufficient for the maintenance of Cao_2 at or above the resting level. The importance of the lactacidosis may lie at the capillary level, where the Bohr-induced right shift of the O_2 equilibrium curve may enable O_2 to be transported into the cell without a decrease in capillary Po_2 below the critical pressure required to sustain diffusion (Wasserman, 1994; Stringer et al., 1994). In addition, a large rise in arterial temperature occurs during intense exercise and would be expected to cause a right-shift of the O_2 equilibrium curve (Butler et al., 1993). Whereas $Paco_2$ in horses and steer exercising at Vo_2Max is at or above the resting level (Kuhlmann et al., 1985; Jones et al., 1989; Butler et al., 1993), in other species, including humans, the decrease in arterial pH stimulates a relative hyperventilation at Vo_2Max such that $Paco_2$ is reduced (Wasserman et al., 1986); ventilation may be limited at high exercise intensities in large mammals by the mechanical coupling between breathing and limb movements (Jones et al., 1989; Butler et al., 1993).

The mobilisation of catecholamines during exhaustive exercise in fish has a significant impact on blood gas transport. In teleosts, circulating catecholamines stimulate splenic contraction through an α-adrenorecep-tor mediated response (Nilsson and Grove, 1974), with the resultant influx of erythrocytes into the circulation elevating blood haemoglobin concentration significantly (Yamamoto et al., 1980; Wells and Weber, 1990); this response appears to be absent in elasmobranch fish (Lowe et al., 1995). The blood haemoglobin concentration may also be increased through haemoconcentration owing to a large net fluid shift from the extracellular into the intracellular compartment in response to the osmotic attraction of elevated intracellular lactate concentrations (Yamamoto et al., 1980; Wood, 1991a). Uniquely in teleost fish, adjustment of the red blood cell intracellular environment to increase Hb-O_2 binding affinity and capacity is also under adrenergic control. The adrenergic sensitivity of the teleost RBC is thought to be linked to the presence in teleost fish of haemoglobins that exhibit a Root effect, that is, haemoglobins in which the maximal Hb-O_2 carrying capacity is reduced by acidification (Tufts and Randall, 1989). Because protons are normally passively distributed across the RBC membrane according to a Donnan equilibrium (see review by Nikinmaa, 1992), the profound exercise-induced extracellular acidosis would, in the absence of adrenergic responsiveness, result in a corresponding reduction in RBC intracellular pH and hence a Root-induced decrease in Hb-O_2 carrying capacity. Catecholamine mobilisation during exhaustive exercise stimulates RBC membrane β-adrenoreceptors and ultimately leads to the activation of a unique cAMP-sensitive Na^+/H^+ antiporter on the RBC membrane. The Na^+/H^+ antiporter extrudes protons from the RBC in exchange for plasma Na^+ with a consequent alkalinisation of the RBC intracellular environment and a lowering of extracellular pH (Nikinmaa and Huestis, 1984; Baroin et al., 1984; Cossins and Richardson, 1985, see also reviews by Nikinmaa and Tufts, 1989; Nikinmaa, 1992; Thomas and Perry, 1992). Stimulation of the RBC β-adrenoreceptors effectively uncouples the RBC intracellular pH from its normal dependence on extracellular pH because the rate of proton extrusion by the Na^+/H^+ antiporter is greater than the rate at which the passive H^+ equilibrium across the erythrocyte membrane can be re-established (Motais et al., 1989). Alkalinisation of RBC will clearly benefit Hb-O_2 binding affinity and capacity through the Bohr and Root effects, respectively, but adrenergic activation of the RBC Na^+/H^+ antiporter can additionally enhance Hb-O_2 binding through RBC swelling and adjustment of the RBC intracellular organic phosphate (NTP) concentrations (Nikinmaa and Tufts, 1989; Nikinmaa, 1992; Thomas and Perry, 1992). Water entry into the RBC is osmotically coupled to the accumulation of Na^+ and results in RBC swelling that, in turn, dilutes RBC haemoglobin and organic phosphates, reducing Hb–NTP complexing and increasing the Hb-O_2 binding affinity (Jensen, 1991). Also, accumulation of Na^+ stimulates the RBC Na^+/K^+ pump, increasing energetic demands and lowering the RBC NTP levels (Ferguson et al., 1989). Thus, the net effect of RBC adrenergic activation by circulating catecholamines in many teleost fish is an increase in the Hb-O_2 binding affinity and capacity produced by the integrated effects of RBC alkalinisation, RBC swelling and a decrease in the RBC intracellular organic phosphate levels.

In addition to the catecholamine-mediated enhancement of the O_2 transport properties of the blood in teleost fish, adrenergic stimulation of teleost RBCs may have an impact on CO_2 transport and excretion (see reviews by Wood and Perry, 1985; Wood, 1991a; Thomas and Perry, 1992; Tufts and Perry, 1998). Alkalinisation of the RBC interior will shift the CO_2 hydration/dehydration equilibrium, $CO_2 + H_2O \leftrightarrow HCO_3^- + H^+$, towards CO_2 hydration, thereby decreasing the intracellular CO_2 tension and producing a temporary reversal of the normal outwardly directed $P\text{CO}_2$ gradient between RBC and plasma. The concomitant increase in intracellular HCO_3^- levels would be expected to impair the passive entry of HCO_3^- into the RBC via the Cl^-/HCO_3^- exchanger. Together, these two factors could diminish HCO_3^- flux through the RBCs and, in vivo, would be predicted to cause inhibition of the net plasma HCO_3^- dehydration rate relative to that which would be observed in the absence of adrenergic stimulation. In support of this 'CO$_2$ retention' theory, Wood (1994) has recently documented a relative reduction in the *in vitro* rate of HCO_3^- flux through RBCs withdrawn from exercised trout in comparison to values for resting trout, despite an increase in the absolute rate of RBC CO_2 excretion induced by exercise. This adrenergically mediated impairment of HCO_3^- flux through the RBCs may contribute significantly to the rise in $Paco_2$ observed following exhaustive exercise in fish (see above).

2.3   Oxygen availability

The levels of oxygen in the natural environment are highly variable. Aquatic ecosystems display particularly unstable levels of oxygen owing to the low solubility of O_2 in water, its poor diffusivity and inadequate convection (see Truchot, 1987). Thus, O_2 levels in poorly mixed bodies of water are significantly influenced by biological activity. The aquatic environment exhibits both temporal and depth-dependent changes in O_2 partial pressures. Small ponds or intertidal pools often exhibit hypoxic conditions during the night and hyperoxic conditions during the day. Stagnant bodies of water in tropical regions may experience gradual depletion of O_2. Even large lakes and oceans may contain stratified zones of hypoxic water. The aerial environment (at any given altitude), on the other hand, is remarkably stable. This reflects the combined effects of a high O_2 solubility coefficient, high diffusivity and excellent atmospheric mixing. Exceptions to the normally constant Po_2 in air can be found in microhabitats including animal burrows and dens that may undergo profound hypoxia. Thus, excluding such microhabitats, the Po_2 of terrestrial habitats is dictated by altitude. Owing to the inverse relationship between barometric pressure and altitude, Po_2 declines with increasing altitude. High-altitude hypoxia, however, is experienced by relatively few species and most are acclimatised to their environment and thus are unlikely to be 'stressed' by the low ambient Po_2. Humans, however, are notable exceptions who choose to experience dramatic reductions in ambient Po_2 during voluntary ascents to high altitude. Such excursions to high altitude offer interesting insights into the cardiovascular and respiratory adjustments of mammals to hypoxia. Another example of restricted oxygen availability occurs during underwater submergence. Species within all classes of air-breathing vertebrates display voluntary submergence, and during such periods of breath holding, the blood becomes progressively hypoxaemic. Many animals have adapted to prolonged submergence and are even able to exercise for extended periods while underwater. In the following discussion, however, we will focus on forced, rather than voluntary submergence, because it is more likely to elicit a 'stress response'.

The physiological limitations imposed by hypoxia are numerous but are minimised by a host of cardiovascular and respiratory responses aimed at maintaining normal rates of metabolism despite the limited availability of O_2. As in exercise, many of these responses occur in the absence of stress hormone elevation while others are partially or wholly dependent on these hormones.

2.3.1   Stress hormones during hypoxia

Table 2.3 summarises the effects of hypoxia on circulating catecholamine levels. Although numerous studies have been performed on fish, relatively few species have been examined and within these species, there is a great deal of variability in the responses to hypoxia. Some of this variability can be attributed to variable methodology, including differences in the severity and duration of hypoxia and the analytical procedures used to measure plasma catecholamines. Nevertheless, it is apparent that fish experience an elevation of catecholamines during hypoxia and that the more active or hypoxia-intolerant species (e.g. salmonids) display a greater catecholamine elevation than the inactive or hypoxia-tolerant species (e.g. carp, eel, hagfish). Additionally, it seems that a greater severity of hypoxia is required to elicit significant catecholamine release in the latter group.

Even amongst the hypoxia-intolerant species, the degree of hypoxia must be severe before there is significant catecholamine release into the circulation (Randall and Perry, 1992). While only a few species have been examined, it is generally believed that the degree of hypoxia must be severe enough to lower blood O_2 content by approximately 50% before significant catecholamine release is initiated (Perry and Reid, 1992a; Thomas and Perry, 1992; Perry and Reid, 1994). Upon reaching this catecholamine release threshold, adrenaline and noradrenaline are abruptly secreted into the blood. Thus, only upon reaching this threshold can plasma catecholamines play a role in the cardiovascular and respiratory responses to hypoxia.

Relatively few studies have addressed the impact of forced submergence on circulating catecholamine levels. However, in the species that have been examined, forced submergence is associated with marked increases in both adrenaline and noradrenaline (Table 2.3). In some instances, it is unclear whether the increase in plasma catecholamines reflects the hypoxaemia or the 'stressful' nature of the forced submergence.

Table 2.3 Levels of plasma catecholamines (nmol l⁻¹) during hypoxia in selected animals. The data are presented as means ± 1 standard error of the mean except in cases where values were estimated from graphs. Except where otherwise stated, the levels of hypoxia are expressed as changes in ambient Po_2

	Normoxia		Hypoxia		Reference
	[adrenaline]	[noradrenaline]	[adrenaline]	[noradrenaline]	
FISH					
Environmental hypoxia					
Gadus morhua; 40 Torr	8.3±3.0	15.5±3.8	108.5±66.7	48.3±10.3	Perry *et al.*, 1991
Gadus morhua; 30–40 Torr	4.5±1.3	7.6±1.9	25.5±7.0	33.5±9.0	Fritsche and Nilsson, 1990
Gadus morhua; 46 Torr	3.5±1.4	4.1±2.1	9.4±5.6	11.0±5.4	Kinkead *et al.*, 1991
Myxine glutinosa;10.5 Torr	0.4±0.1	1.8±0.4	1.0±0.5	10.8±2.4	Perry *et al.*, 1993
Eptatretus stouti; 25 Torr	1	2	40	28	Bernier *et al.*, 1996
Eptatretus stouti; 10 Torr	1.8	3.8	3.0	10.2	Bernier *et al.*, 1996
Oncorhynchus mykiss; 60 Torr	10±1	2±0.2	320±100	3.8±0.4	Thomas *et al.*, 1991
Oncorhynchus mykiss; 45 Torr	10.0±5.4	4.0±0.8	150.3±44.9	22.6±4.4	Perry and Gilmour, 1996
Oncorhynchus mykiss; 25–45 Torr	5	<5	150	60	Thomas *et al.*, 1992
O. mykiss; Pao_2 = 12–15 Torr	3.9±0.6	1.0±0.2	98.9±18.2	16.3±3.1	Fievet *et al.*, 1990
Oncorhynchus mykiss; 47 Torr	3.8±0.4	5.9±0.7	14.7±4.2	20.5±3.6	Ristori and Laurent, 1989
Oncorhynchus mykiss; 50 Torr	0.4±0.1	0.2±0.1	7.1±2.7	4.4±2.8	Boutilier *et al.*, 1988
Oncorhynchus mykiss; 40 Torr	0.6±0.3	1.2±0.2	18.3	28.5	Tetens and Christensen, 1987
Oncorhynchus mykiss; 40 Torr	5.0 V 0.9	11.6±2.4	25.2±2.0	17.0±3.0	Fievet *et al.*, 1987
Oncorhynchus mykiss; 36 Torr	0.9±0.5	3.3±1.2	68.1±55.7	50.8±21.0	Van Raaij *et al.*, 1996
Cyprinus carpio; 2 Torr	0.2±0.1	1.5±0.4	9.9±2.2	289.3±62.4	Van Raaij *et al.*, 1996
Anguilla rostrata; 20 Torr	0.8±0.1	0.5±0.1	4.5	2.8	Perry and Reid, 1992a
Scyliorhinus canicula; 35 Torr	25.6±6.5	32.1±19.3	288.4±86.2	446.5±117.6	Butler *et al.*, 1978
Scyliorhinus canicula; 55 Torr	19.4±5.4	18.5±2.7	42.1±17.1	62.7±15.5	Butler *et al.*, 1979
Squalus acanthias; 35 Torr	3.0±1.1	3.4±0.8	6.4±4.7	7.1±1.9	Perry and Gilmour, 1996
Scyliorhinus canicula; 56 Torr	62±22	46±16	212±120	387±40	Metcalfe and Butler, 1989
Acipenser baeri; 10 Torr	3.9	1.2	301±50	196±33	Maxime *et al.*, 1995

AMPHIBIANS					
Xenopus laevis; submergence	2.5	7	7	25	Boutilier and Lantz, 1989
Ambystoma tigrinum; 24 Torr	2	2.2	140	420	Talbot and Stiffler, 1991
REPTILES					
Chrysemys picta; anoxia	0.2	0.2	5.9	22.2	Keiver et al., 1992
BIRDS					
Anas platyrhynchos; submergence	1.3 ± 0.3	5.1 ± 0.8	2312 ± 713	5049 ± 1309	Lacombe and Jones, 1991b
Anas platyrhynchos; submergence	7.5 ± 3.9	3.7 ± 1.2	2260 ± 497	1720 ± 407	Hudson and Jones, 1982
MAMMALS					
Homo sapiens; 6,000 M	0.5 ± 0.1	1.6 ± 0.2	0.6 ± 0.2	4.6 ± 0.8	Anand et al., 1993
Cavia porcellus; 50% decrease in P_{O_2}	0.2 ± 0.1	2.6 ± 0.3	18.5 ± 9.0	9.2 ± 2.7	Jelinek and Jensen, 1991
Homo sapiens; 60 Torr (hypobaric)	0.2 ± 0.02	~2.0	NC	6.0 ± 0.8	Young et al., 1989
Phoca vitulina; submergence	1.0 ± 0.6	1.9 ± 1.0	9.7 ± 8.1	6.6 ± 2.6	Hance et al., 1982

NC, no change.

At high altitude or simulated high altitude, plasma catecholamine levels become elevated in humans although the changes are modest and thus may have little physiological impact. As with exercise, a portion of the increase in noradrenaline levels may simply reflect neuronal spillover rather than adrenal secretion.

The effects of hypoxia on plasma cortisol levels are summarised in Table 2.4. In fish, hypoxia (if sufficiently severe) elicits a pronounced rise in circulating cortisol levels. Although cortisol is normally considered a chronic stress hormone, the majority of the studies performed using fish have examined the effects of acute hypoxia exposures (0.5–4 h). Currently, it is unknown whether elevated cortisol levels are sustained in fish during chronic exposure to hypoxia. A particularly interesting result is the decline in plasma corticosterone levels in the turtle, *Chyrsemys picta*, during prolonged anoxia (Keiver *et al.*, 1992); in the same study, plasma catecholamine levels were significantly elevated. Generally, exposure of humans to high altitude causes a pronounced increase in cortisol levels. However, in certain instances, the response is transient with plasma cortisol levels returning to baseline levels as the duration of exposure is increased. Furthermore, gradual acclimatisation of subjects to high altitude results in lower plasma cortisol levels when compared to abrupt transfer (Frayser *et al.*, 1975).

2.3.2   Cardiovascular responses to altered oxygen availability

2.3.2.1   Aquatic hypoxia

Several detailed reviews have been written on the cardiovascular responses of aquatic animals (principally fish) to hypoxia (Taylor, 1982; Randall, 1982; Butler and Metcalfe, 1988; Forster *et al.*, 1991; Bushnell and Jones, 1992; Fritsche and Nilsson, 1993; Olson, 1998). Thus, rather than re-addressing the cardiovascular responses of aquatic organisms in detail, the following discussion will focus predominantly on the relative involvement of the 'stress hormones'. Numerous studies have examined the circulatory responses of cephalopod molluscs, crustaceans and fish to lowered ambient O_2 and from these, several general conclusions can be reached.

(i) Bradycardia: One of the most widely conserved responses to hypoxia is a reflex bradycardia (Holeton and Randall, 1967; Taylor and Barrett, 1985; Peyreaud-Waitzenegger and Soulier, 1989; Fritsche and Nilsson, 1989; Fritsche, 1990; Gamperl *et al.*, 1994b; Maxime *et al.*, 1995) that originates from stimulation of branchial chemoreceptors. The bradycardia arises principally as a consequence of a marked increase in parasympathetic tone (e.g. Wood and Shelton, 1980) that is often opposed by enhanced

Table 2.4 Levels of plasma cortisol or [a]corticosterone (nmol l^{-1}) during hypoxia in selected animals. The data are presented as means $\pm$ 1 standard error of the mean except in cases where values were estimated from graphs. Except where otherwise stated, the levels of hypoxia are expressed as changes in ambient Po_2

	Normoxia	Hypoxia	Reference
FISH			
Oncorhynchus mykiss; 75 Torr—1 h	65.7 ± 33.4	156.1 ± 76.7	Swift, 1981
Oncorhynchus mykiss; 51 Torr—1 h	46.5 ± 8.2	63.0 ± 13.7	Swift, 1981
Oncorhynchus mykiss; 42 Torr—1 h	30.4 ± 2.8	112.3 ± 13.7	Swift, 1981
Oncorhynchus mykiss; 35 Torr—1 h	46.5 ± 27.4	169.8 ± 21.9	Swift, 1981
Oncorhynchus mykiss; 26 Torr—1 h	68.5 ± 8.2	197.2 ± 43.8	Swift, 1981
Oncorhynchus mykiss; 60 Torr—48 h	89	NC	Reid and Perry, 1995
Oncorhynchus mykiss; 36 Torr—1.5 h	257 ± 71	2013 ± 1161	Van Raaij et al., 1996
Oncorhynchus mykiss; 32 Torr—4 h	151 ± 49	383 ± 79	Swift, 1982
Cyprinus carpio; 2 Torr—1.5 h	731 ± 184	2062 ± 438	Van Raaij et al., 1996
Acipenser baeri; 30 Torr—30 mim	16.4	87.0	Maxime et al., 1995
REPTILES			
[a]*Chyrsemys picta*; anoxia—28 days	4.7 ± 2.2	1.3 ± 0.5	Keiver et al., 1992
MAMMALS			
Homo sapiens; >6,000 M—>10 weeks	202.6 ± 87.6	646.2 ± 64.1	Anand et al., 1993
Homo sapiens; 120 Torr—10 days	290 ± 55	518 ± 47	Humpeler et al., 1980
Homo sapiens; 5833 M—1 day (no acclimatisation)	219	1232	Frayser et al., 1975
Homo sapiens; 5833 M—4 day (no acclimatisation)	219	500	Frayser et al., 1975
Homo sapiens; 5833 M—3 day (8 days acclimatisation)	274	575	Frayser et al., 1975
Homo sapiens; 5833 M—10 day (no acclimatisation)	274	280	Frayser et al., 1975

NC, no change.

adrenergic stimulation via an increase in sympathetic tone or an elevation of plasma catecholamine levels (Table 2.3). Despite the bradycardia, cardiac output usually is maintained (e.g. Wood and Shelton, 1980) owing to a concurrent increase in cardiac stroke volume (H_{sv}). The physiological significance of the hypoxic bradycardia has been the topic of considerable debate and will be addressed below.

The exact mechanisms underlying the increase in H_{sv} are unclear but are thought to include positive inotropic effects of adrenergic stimulation and increased diastolic filling. Only a few studies have directly evaluated the contribution of circulating catecholamines to cardiac function during hypoxia and these have focused exclusively on elasmobranchs (Metcalfe and Butler, 1988, 1989). It has generally been considered that the elasmobranch heart may have a greater reliance on circulating catecholamines than in other fish owing to its absence of adrenergic innervation. However, the studies by Metcalfe and Butler (1988, 1989) could provide no evidence that circulating catecholamines have any cardiovascular role during hypoxia in *Scyliorhinus canicula*. It would appear that in elasmobranchs during hypoxia, cardiac frequency is controlled largely by parasympathetic nerves.

Although widespread, bradycardia is not a universal response to hypoxia in fish and, moreover, within any given species there can be significant variability in the degree of hypoxic bradycardia that is exhibited. For example, the hypoxia-tolerant hagfish (Axelsson *et al.*, 1990; Forster *et al.*, 1992) and sea raven (Saunders and Sutterlin, 1970) do not exhibit bradycardia during severe hypoxia nor does the five-bearded rockling, *Ciliata mustela* (Fritsche, 1990). Several studies have failed to observe significant changes in H_f in species that are generally thought to respond to hypoxia by exhibiting bradycardia (e.g. *Scyliorhinus canicula* (Metcalfe and Butler, 1988), *Gadus morhua* (Sundin, 1995)). Reasons for the discrepancies are unknown but may include differences in the degree of hypoxia and the rapidity with which the hypoxia is imposed.

(ii) Systemic and branchial vascular resistance: There is tremendous variation in the response of the systemic vasculature of fish to hypoxia (Bushnell and Jones, 1992) and thus it is difficult to draw general conclusions. However, in elasmobranchs, systemic resistance (R_s) decreases during hypoxia (Piiper *et al.*, 1970; Butler and Metcalfe, 1988; Metcalfe and Butler, 1988, 1989), while in hagfish, R_s is unaffected (Axelsson *et al.*, 1990; Forster *et al.*, 1992). The lack of an increase in R_s during hypoxia in elasmobranchs and hagfish may reflect the absent or sparse adrenergic innervation of the systemic peripheral vasculature. In teleosts, responses of R_s to hypoxia range from little or no change (Peyreaud-Waitzenegger and Soulier, 1989; Axelsson and Fritsche, 1991;

Bushnell and Brill, 1992; Gamperl *et al.*, 1994b) to large increases (Fritsche and Nilsson, 1989, 1990; Axelsson and Farrell, 1993; Sundin, 1995). The mechanisms underlying the influence of hypoxia on R_s have been examined thoroughly in the Atlantic cod, *Gadus morhua* (Fritsche and Nilsson, 1990; Axelsson and Fritsche, 1991). Essentially, the net effect on R_s in cod during hypoxia reflects the stimulation of systemic α-adrenoreceptors by sympathetic nerves and circulating catecholamines that is opposed by unidentified vasodilator substances; generally the vasoconstrictor effect predominates.

The effects of hypoxia on branchial vascular resistance (R_g) also are variable amongst the species although the most common response appears to be an increase of R_g (Holeton and Randall, 1967; Butler and Metcalfe, 1988; Metcalfe and Butler, 1989; Peyreaud-Waitzenegger and Soulier, 1989; Forster *et al.*, 1992). The factors influencing R_g are numerous and include β-adrenergic vasodilatation, α-adrenergic vasoconstriction, serotonergic vasoconstriction (Sundin, 1995) and direct constrictor effects of localised hypoxia (Pettersson and Johansen, 1982).

(iii) Re-distribution of blood flow: Few studies have examined blood flow re-distribution during hypoxia in fish. In *G. morhua*, blood flow to the gut is reduced during hypoxia owing to increases in visceral vascular resistance (Axelsson and Fritsche, 1991). The increases in visceral resistance during hypoxia reflect the combined actions of sympathetic nerves and circulating catecholamines. Reduced blood flow to the gut during hypoxia will enable a greater percentage of $\dot{V}b$ to be directed toward vital tissues. In particular, there is a need for increased coronary blood flow during hypoxia because the reduced levels of O_2 in venous blood may prevent adequate delivery of O_2 to the myocardial tissue. Indeed, coronary blood flow increases during hypoxia in *O. mykiss* (Gamperl *et al.*, 1994b) and *O. kisutch* (Axelsson and Farrell, 1993). As in exercising fish, coronary blood flow during hypoxia is probably under metabolic control and in particular is likely to be increased owing to vasodilator effects of lowered O_2 and/or increased levels of adenosine.

2.3.2.2 Aquatic hyperoxia

The cardiovascular responses to hyperoxia have been examined in only two teleost species, *Catostomus commersoni* (Wilkes *et al.*, 1981) and *Cyprinus carpio* (Takeda, 1990). In *C. commersoni*, hyperoxia elicits a gradual reduction in dorsal aortic pressure and a fall in H_f. In *C. carpio*, severe hypoxia is associated with an increase in $\dot{V}b$. Circulating catecholamines are unlikely to be involved in mediating these response because plasma levels are unaltered (at least in trout) during hyperoxia (Perry *et al.*, 1989; Aota *et al.*, 1990).

2.3.2.3   High-altitude hypoxia

The cardiovascular responses to high-altitude hypoxia have been studied extensively in birds and mammals (West, 1982; Faraci, 1991). In both groups, acute hypoxia is associated with pronounced increases in H_f and $\dot{V}b$ (Jones and Holeton, 1972; Faraci *et al.*, 1984; Koller *et al.*, 1991). The increases in $\dot{V}b$ are believed to be important to increase respiratory gas transfer. The changes in cardiac function during hypoxia reflect the combined actions of a withdrawal of parasympathetic tone and an increased sympathetic tone. At extreme altitudes, increases in circulating catecholamines (Table 2.3) may supplement the enhanced sympathetic activity. The increased levels of corticosteroids that occur in mammals at altitude may also have an important role. Indeed, it was shown (Roosevelt *et al.*, 1972) that survival time of rats during exposure to acute severe hypoxia (40 Torr) was significantly reduced by adrenalectomy or hypophysectomy and enhanced by administration of exogenous cortisol. The protective effects of corticosteroids may reflect their permissive role in β-adrenergically mediated events (see above) and thus an increased responsiveness of the heart to neuronal and circulating catecholamines.

Although $\dot{V}b$ increases during hypoxia, mean systemic blood pressure does not change. The constant blood pressure probably reflects a generalised systemic vasodilatation owing to the lowered blood P_{O_2} and likely is the cause of a reduced diastolic pressure during high-altitude hypoxia. Pulmonary blood pressure, however, may increase markedly during acute high-altitude hypoxia as a result of hypoxic pulmonary vasoconstriction (West, 1982; Smith and Kampine, 1990) and may contribute to pulmonary oedema. Increased $\dot{V}b$, pulmonary vasoconstriction and polycythaemia contribute to increase the work performed by the heart at high altitude. Polycythaemia traditionally has been considered an adaptive response to high-altitude hypoxia. This view has been challenged however, (West, 1982) because the presumed benefits for blood O_2 transport (see below) may be outweighed by the deleterious effects of increased viscosity. Indeed, the ability to perform exercise at altitude appears to be largely unrelated to haematocrit (West, 1982).

Some birds are remarkable in their tolerance of hypoxia and indeed there are reports of certain species (e.g. bar-headed goose) flying over Mt. Everest (Faraci, 1991). Numerous physiological adaptations presumably act in concert to allow birds to exercise at such severe levels of hypoxia and include unusually high cardiac outputs and highly effective gas transfer (see below). However, one particularly important adaptation is the insensitivity of the avian cerebral circulation to hypocapnia (Faraci *et al.*, 1984). In mammals, a lowering of blood P_{CO_2} causes a pronounced vasoconstriction of cerebral blood vessels (Smith and Kampine, 1990). At high altitude, hyperventilation causes large reductions in blood P_{CO_2} (see below) and in mammals this hypocapnia counteracts the vasodilator influence of blood hypoxia on the cerebral circulation. The vasoconstrictor effect of hypocapnia in mammals may severely constrain O_2 delivery to the brain during high-altitude hypoxia. Birds, however, display an intense vasodilatation of the cerebral circulation during hypocapnic hypoxia owing to their insensitivity to lowered P_{CO_2}.

2.3.2.4   Forced submergence

The cardiovascular responses of animals to forced submergence have been studied extensively (for reviews see Butler, 1982; Shelton and Boutilier, 1982). Although the intensity of the physiological responses to forced versus voluntary submergence vary tremendously, the studies on forced submergence have provided interesting examples of the involvement of stress hormones in the cardiovascular responses to reduced O_2 availability. Vertebrates respond to forced submergence by exhibiting a marked peripheral vasoconstriction that is accompanied by profound bradycardia (Jones, 1968; Butler and Taylor, 1983). The net result is shunting of blood away from the periphery and its preferential distribution to the brain and heart. Changes in blood pressure are minimised by reductions in $\dot{V}b$ that are associated with the bradycardia. During voluntary submergence, the changes in peripheral resistance and H_f are much less pronounced and only approach the changes observed during forced submergence during unusually long periods underwater or when re-emergence is prevented (Butler, 1989).

The principal cause of the bradycardia during submergence is an increase in parasympathetic activity to the heart. The peripheral vasoconstriction reflects stimulation of vascular α-adrenoreceptors by sympathetic nerves and circulating catecholamines. The involvement of circulating catecholamines may be particularly important in submerged birds that experience massive increases in both adrenaline and noradrenaline levels (Hudson and Jones, 1982; Lacombe and Jones, 1991b). Indeed, Lacombe and Jones (1991a) demonstrated that adrenalectomy or adrenal denervation significantly reduced maximum underwater tolerance times in ducks that could be restored by intravenous infusion of exogenous catecholamines. The importance of circulating catecholamines during submergence probably reflects the depressant effect of hypercapnia on neuronal peripheral vasoconstriction (Lacombe and Jones, 1991a). Thus, as CO_2 levels increase in the blood during submergence, the neuronally mediated systemic vasoconstriction is inhibited and must be supplemented by humoral catecholamines if peripheral vasoconstriction (and hence adequate O_2 delivery to the brain and heart) is to be maintained.

2.3.3 Respiratory responses to altered oxygen availability

2.3.3.1 Aquatic hypoxia

A number of comprehensive reviews that detail or deal with aspects of the respiratory responses of fish and invertebrate water-breathers to aquatic hypoxia or hyperoxia are available (Randall, 1982; Taylor, 1982; Randall and Daxboeck, 1984; Shelton et al., 1986; Perry and Wood, 1989; Thomas and Motais, 1990; Jensen, 1991; Nikinmaa, 1992; Jensen et al., 1993; Fritsche and Nilsson, 1993; Burleson, 1995). Thus, the present discussion will focus largely on the role of 'stress hormones' in the response of water-breathers to changes in the environmental O_2 tension.

An increase in gill ventilation volume effected through increases in ventilatory stroke volume and/or frequency is the immediate response to hypoxia in both fish (e.g. Piiper et al., 1970; Wood and Johansen, 1973; Thomas and Hughes, 1982; Forgue et al., 1989; Metcalfe and Butler, 1989; Kinkead and Perry, 1990, 1991; Perry and Thomas, 1991; Kinkead et al., 1991; McKenzie et al., 1991; Nonnotte et al., 1993; Bindon et al., 1994b; Greco et al., 1995; Maxime et al., 1995; Perry and Gilmour, 1996) and aquatic crustaceans (e.g. Batterton and Cameron, 1978; Burnett, 1979; Wheatly and Taylor, 1981; Taylor and Spicer, 1991), and serves to increase the rate of delivery of O_2 to the gills in the face of lowered environmental O_2 availability. This hyperventilatory reflex is probably mediated by O_2-sensitive chemoreceptors that, in fish, are thought to be distributed throughout all of the gill arches and are responsive to both external hypoxia and internal hypoxaemia (see review by Burleson, 1995); a similar reflex probably operates in crustaceans but the location of the O_2-sensitive receptors is not yet clear (Taylor, 1982). Percentage utilisation of O_2 from the ventilatory water generally remains high despite the hyperventilation-induced reduction in the residence time of water at the gills (Holeton and Randall, 1967; Itazawa and Takeda, 1978; Lomholt and Johansen, 1979; Burnett, 1979; Wheatly and Taylor, 1981; Metcalfe and Butler, 1988), and therefore, the O_2 diffusive conductance across the gills must be increased during hypoxia, presumably through the mechanisms described above for exercise-related increases in gill O_2 diffusive conductance. The hypoxic bradycardia (see above) may be of physiological significance in this regard, in that it is thought to enhance gas transfer (Taylor and Barrett, 1985). Several mechanisms are likely to be involved, including improvement in the efficiency of gas exchange achieved through synchronisation of breathing and heart rates, increased functional surface area of the gill owing to the effect of elevated pulsatility in promoting lamellar recruitment, and increased residence time of blood in the gills (Randall, 1982; Davie and Daxboeck, 1982; Randall and Daxboeck, 1984). An additional or alternative strategy employed by fish which are bimodal breathers and some crustaceans is to increase O_2 uptake from the air or switch to air breathing during hypoxia (e.g. Taylor, 1982; Fritsche *et al.*, 1993; Brauner *et al.*, 1995; Val, 1996). Crustaceans which are facultative air-breathers, such as the shore crab *Carcinus meanas*, experience a respiratory acidosis when in air and accumulate buffer base in the haemolymph in compensation (Taylor, 1982). Similarly, a reduction in gill perfusion during hypoxia in facultatively air-breathing fish to minimise O_2 loss to the O_2-deficient aquatic environment may also result in CO_2 retention in some species (Val, 1996).

The hyperventilatory response is insufficient to defend Pao_2, which decreases during hypoxia (e.g. Itazawa and Takeda, 1978; Burnett, 1979; Wheatly and Taylor, 1981; Thomas *et al.*, 1988; Metcalfe and Butler, 1988, 1989; Perry and Thomas, 1991; Forgue *et al.*, 1992; Perry and Reid, 1992a; Thomas *et al.*, 1992, 1994; Maxime *et al.*, 1995). In crustaceans (Wheatly and Taylor, 1981) and dogfish (Butler *et al.*, 1979; Metcalfe and Butler, 1988, 1989), venous Po_2 also decreases, whereas Pvo_2 in teleost fish has been found to be maintained at near normoxic levels during moderate hypoxia, declining only during severe or prolonged hypoxia (Holeton and Randall, 1967; Itazawa and Takeda, 1978; Perry *et al.*, 1991; Thomas *et al.*, 1994). Assuming constant cardiac output (see above), an increase in the O_2 carrying capacity of the blood and/or an increase in the O_2 affinity of the respiratory pigment is therefore required to sustain O_2 extraction from the blood by the tissues in the face of the reductions in blood O_2 content which tend to accompany the lower blood Po_2 values. Arterial Pco_2 decreases during hypoxia because of the hyperventilation, and the corresponding respiratory alkalosis (e.g. Wheatly and Taylor, 1981; Thomas and Hughes, 1982; Thomas *et al.*, 1988, 1992; Claireaux *et al.*, 1988; Fievet *et al.*, 1990; Perry and Thomas, 1991; Taylor and Spicer, 1991; Forgue *et al.*, 1992; Nonnotte *et al.*, 1993; Maxime *et al.*, 1995; Perry and Gilmour, 1996), in turn, causes a left-shift of the O_2 equilibrium curve through the Bohr effect, with a resultant increase in haemocyanin- or Hb-O_2 binding affinity (Burnett, 1979; Tetens and Lykkeboe, 1985; Bouchet and Truchot, 1985; Jensen, 1991). The Hb-O_2 binding affinity may be further increased in teleost fish by alkalinisation of the RBC interior owing to oxygenation-linked proton binding by haemoglobin, i.e. the Haldane effect (Weber and Jensen, 1988). In both rainbow trout (Brauner *et al.*, 1996) and tench (Jensen, 1986), the majority of the increase in RBC intracellular pH occurs for decreases in Hb-O_2 saturation from 100 to 60%; elasmobranch erythrocytes, on the other hand, do not exhibit a Haldane effect (Wood *et al.*, 1994). During prolonged hypoxia (hours to days), the respiratory alkalosis may be partially or fully compensated by a simultaneous lactacidosis stemming from increased reliance on anaerobic metabolism (Butler *et al.*, 1979; Thomas and Hughes, 1982; Boutilier *et al.*, 1988). However, concentrations of RBC intracellular organic phosphates are normally reduced during prolonged hypoxia (Wood *et al.*, 1975; Weber and Lykkeboe, 1978; Soivio *et al.*, 1980; Tetens and Lykkeboe, 1981; Boutilier *et al.*, 1988); these reductions will enhance Hb-O_2 binding affinity directly, but also indirectly through RBC swelling and increases in the RBC intracellular pH, both of which are mediated by changes in the Donnan distribution ratios across the RBC membrane (Weber and Jensen, 1988; Jensen, 1991). In crustaceans, elevated lactate levels have a direct effect in increasing haemocyanin-O_2 binding affinity (Bouchet and Truchot, 1985).

The mobilisation of stress hormones into the circulation during severe hypoxia initiates a series of integrated responses that acts to optimise blood O_2 transport in teleost fish. As during exhaustive exercise, injection of RBCs into the circulation via adrenergically stimulated splenic contraction increases the blood O_2 carrying capacity (Tetens and Lykkeboe, 1985; Yamamoto *et al.*, 1985; Claireaux *et al.*, 1988; Wells and Weber, 1990), while stimulation of the RBC β-adrenoreceptors enhances the Hb-O_2 binding affinity through the RBC alkalinisation and swelling and the reduction in RBC organic phosphate concentrations that result from activation of the Na^+/H^+ antiporter (Tetens and Lykkeboe, 1985; Tetens and Christensen, 1987; Claireaux *et al.*, 1988). Indeed, the adrenergically induced increase in Hb-O_2 binding affinity is reflected in a detectable decrease in Pv_{O_2} as augmented binding of O_2 to haemoglobin lowers the RBC intracellular Po_2, aspirating O_2 into the erythrocytes (Perry and Thomas, 1993; Thomas *et al.*, 1994). Furthermore, the RBC response to adrenergic stimulation is enhanced by hypoxia (Motais *et al.*, 1987; Salama and Nikinmaa, 1988, 1990; Reid and Perry, 1991; Perry and Reid, 1992b; Reid *et al.*, 1993); hypoxic exposure increases the number of RBC membrane β-adrenoreceptors, resulting in greater cAMP accumulation, and hence increased activity of the RBC Na^+/H^+ exchanger (Salama and Nikinmaa, 1990; Reid and Perry, 1991; Reid *et al.*, 1993). In contrast to the situation in teleost fish, the mobilisation of catecholamines during severe hypoxia in dogfish does not appear to have significant benefits for blood O_2 transport. Neither pharmacological blockade of α- and β-adrenoreceptors during hypoxia (Metcalfe and Butler, 1988), nor treatment of dogfish with alpha-methyl-*p*-tyrosine to inhibit catecholamine synthesis and hence impede the elevation of circulating catecholamines during hypoxia (Metcalfe and Butler, 1989) impacted significantly upon the respiratory responses of dogfish to hypoxia. In agreement with these findings, RBC intracellular pH is not affected by adrenergic stimulation in elasmobranchs (Tufts and Randall, 1989).

Much interest has been focused on the potential of catecholamines to promote O_2 uptake at the gill during severe hypoxia. There is little disagreement that the O_2 diffusive conductance of the gill is enhanced by the mobilisation of catecholamines through increases in the permeability of the respiratory epithelium and functional surface area of the gill, as in exhaustive exercise (see above). Considerable debate has occurred, however, over the possible role of catecholamines in stimulating ventilation during hypoxia or other stresses such as hypercapnia or exercise (reviewed by Perry et al., 1992). While catecholamine adminis- tration has been demonstrated to have hyperventilatory effects in eels (Peyraud-Waitzenegger, 1979; Peyraud-Waitzenegger et al., 1980), dog- fish (Taylor and Wilson, 1989), trout (Aota and Randall, 1993) and bowfin (McKenzie et al., 1991), decreases in ventilation or no response following the injection of catecholamines were also observed in several of these studies. Either hypoventilatory responses or no changes in ventilation were also documented in a number of studies in which physiological doses of catecholamines were injected or infused into resting fish or into fish during exposure to hypoxia or hypercapnia (Playle et al., 1990; Kinkead and Perry, 1990, 1991; Kinkead et al., 1991; Burleson and Milsom, 1995; Perry and Gilmour, 1996). Moreover, reductions in both ventilation frequency and amplitude have been reported in rainbow trout following the release of endogenous catecholamines during severe hypoxia (Perry et al., 1992), while the hyperventilatory response to hypoxia was not impaired in dogfish treated with alpha-methyl-p-tyrosine to inhibit catecholamine release during hypoxia (Metcalfe and Butler, 1989). Thus, increasingly, the balance of experimental evidence indicates that elevated levels of circulating catecholamines do not contribute to hyperventilatory responses to stressors in fish.

2.3.3.2 *Aquatic hyperoxia*

In accordance with the primary ventilatory drive in water-breathers being keyed to O_2, exposure to hyperoxic conditions elicits a marked hypoventilatory response in both fish (Wood and Jackson, 1980; Wilkes et al., 1981; Kinkead and Perry, 1990; Takeda, 1990) and crustaceans (Truchot, 1975; Sinha and Dejours, 1980; Wheatly, 1989). Percentage utilisation of O_2 from the ventilatory water tends to be maintained or increased during hyperoxia, and both arterial and venous Po_2 increase in parallel with increasing Po_2 of the inspired water (Wood and Jackson, 1980; Wilkes et al., 1981; Takeda, 1990). However, significant increases in arterial and venous Pco_2 accompany the hypoventilation and result in a depression of arterial and venous pH (Truchot et al., 1980; Wood and Jackson, 1980; Wilkes et al., 1981; Höbe et al., 1984; Wheatly, 1987, 1989;

Takeda, 1990; Wood and LeMoigne, 1991); the CO_2 retention has been attributed to both external convective limitations (i.e. hypoventilation) and internal diffusive and/or perfusive limitations (Wood and Jackson, 1980; Wheatly, 1987; Takeda, 1990). While the respiratory acidosis must decrease the Hb-O_2 binding affinity through the Bohr effect, the elevated blood Po_2 ensures that blood O_2 content is maintained (Perry et al., 1989; Takeda, 1990). Indeed, increasing percentage saturation of haemoglobin in the venous blood as Pvo_2 increases will place increasing importance on O_2 transport in physical solution (Wilkes et al., 1981; Takeda, 1990). Presumably because blood O_2 content is maintained, catecholamines are not mobilised during hyperoxia despite the respiratory acidosis and consequent reductions in RBC intracellular pH (Perry et al., 1989; Kinkead and Perry, 1990), nor are elevated cortisol levels observed (Wood and LeMoigne, 1991; Wood, 1991b). During prolonged hyperoxia, the respiratory acidosis may be compensated by the excretion of acidic equivalents across the gills such that the HCO_3^- concentration of the blood rises and blood pH recovers to its normoxic level even though blood Pco_2 remains elevated (Wheatly, 1989; Wood, 1991b).

2.3.3.3   High-altitude hypoxia

The respiratory responses of mammals, particularly humans, and birds to high-altitude hypoxia have been the focus of much research effort and are the subject of numerous reviews (e.g. West, 1982, 1989; Fedde et al., 1985; Weil, 1986; Faraci, 1991; Butler, 1991; Monge and León-Velarde, 1991; Hochachka, 1992; Weber, 1995). As with water-breathers experiencing aquatic hypoxia, high-altitude hypoxia elicits a marked increase in ventilation in both birds and mammals (Black and Tenney, 1980; West et al., 1983; Kiley et al., 1985; Shams and Scheid, 1987; Sutton et al., 1988; Fedde et al., 1989). Increased tidal volume appears to be the more important contributor to the hyperventilatory response of mammals (Weil, 1986), while increases in both breathing frequency and tidal volume occur in birds (Shams and Scheid, 1987; Fedde et al., 1989). The hyperventilation is mediated by the peripheral chemoreceptors, which respond to a fall in Pao_2 (Weil, 1986), and results in both hypocapnia and a respiratory alkalosis (Lutz and Schmidt-Nielson, 1977; Black and Tenney, 1980; West et al., 1983; Shams and Scheid, 1987; Sutton et al., 1988; Fedde et al., 1989; Samaja et al., 1997) that tend to attenuate the hyperventilatory response owing to the primary CO_2/H^+-based ventilatory drive in air-breathers (Weil, 1986). Over several days at high altitude, a process of ventilatory acclimatisation occurs in which ventilation gradually rises while $Paco_2$ decreases; the mechanisms responsible for this process are not yet understood (West, 1982; Weil, 1986). Birds appear to be more tolerant of low Pco_2 than mammals, perhaps because of the insensitivity of cerebral blood flow to hypocapnia (see above), and consequently can elevate ventilation to the point where Pao_2 approaches the inspired Po_2 (Lutz and Schmidt-Nielson, 1977; Shams and Scheid, 1987; Butler, 1991).

The decrease in $Paco_2$ and respiratory alkalosis associated with the hyperventilatory response to hypoxia serve to increase Hb-O_2 binding affinity through the Bohr effect in both birds and mammals (Lutz and Schmidt-Nielson, 1977; Winslow et al., 1984; West, 1989; Monge and León-Velarde, 1991; Weber, 1995). A hypoxia-induced hypothermia may also play a role in enhancing Hb-O_2 binding affinity in birds (Maginniss et al., 1997). In mammals, however, the alkalosis also results in stimulation of the synthesis of 2,3-diphosphoglycerate (2,3-DPG) within the erythrocytes, and elevated levels of this organic phosphate decrease Hb-O_2 binding affinity (Weber, 1995). Thus, the initial left-shift of the O_2 equilibrium curve in response to exposure to hypoxia is succeeded (over hours to days) by a rightward shift as the RBC 2,3-DPG levels increase. While traditionally this right-shift of the O_2 equilibrium curve was thought to be adaptive in that it secured O_2 delivery to the tissues, recent models (Samaja et al., 1986) suggest that it may be considered advantageous only at altitudes below 5400 m and during rest or moderate exercise. At extreme altitudes or during severe exercise, an enhanced Hb-O_2 binding affinity (left-shifted O_2 equilibrium curve) favouring O_2 loading at the pulmonary capillary would be of greater benefit, and hence the right-shift of the O_2 equilibrium curve should be considered maladaptive (Winslow et al., 1984; Samaja et al., 1986, 1997; see reviews by West, 1982; Monge and León-Velarde, 1991). In this respect, it is significant that mammals and birds that are genotypically adapted to high altitude (e.g. llama, vicuna, bar-headed goose) exhibit high Hb-O_2 binding affinity (Fedde et al., 1985; Monge and León-Velarde, 1991).

An additional difference in the respiratory response to high-altitude hypoxia between lowland birds and mammals and those that are genotypically adapted to high altitude is the polycythemia exhibited by the former (Monge and León-Velarde, 1991). Prolonged exposure to high-altitude hypoxia elicits a haematopoietic response in lowland birds and mammals that increases the blood haemoglobin concentration and hence elevates blood O_2 carrying capacity (Black and Tenney, 1980; West et al., 1983; Winslow et al., 1984; Sutton et al., 1988; Maginniss et al., 1997). The mechanism responsible for the haematopoietic response probably involves a hypoxaemia-induced stimulation of erythropoietin production by the kidney (Monge and León-Velarde, 1991). By increasing the blood O_2 content for a given Po_2, polycythemia would be expected to be of benefit in securing O_2 delivery to the tissues during hypoxaemia, provided that cardiac output is maintained. However, the increased blood viscosity associated with polycythemia may compromise cardiac output (see above) and hence, increasingly, this haematopoietic response to high altitude is considered maladaptive (Black and Tenney, 1980; West, 1982; Winslow *et al.*, 1984; Monge and León-Velarde, 1991).

2.3.3.4   Forced submergence

Forced submergence elicits a similar suite of respiratory responses in a wide variety of air-breathing animals (see reviews by Butler and Jones, 1982; Butler, 1982, 1991; Burggren, 1988). Aerobic metabolism declines, and despite the potential to supplement metabolism anaerobically, the total metabolic rate is also depressed (Jones, 1967, 1972a,b; Jones and Mustafa, 1973). Because ventilation is suspended during forced submergence, the blood becomes progressively hypoxaemic and hypercapnic (Clausen and Ersland, 1970; Butler and Jones, 1971; Butler and Taylor, 1973; Lillo, 1978; Boutilier and Shelton, 1986b; Lacombe and Jones, 1991b; Wasser and Jackson, 1991; Wasser *et al.*, 1991). The reflex inhibition of respiratory activity initiated by stimulation of the trigeminal nerve via cold and/or mechanoreceptors dominates the stimulatory inputs of the chemoreceptors so that apnoea is maintained throughout the enforced dive (Butler, 1982). The elevated $Pa\text{CO}_2$ causes a respiratory acidosis that may be compounded by a metabolic acidosis resulting from increasing reliance on anaerobic metabolism and consequent elevation of blood lactate levels (Clausen and Ersland, 1970; Jones and Mustafa, 1973; Boutilier and Shelton, 1986a,b; Lacombe and Jones, 1991b; Wasser and Jackson, 1991; Wasser *et al.*, 1991). It is noteworthy in this regard that the selective peripheral vasoconstriction (see above) tends to minimise the blood acidosis by sequestering both CO_2 and lactic acid within the tissues; blood lactate levels increase substantially following emergence concomitant with a fall in blood pH (Clausen and Ersland, 1970; Boutilier and Shelton, 1986a). The right shift of the O_2 equilibrium curve induced by the compound acidosis via the Bohr effect lowers the Hb-O_2 binding affinity, enabling the venous O_2 reserve to be tapped to supply the essential (perfused) tissues with O_2 (Boutilier and Shelton, 1986a). Upon emergence from an enforced dive, hyperventilation is observed and O_2 uptake is elevated above the pre-submergence level to repay the O_2 debt accumulated during the apnoeic period (Jones, 1967; Boutilier and Shelton, 1986b). The O_2 debt has three components; the cost of replenishing the blood O_2 stores and other O_2 stores depleted during submergence, the cost of metabolising the lactate that accumulated during submergence, and the energetic cost of the post-submergence hyperventilation which serves to restore O_2 stores and eliminate the CO_2 retained during the enforced dive (Jones, 1972a; Jones and Mustafa, 1973).

References

Ainsworth, D.M., Smith, C.A., Eicker, S.W., Ducharme, N.G., Henderson, K.S., Snedden, K. and Dempsey, J.A. (1997) Pulmonary-locomotory interactions in exercising dogs and horses. *Respiration Physiology*, **110** 287-294.

Anand, I.S., Chandrashekhar, Y., Rao, S.K., Malhotra, R.M., Ferrari, R., Chandana, J., Ramesh, B., Shetty, K.J. and Boparai, M.S. (1993) Body fluid compartments, renal blood flow, and hormones at 6,000 m in normal subjects. *Journal of Applied Physiology*, **74** 1234-1239.

Aota, S. and Randall, D.J. (1993) The effect of exogenous catecholamines on the ventilatory and cardiac responses of normoxic and hyperoxic rainbow trout, *Oncorhynchus mykiss*. *Journal of Comparative Physiology*, **163** 138-146.

Aota, S., Holmgren, K.D., Gallaugher, P. and Randall, D.J. (1990) A possible role for catecholamines in the ventilatory responses associated with internal acidosis or external hypoxia in rainbow trout *Oncorhynchus mykiss*. *Journal of Experimental Biology*, **151** 57-70.

Axelsson, M. (1995) The coronary circulation: A fish perspective. *Brazilian Journal of Medical Biological Research*, **28** 1167-1177.

Axelsson, M. and Farrell, A.P. (1993) Coronary blood flow in vivo in the coho salmon (*Oncorhynchus kisutch*). *American Journal of Physiology*, **264** R963-R971.

Axelsson, M. and Fritsche, R. (1991) Effects of exercise, hypoxia and feeding on the gastrointestinal blood flow in the Atlantic cod *Gadus morhua*. *Journal of Experimental Biology*, **158** 181-198.

Axelsson, M. and Nilsson, S. (1986) Blood pressure control during exercise in the Atlantic cod, *Gadus morhua*. *Journal of Experimental Biology*, **126** 225-236.

Axelsson, M., Ehrenström, F. and Nilsson, G.E. (1987) Cholinergic and adrenergic influence on the teleost heart in vivo. *Experimental Biology*, **46** 179-186.

Axelsson, M., Farrell, A.P. and Nilsson, S. (1990) Effects of hypoxia and drugs on the cardiovascular dynamics of the Atlantic hagfish, *Myxine glutinosa*. *Journal of Experimental Biology*, **151** 297-316.

Axelsson, M., Davison, W., Forster, M.E. and Farrell, A.P. (1992) Cardiovascular responses of the red-blooded Antarctic fishes *Pagothenia bernacchii* and *P. borchgrevinki*. *Journal of Experimental Biology*, **167** 179-201.

Axelsson, M., Davison, B., Forster, M. and Nilsson, S. (1994) Blood pressure control in the Antarctic fish *Pagothenia borchgrevinki*. *Journal of Experimental Biology*, **190** 265-279.

Baroin, A., Garcia-Romeu, F., Lamarre, T. and Motais, R. (1984) A transient sodium-hydrogen exchange system induced by catecholamines in erythrocytes of rainbow trout, *Salmo gairdneri*. *Journal of Physiology*, **356** 21-31.

Batterton, C.V. and Cameron, J.N. (1978) Characteristics of resting ventilation and response to hypoxia, hypercapnia and emersion in the blue crab *Callinectes sapidus* (Rathbun). *Journal of Experimental Zoology*, **203** 403-418.

Baudinette, R.V. (1991) The energetics and cardiorespiratory correlates of mammalian terrestrial locomotion. *Journal of Experimental Biology*, **160** 209-231.

Beamish, F.W.H. (1978) Swimming capacity, in *Locomotion* (eds. W.S. Hoar and D.J. Randall), Academic Press, New York, pp 101-187.

Bernier, N.J. and Perry, S.F. (1998a) Cardiovascular effects of angiotensin II-mediated adrenaline release in rainbow trout. *Journal of Experimental Biology*, in press.

Bernier, N.J. and Perry, S.F. (1998b) The control of catecholamine secretion in hagfish, in *The Biology of Hagfishes* (eds. J.M. Jorgensen, J.P. Lomholt, R.E. Weber and H. Malte), Chapman and Hall, London, pp 413-427.

Bernier, N.J., Fuentes, J. and Randall, D.J. (1996) Adenosine receptor blockade and hypoxia-tolerance in rainbow trout and Pacific hagfish II. Effects on plasma catecholamines and erythrocytes. *Journal of Experimental Biology*, **199** 497-507.

Betito, K., Diorio, J. and Boksa, P. (1993) Brief cortisol exposure elevates adrenal phenylethanolamine n-methyltransferase after a necessary lag period. *European Journal of Pharmacology*, **238** 273-282.

Bindon, S.D., Fenwick, J.C. and Perry, S.F. (1994a) Branchial chloride cell proliferation in the rainbow trout, *Oncorhynchus mykiss*: implications for gas transfer. *Canadian Journal of Zoology*, **72** 1395-1402.

Bindon, S.D., Gilmour, K.M., Fenwick, J.C. and Perry, S.F. (1994b) The effects of branchial chloride cell proliferation on respiratory function in the rainbow trout *Oncorhynchus mykiss*. *Journal of Experimental Biology*, **197** 47-63.

Black, C.P. and Tenney, S.M. (1980) Oxygen transport during progressive hypoxia in high-altitude and sea-level waterfowl. *Respiration Physiology*, **39** 217-239.

Boesgaard, L., Nielsen, M.E. and Rosenkilde, P. (1993) Moderate exercise decreases plasma cortisol levels in Atlantic salmon (*Salmo salar*). *Comparative Biochemistry and Physiology*, **106A** 641-643.

Boggs, D.F., Seveyka, J.J., Kilgore, D.L. and Dial, K.P. (1997) Coordination of respiratory cycles with wingbeat cycles in the black-billed magpie (*Pica pica*). *Journal of Experimental Biology*, **200** 1413-1420.

Booth, J.H. (1979) The effects of oxygen supply, epinephrine and acetylcholine on the distribution of blood flow in trout gills. *Journal of Experimental Biology*, **83** 31-39.

Bouchet, J.Y. and Truchot, J.-P. (1985) Effects of hypoxia and L-lactate on the haemocyanin-oxygen affinity of the lobster, *Homarus vulgaris*. *Comparative Biochemistry and Physiology*, **80A** 69-73.

Boutilier, R.G. and Lantz, C.J. (1989) The effects of forced and voluntary diving on plasma catecholamines and erythrocyte pH in the aquatic anuran, *Xenopus laevis*. *Experimental Biology*, **48** 83-88.

Boutilier, R.G. and Shelton, G. (1986a) Respiratory properties of blood from voluntarily and forcibly submerged *Xenopus laevis*. *Journal of Experimental Biology*, **121** 285-300.

Boutilier, R.G. and Shelton, G. (1986b) The effects of forced and voluntary diving on ventilation, blood gases and pH in the aquatic amphibian, *Xenopus laevis*. *Journal of Experimental Biology*, **122** 209-222.

Boutilier, R.G., Dobson, G.P., Hoeger, U. and Randall, D.J. (1988) Acute exposure to graded levels of hypoxia in rainbow trout (*Salmo gairdneri*): metabolic and respiratory adaptations. *Respiration Physiology*, **71** 69-82.

Brauner, C.J., Ballantyne, C.L., Randall, D.J. and Val, A.L. (1995) Air breathing in the armoured catfish (*Hoplosternum littorale*) as an adaptation to hypoxic, acidic and hydrogen sulphide rich waters. *Canadian Journal of Zoology*, **73** 739-744.

Brauner, C.J., Gilmour, K.M. and Perry, S.F. (1996) Effect of haemoglobin oxygenation on Bohr proton release and CO_2 excretion in the rainbow trout. *Respiration Physiology*, **106** 65-70.

Brenner, I.K., Zamecnik, J., Shek, P.N. and Shephard, R.J. (1997) The impact of heat exposure and repeated exercise on circulating stress hormones. *European Journal of Applied Physiology*, **76** 445-454.

Burggren, W.W. (1988) Cardiovascular responses to diving and their relation to lung and blood oxygen stores in vertebrates. *Canadian Journal of Zoology*, **66** 20-28.

Burleson, M.L. (1995) Oxygen availability: Sensory systems, in *Biochemistry and Molecular Biology of Fishes, 5. Environmental and Ecological Biochemistry* (eds. P.W. Hochachka and T.P. Mommsen), Elsevier, Amsterdam, pp 1-18.

Burleson, M.L. and Milsom, W.K. (1995) Cardio-ventilatory control in rainbow trout: II. Reflex effects of exogenous neurochemicals. *Respiration Physiology*, **101** 289-299.

Burnett, L.E. (1979) The effects of environmental oxygen levels on the respiratory function of hemocyanin in the crabs, *Libinia emarginata* and *Ocypode quadrata*. *Journal of Experimental Zoology*, **210** 289-300.

Bushnell, P.G. and Brill, R.W. (1992) Oxygen transport and cardiovascular responses in skipjack tuna (*Katsuwonus pelamis*) and yellowfin tuna (*Thunnus albacares*) exposed to acute hypoxia. *Journal of Comparative Physiology B*, **162** 131-143.

Bushnell, P.G. and Jones, D.R. (1992) The arterial system, in *The Cardiovascular System* (eds. W.S. Hoar, D.J. Randall and A.P. Farrell), Academic Press, New York, pp 89-139.

Butler, P.J. (1982) Respiratory and cardiovascular control during diving in birds and mammals. *Journal of Experimental Biology*, **100** 195-221.

Butler, P.J. (1986) Exercise, in *Fish Physiology: Recent Advances* (eds. S. Nilsson and S. Holmgren), Croom Helm, London, pp 102-118.

Butler, P.J. (1989) Metabolic adjustments to breath holding in higher vertebrates. *Can. J. Zool.*, **67** 3024-3031.

Butler, P.J. (1991) Exercise in birds. *Journal of Experimental Biology*, **160** 233-262.

Butler, P.J. and Jones, D.R. (1971) The effect of variations in heart rate and regional distribution of blood flow on the normal pressor response to diving in ducks. *Journal of Physiology*, **214** 457-479.

Butler, P.J. and Jones, D.R. (1982) The comparative physiology of diving in vertebrates. *Advances in Comparative Physiology and Biochemistry*, **8** 179-364.

Butler, P.J. and Metcalfe, J.D. (1988) Cardiovascular and respiratory systems, in *Physiology of Elasmobranch Fishes*, (ed. T.J. Shuttleworth), Springer-Verlag, Berlin, pp 1-47.

Butler, P.J. and Taylor, E.W. (1973) The effect of hypercapnic hypoxia, accompanied by different levels of lung ventilation, on heart rate in duck. *Respiration Physiology*, **19** 176-187.

Butler, P.J. and Taylor, E.W. (1983) Factors affecting the respiratory and cardiovascular responses to hypercapnic hypoxia, in mallard ducks. *Respiration Physiology*, **53** 109-127.

Butler, P.J., West, N.H. and Jones, D.R. (1977) Respiratory and cardiovascular responses of the pigeon to sustained, level flight in a wind-tunnel. *Journal of Experimental Biology*, **71** 7-26.

Butler, P.J., Taylor, E.W., Capra, M.F. and Davison, W. (1978) The effect of hypoxia on the levels of circulating catecholamines in the dogfish *Scyliorhinus canicula*. *Journal of Comparative Physiology*, **127** 325-330.

Butler, P.J., Taylor, E.W. and Davison, W. (1979) The effect of long term, moderate hypoxia on acid-base balance, plasma catecholamines and possible anaerobic end products in the unrestrained dogfish *Scyliorhinus canicula*. *Journal of Comparative Physiology*, **132** 297-303.

Butler, P.J., Metcalfe, J.D. and Ginley, S.A. (1986) Plasma catecholamines in the lesser spotted dogfish and rainbow trout at rest and during different levels of exercise. *Journal of Experimental Biology*, **123** 409-421.

Butler, P.J., Axelsson, M., Ehrenström, F., Metcalfe, J.D. and Nilsson, S. (1989) Circulating catecholamines and swimming performance in the Atlantic cod, *Gadus morhua*. *Journal of Experimental Biology*, **141** 377-387.

Butler, P.J., Woakes, A.J., Smale, K., Roberts, C.A., Hillidge, C.J., Snow, D.H. and Marlin, D.J. (1993) Respiratory and cardiovascular adjustments during exercise of increasing intensity and during recovery in thoroughbred racehorses. *Journal of Experimental Biology*, **179** 159-180.

Claireaux, G., Thomas, S., Fievet, B. and Motais, R. (1988) Adaptive respiratory responses of trout to acute hypoxia. II. Blood oxygen carrying properties during hypoxia. *Respiration Physiology*, **74** 91-98.

Clausen, G. and Ersland, A. (1970) Blood O_2 and acid-base changes in the beaver during submersion. *Respiration Physiology*, **11** 104-112.

Cossins, A.R. and Richardson, P.A. (1985) Adrenalin-induced Na^+/H^+ exchange in trout erythrocytes and its effects upon oxygen-carrying capacity. *Journal of Experimental Biology*, **118** 229-246.

Davie, P.S. and Daxboeck, C. (1982) Effect of pulse pressure on fluid exchange between blood and tissues in trout gills. *Canadian Journal of Zoology*, **60** 1000-1006.

Davie, P.S. and Farrell, A.P. (1991) The coronary and luminal circulations of the myocardium of fishes. *Canadian Journal of Zoology*, **69** 1993-2001.

Davies, C.T.M. and Few, J.D. (1973) Effects of exercise on adrenocortical function. *Journal of Applied Physiology*, **35** 887-891.

Davison, W., Axelsson, M., Nilsson, S. and Forster, M.E. (1997) Cardiovascular control in Antarctic Notothenioid fishes. *Comparative Biochemistry and Physiology*, **118A** 1001-1008.

Driedzic, W.R. and Hochachka, P.W. (1978) Metabolism in fish during exercise, in *Locomotion* (eds. W.S. Hoar and D.J. Randall), Academic Press, New York, pp 503-543.

Egginton, S. (1997) A comparison of the response to induced exercise in red- and white- blooded Antarctic fishes. *Journal of Comparative Physiology B*, **167** 129-134.

Eros, S.K. and Milligan, C.L. (1996) The effect of cortisol on recovery from exhaustive exercise in rainbow trout (*Oncorhynchus mykiss*): Potential mechanisms of action. *Physiological Zoology*, **69** 1196-1214.

Evans, D.L. and Rose, R.J. (1988a) Cardiovascular and respiratory responses in thoroughbred horses during treadmill exercise. *Journal of Experimental Biology*, **134** 397-408.

Evans, D.L. and Rose, R.J. (1988b) Dynamics of cardiorespiratory function in Standardbred horses during different intensities of constant-load exercise. *Journal of Comparative Physiology B*, **157** 791-799.

Evinger, M.J., Towle, A.C., Park, D.H., Lee, P. and Joh, T.H. (1992) Glucocorticoids stimulate transcription of the rat phenylethanolamine n-methyltransferase (PNMT) gene in vivo and in vitro. *Cell Molecular Neurobiology*, **12** 193-215.

Faraci, F.M. (1991) Adaptations to hypoxia in birds: how to fly high. *Annual Review of Physiology*, **53** 59-70.

Faraci, F.M., Kilgore, D.L. Jr. and Fedde, M.R. (1984) Oxygen delivery to the heart and brain during hypoxia: Pekin duck vs. bar-headed goose. *American Journal of Physiology*, **247** R69-R75.

Farmer, C.G. and Jackson, D.C. (1998) Air-breathing during activity in the fishes *Amia calva* and *Lepisosteus oculatus*. *Journal of Experimental Biology*, **201** 943-948.

Farrell, A.P. (1987) Coronary flow in a perfused rainbow trout heart. *Journal of Experimental Biology*, **129** 107-123.

Farrell, A.P. (1993) Cardiovascular system, in *The Physiology of Fishes* (ed. D.H. Evans), CRC Press, Boca Ratan, pp 219-250.

Farrell, A.P. (1996) Features heightening cardiovascular performance in fishes, with special reference to tunas. *Comparative Biochemistry and Physiology*, **113A** 61-67.

Farrell, A.P. and Steffensen, J.F. (1987) Coronary ligation reduces maximum sustained swimming speed in the Chinook salmon, *Oncorhynchus tshawytscha*. *Comparative Biochemistry and Physiology*, **87A** 35-37.

Farrell, A.P., Daxboeck, C. and Randall, D.J. (1979) The effect of input pressure and flow on the pattern and resistance to flow in the isolated perfused gill of a teleost fish. *Journal of Comparative Physiology*, **133** 233-240.

Farrell, A.P., Sobin, S.S., Randall, D.J. and Crosby, S. (1980) Intralamellar blood flow patterns in fish gills. *American Journal of Physiology*, **239** R428-R436.

Fedde, M.R., Faraci, F.M., Kilgore, D.L., Cardinet, G.H. and Chatterjee, A. (1985) Cardiopulmonary adaptations in birds for exercise at high altitude, in *Circulation, Respiration and Metabolism* (ed. R. Gilles), Springer-Verlag, Berlin, pp 149-163.

Fedde, M.R., Orr, J.A., Shams, H. and Scheid, P. (1989) Cardiopulmonary function in exercising bar-headed geese during normoxia and hypoxia. *Respiration Physiology*, **77** 239-262.

Ferguson, R.A., Tufts, B.L. and Boutilier, R.G. (1989) Energy metabolism in trout red cells: consequences of adrenergic stimulation *in vivo* and *in vitro*. *Journal of Experimental Biology*, **143** 133-147.

Few, J.D. (1974) Effect of exercise on the secretion and metabolism of cortisol in man. *Journal of Endocrinology*, **62** 341-353.

Fievet, B., Motais, R. and Thomas, S. (1987) Role of adrenergic-dependent H^+ release from red cells in acidosis induced by hypoxia in trout. *American Journal of Physiology*, **252** R269-R275.

Fievet, B., Caroff, J. and Motais, R. (1990) Catecholamine release controlled by blood oxygen tension during deep hypoxia in trout: effect on red blood cell Na/H exchanger activity. *Respiration Physiology*, **79** 81-90.

Forgue, J., Burtin, B. and Massabuau, J.-C. (1989) Maintenance of oxygen consumption in resting *Silurus glanis* at different levels of ambient oxygenation. *Journal of Experimental Biology*, **143** 305-319.

Forgue, J., Massabuau, J.-C. and Truchot, J.-P. (1992) When are resting water-breathers lacking O_2? Arterial PO_2 at the anaerobic threshold in crab. *Respiration Physiology*, **88** 247-256.

Forster, M.E., Axelsson, M. and Farrell, A.P. (1991) Cardiac function and circulation in hagfishes. *Canadian Journal of Zoology*, **69** 1985-1992.

Forster, M.E., Davison, W., Axelsson, M. and Farrell, A.P. (1992) Cardiovascular responses to hypoxia in the hagfish, *Eptatretus cirrhatus*. *Respiration Physiology*, **88** 373-386.

Frayser, R., Rennie, I.D., Gray, G.W. and Houston, C.S. (1975) Hormonal and electrolyte response to exposure to 17,500 ft. *Journal of Applied Physiology*, **38** 636-642.

Fritsche, R. (1990) Effects of hypoxia on blood pressure and heart rate in three marine teleosts. *Fish Physiology and Biochemistry*, **8** 85-92.

Fritsche, R. and Nilsson, S. (1989) Cardiovascular responses to hypoxia in the Atlantic cod, *Gadus morhua*. *Experimental Biology*, **48** 153-160.

Fritsche, R. and Nilsson, S. (1990) Autonomic nervous control of blood pressure and heart rate during hypoxia in the cod, *Gadus morhua*. *Journal of Comparative Physiology B*, **160** 287-292.

Fritsche, R. and Nilsson, S. (1993) Cardiovascular and ventilatory control during hypoxia, in *Fish Ecophysiology* (eds. J.C. Rankin and F.B. Jensen), Chapman & Hall, London, pp 180-206.

Fritsche, R., Axelsson, M., Franklin, C.E., Grigg, G.G., Holmgren, S. and Nilsson, S. (1993) Respiratory and cardiovascular responses to hypoxia in the Australian lungfish. *Respiration Physiology*, **94** 173-187.

Gaesser, G.A., Ward, S.A., Baum, V.C. and Whipp, B.J. (1994) Effects of infused epinephrine on slow phase of O_2 uptake kinetics during heavy exercise in humans. *Journal of Applied Physiology*, **77** 2413-2419.

Gallaugher, P., Axelsson, M. and Farrell, A.P. (1992) Swimming performance and haematological variables in splenectomized rainbow trout, *Oncorhynchus mykiss*. *Journal of Experimental Biology*, **171** 301-314.

Gamperl, A.K., Pinder, A.W. and Boutilier, R.G. (1994a) Effect of coronay ablation and adrenergic stimulation on *in vivo* cardiac performance in trout (*Oncorhynchus mykiss*). *Journal of Experimental Biology*, **186** 127-143.

Gamperl, A.K., Pinder, A.W., Grant, R.R. and Boutilier, R.G. (1994b) Influence of hypoxia and adrenaline administration on coronary blood flow and cardiac performance in seawater rainbow trout (*Oncorhynchus mykiss*). *Journal of Experimental Biology*, **1983** 209-232.

Gamperl, A.K., Vijayan, M.M. and Boutilier, R.G. (1994c) Experimental control of stress hormone levels in fishes: techniques and applications. *Review of Fish Biology and Fisheries*, **4** 215-255.

Gamperl, A.K., Wilkinson, M. and Boutilier, R.G. (1994d) β-adrenoreceptors in the trout (*Oncorhynchus mykiss*) heart: characterisation, quantification and effects of repeated catecholamine exposure. *General and Comparative Endocrinology*, **95** 259-272.

Gfell, B., Kloas, W. and Hanke, W. (1997) Neuroendocrine effects of adrenal hormone secretion in carp (*Cyprinus carpio*). *General and Comparative Endocrinology*, **106** 310-319.

Gilmour, K.M., Didyk, N.E., Reid, S.G. and Perry, S.F. (1994) Down-regulation of red blood cell β-adrenoreceptors in response to chronic elevation of plasma catecholamines in the rainbow trout. *Journal of Experimental Biology*, **186** 309-314.

Gleeson, T.T. (1991) Patterns of metabolic recovery from exercise in amphibians and reptiles. *Journal of Experimental Physiology*, **160** 187-207.

Gleeson, T.T. (1996) Post-exercise lactate metabolism: A comparative review of sites, pathways and regulation. *Annual Review of Physiology*, **58** 565-581.

Gleeson, T.T. and Bennett, A.F. (1985) Respiratory and cardiovascular adjustments to exercise in reptiles, in *Circulation, Respiration, and Metabolism* (ed. R. Gilles), Springer-Verlag, Berlin, pp 23-38.

Gleeson, T.T., Dalessio, P.M., Carr, J.A., Wickler, S.J. and Mazzeo, R.S. (1993) Plasma catecholamine and corticosterone and their in vitro effects on lizard skeletal muscle lactate metabolism. *American Journal of Physiology*, **265** R632-R639.

Gonzalez, R.J. and McDonald, D.G. (1992) The relationship between oxygen consumption and ion loss in a freshwater fish. *Journal of Experimental Biology*, **163** 317-332.

Greco, A.M., Gilmour, K.M., Fenwick, J.C. and Perry, S.F. (1995) The effects of softwater acclimation on respiratory gas transfer in the rainbow trout *Oncorhynchus mykiss*. *Journal of Experimental Biology*, **198** 2557-2567.

Hadcock, J.R. and Malbon, C.C. (1988) Regulation of β-adrenergic receptors by "permissive" hormones: Glucocorticoids increase steady-state levels of receptor mRNA. *Proceedings of the National Academy of Sciences, USA*, **85** 8415-8419.

Hamilton, N.M. and Houlihan, D.F. (1992) Respiratory and circulatory adjustments during aquatic treadmill exercise in the European shore crab *Carcinus maenas*. *Journal of Experimental Biology*, **162** 37-54.

Hance, A.J., Robin, E.D., Halter, J.R., Lewiston, N., Robin, D.A., Cornell, L., Caligiuri, M. and Theodore, J. (1982) Hormonal changes and enforced diving in the harbor seal *Phoca vitulina*. II. Plasma catecholamines. *American Journal of Physiology*, **242** R528-R532.

Haouzi, P., Hirsh, J.J., Gille, J.P., Marchal, F., Crance, J.P. and Huszczuk, A. (1996) Papaverine injection into the hindlimb circulation stimulates ventilation in sheep. *Respiration Physiology*, **105** 143-153.

Hausdorff, W.P., Caron, M.G. and Lefkowitz, R.J. (1990) Turning off the signal - Desensitization of beta-adrenergic receptor function. *FASEB Journal*, **4:11** 2881-2889.

Hipkins, S.F., Smith, D.G. and Evans, B.K. (1986) Lack of adrenergic control of dorsal aortic blood pressure in the resting eel, *Anguilla australis*. *Journal of Experimental Zoology*, **238** 155-166.

Hōbe, H., Wood, C.M. and Wheatly, M.G. (1984) The mechanisms of acid-base and ionoregulation in the freshwater rainbow trout during environmental hyperoxia and subsequent normoxia. I. Extra- and intracellular acid-base status. *Respiration Physiology*, **55** 139-154.

Hochachka, P.W. (1992) Principles of physiological and biochemical adaptation, high-altitude man as a case study, in *Physiological Adaptations in Vertebrates, Respiration, Circulation, and Metabolism* (eds. S.C. Wood, R.E. Weber, A.R. Hargens and R.W. Millard), Marcel Dekker, New York, pp 21-35.

Holbert, P.W., Boland, E.J. and Olson, K.R. (1979) The effect of epinephrine and acetylcholine on the distribution of red cells within the gills of the channel catfish (*Ictalurus punctatus*). *Journal of Experimental Biology*, **79** 135-146.

Holeton, G.F. and Randall, D.J. (1967) The effect of hypoxia upon the partial pressure of gases in the blood and water afferent and efferent to the gills of rainbow trout. *Journal of Experimental Biology*, **46** 317-327.

Hopkins, S.R., McKenzie, D.C., Schoene, R.B., Glenny, R.B. and Robertson, H.T. (1994) Pulmonary gas exchange during exercise in athletes I. Ventilation-perfusion mismatch and diffusion limitation. *Journal of Applied Physiology*, **77** 912-917.

Hopkins, S.R., Hicks, J.W., Cooper, T.K. and Powell, F.L. (1995) Ventilation and pulmonary gas exchange during exercise in the savannah monitor lizard (*Varanus exanthematicus*). *Journal of Experimental Biology*, **198** 1783-1789.

Hudson, D.M. and Jones, D.R. (1982) Remarkable blood catecholamine levels in forced dived ducks. *Journal of Experimental Zoology*, **224** 451-456.

Hughes, G.M., Pennec-Le Bras, Y. and Pennec, J.P. (1988) Relationships between swimming speed, oxygen consumption, plasma catecholamines and heart performance in rainbow trout (*S. gairdneri* R.). *Experimental Biology*, **48** 45-49.

Humpeler, E., Skrabal, F. and Bartsch, G. (1980) Influence of exposure to moderate altitude on the plasma concentration of cortisol, aldosterone, renin, testosterone, and gonadotropins. *European Journal of Applied Physiology*, **45** 167-176.

Isaia, J., Girard, J.P. and Payan, P. (1978a) Kinetic study of gill epithelium permeability to water diffusion in the fresh water trout, *Salmo gairdneri*: effect of adrenaline. *Journal of Membrane Biology*, **41** 337-347.

Isaia, J., Maetz, J. and Haywood, G.P. (1978b) Effects of epinephrine on branchial non-electrolyte permeability in rainbow trout. *Journal of Experimental Biology*, **74** 227-237.

Itazawa, Y. and Takeda, T. (1978) Gas exchange in the carp gills in normoxic and hypoxic conditions. *Respiration Physiology*, **35** 263-269.

Jelinek, J. and Jensen, A. (1991) Catecholamine concentrations in plasma and organs of the fetal guinea pig during normoxemia, hypoxemia, and asphyxia. *Journal of Developmental Physiology*, **15** 145-152.

Jensen, F.B. (1986) Pronounced influence of Hb-O_2 saturation on red cell pH in tench blood in vivo and in vitro. *Journal of Experimental Zoology*, **238** 119-124.

Jensen, F.B. (1991) Multiple strategies in oxygen and carbon dioxide transport by haemoglobin, in *Physiological Strategies for Gas Exchange and Metabolism* (eds. A.J. Woakes, M.K. Grieshaber and C.R. Bridges), Cambridge University Press, Cambridge, pp 55-78.

Jensen, F.B., Nikinmaa, M. and Weber, R.E. (1993) Environmental perturbations of oxygen transport in teleost fishes: causes, consequences and compensations, in *Fish Ecophysiology* (eds. J.C. Rankin and F.B. Jensen), Chapman & Hall, London, pp 161-179.

Jones, D.R. (1967) Oxygen consumption and heart rate of several species of anuran amphibian during submergence. *Comparative Biochemistry and Physiology*, **20** 691-707.

Jones, D.R. (1968) Specific and seasonal variations in development of diving bradycardia in anuran amphibia. *Comparative Biochemistry and Physiology*, **25** 821-834.

Jones, D.R. (1972a) Anaerobiosis and the oxygen debt in an anuran amphibian, *Rana esculenta* (L.). *Journal of Comparative Physiology*, **77** 356-382.

Jones, D.R. (1972b) The effect of thermal acclimation on heart rate and oxygen consumption of frogs during submergence. *Comparative Biochemistry and Physiology*, **41A** 97-104.

Jones, D.R. and Holeton, G.F. (1972) Cardiovascular and respiratory responses of ducks to progressive hypocapnic hypoxia. *Journal of Experimental Biology*, **56** 657-666.

Jones, D.R. and Mustafa, T. (1973) The lactacid oxygen debt in frogs after one hour's apnoea in air. *Journal of Comparative Physiology*, **85** 15-24.

Jones, D.R. and Randall, D.J. (1978) The respiratory and circulatory systems during exercise, in *Fish Physiology* (eds. W.S. Hoar and D.J. Randall), Academic Press, Inc., London, pp 425-501.

Jones, J.H., Longworth, K.E., Lindholm, A., Conley, K.E., Karas, R.H., Kayar, S.R. and Taylor, C.R. (1989) Oxygen transport during exercise in large mammals I. Adaptive variation in oxygen demand. *Journal of Applied Physiology*, **67** 862-870.

Jönsson, A.C., Wahlqvist, I. and Hansson, T. (1983) Effects of hypophysectomy and cortisol on the catecholamine biosynthesis and catecholamine content in chromaffin tissue from rainbow trout, *Salmo gairdneri*. *General and Comparative Endocrinology*, **51** 278-285.

Keiver, K.M., Weinberg, J. and Hochachka, P.W. (1992) Roles of catecholamines and corticosterone during anoxia and recovery at 5°C in turtles. *American Journal of Physiology*, **263** R770-R774.

Kiceniuk, J.W. and Jones, D.R. (1977) The oxygen transport system in trout (*Salmo gairdneri*) during sustained exercise. *Journal of Experimental Biology*, **69** 247-260.

Kiley, J.P., Faraci, F.M. and Fedde, M.R. (1985) Gas exchange during exercise in hypoxic ducks. *Respiration Physiology*, **59** 105-115.

Kinkead, R. and Perry, S.F. (1990) An investigation of the role of circulating catecholamines in the control of ventilation during acute moderate hypoxia in rainbow trout (*Oncorhynchus mykiss*). *Journal of Comparative Physiology*, **160B** 441-448.

Kinkead, R. and Perry, S.F. (1991) The effects of catecholamines on ventilation in rainbow trout during hypoxia or hypercapnia. *Respiration Physiology*, **84** 77-92.

Kinkead, R., Fritsche, R., Perry, S.F. and Nilsson, S. (1991) The role of circulating catecholamines in the ventilatory and hypertensive responses to hypoxia in the Atlantic cod (*Gadus morhua*). *Physiological Zoology*, **64** 1087-1109.

Kinugawa, T., Ogino, K., Kitamura, H., Saitoh, M., Omodani, H., Osaki, S., Hisatome, I. and Miyakoda, H. (1996) Catecholamines, renin-angiotensin-aldosterone system, and atrial natriuretic peptide at rest and during submaximal exercise in patients with congestive heart failure. *American Journal of Medical Science*, **312** 110-117.

Koller, E.A., Bischoff, M., Buhrer, A., Felder, L. and Schopen, M. (1991) Respiratory, circulatory and neuropsychological responses to acute hypoxia in acclimatized and non-acclimatized subjects. *European Journal of Applied Physiology*, **62** 67-72.

Kolok, A.S., Spooner, R.M. and Farrell, A.P. (1993) The effect of exercise on the cardiac output and blood flow distribution of the large-scale sucker *Catostomus macrocheilus*. *Journal of Experimental Biology*, **183** 301-321.

Korsmeyer, K.E., Lai, N.C., Shadwick, R.E. and Graham, J.B. (1997) Oxygen transport and cardiovascular responses to exercise in the yellowfin tuna *Thunnus albacares*. *Journal of Experimental Biology*, **200** 1987-1997.

Kuhlmann, W.D., Hodgson, D.S. and Fedde, M.R. (1985) Respiratory, cardiovascular, and metabolic adjustments to exercise in the Hereford calf. *Journal of Applied Physiology*, **58** 1273-1280.

Lacombe, A.M.A. and Jones, D.R. (1991a) Neural and humoral effects on hindlimb vascular resistance of ducks during forced submergence. *American Journal of Physiology*, **261** R1579-R1586.

Lacombe, A.M.A. and Jones, D.R. (1991b) Role of adrenal catecholamines during forced submergence in ducks. *American Journal of Physiology*, **261** R1364-R1372.

Laub, M., Hvid-Jacobsen, K., Hovind, P., Kanstrup, I.-L., Christensen, N.J. and Nielsen, S.L. (1993) Spleen emptying and venous hematocrit in humans during exercise. *Journal of Applied Physiology*, **74** 1024-1026.

Lillo, R.S. (1978) The effect of arterial blood PO_2, PCO_2, and pH on diving bradycardia in the bullfrog *Rana catesbeiana*. *Physiological Zoology*, **51** 340-346.

Lomholt, J.P. and Johansen, K. (1979) Hypoxia acclimation in carp - How it affects O_2 uptake, ventilation, and O_2 extraction from water. *Physiological Zoology*, **52** 38-49.

Longworth, K.E., Jones, J.H., Bicudo, J.E.P.W., Taylor, C.R. and Weibel, E.R. (1989) High rate of O_2 consumption in exercising foxes: large PO_2 difference drives diffusion across the lung. *Respiration Physiology*, **77** 263-276.

Lowe, T.E., Wells, R.M.G. and Baldwin, J. (1995) Absence of regulated blood-oxygen transport in response to strenuous exercise by the shovelnosed ray, *Rhinobatos typus*. *Marine and Freshwater Research*, **46** 441-446.

Lutz, P.L. and Schmidt-Nielson, K. (1977) Effect of simulated altitude on blood gas transport in the pigeon. *Respiration Physiology*, **30** 383-388.

Maginniss, L.A., Bernstein, M.H., Deitch, M.A. and Pinshow, B. (1997) Effects of chronic hypobaric hypoxia on blood oxygen binding in pigeons. *Journal of Experimental Zoology*, **277** 293-300.

Mateika, J.H. and Duffin, J. (1995) A review of the control of breathing during exercise. *European Journal of Applied Physiology*, **71** 1-27.

Maxime, V., Nonnotte, G., Peyraud, C., Williot, P. and Truchot, J.P. (1995) Circulatory and respiratory effects of an hypoxic stress in the Siberian sturgeon. *Respiration Physiology*, **100** 203-212.

Mazzeo, R.S. (1991) Catecholamine responses to acute and chronic exercise. *Medicine and Science in Sports and Exercise*, **23** 839-845.

Mazzeo, R.S. and Marshall, P. (1989) Influence of plasma catecholamines on the lactate threshold during graded exercise. *Journal of Applied Physiology*, **67** 1319-1322.

Mazzocchi, G., Gottardo, G. and Nussdorfer, G.G. (1998) Paracrine control of steroid hormone secretion by chromaffin cells in the adrenal gland of lower vertebrates. *Histology and Histopathology*, **13** 209-220.

McDermott, J.C., Elder, G.C.B. and Bonen, A. (1987) Adrenal hormones enhance glycogenolysis in non-Expercising muscle during exercise. *Journal of Applied Physiology*, **63** 1275-1283.

McDonald, D.G., Boutilier, R.G. and Toews, D. (1980) The effects of enforced activity on ventilation, circulation and blood acid-base balance in the semi-terrestrial anuran, *Bufo marinus*. *Journal of Experimental Biology*, **84** 273-287.

McKenzie, D.J., Aota, S. and Randall, D.J. (1991) Ventilatory and cardiovascular responses to blood pH, plasma PCO_2, blood O_2 content and catecholamines in an air-breathing fish, the bowfin (*Amia calva*). *Physiological Zoology*, **64** 432-450.

McMahon, B.R., McDonald, D.G. and Wood, C.M. (1979) Ventilation, oxygen uptake and haemolymph oxygen transport, following enforced exhausting activity in the Dungeness crab *Cancer magister*. *Journal of Experimental Biology*, **80** 271-285.

Metcalfe, J.D. and Butler, P.J. (1988) The effects of alpha- and beta-adrenergic receptor blockade on gas exchange in the dogfish (*Scyliorhinus canicula* L.) during normoxia and hypoxia. *Journal of Comparative Physiology B*, **158** 39-44.

Metcalfe, J.D. and Butler, P.J. (1989) The use of alpha-methyl-*p*-tyrosine to control circulating catecholamines in the dogfish *Scyliorhinus canicula*: The effects on gas exchange in normoxia and hypoxia. *Journal of Experimental Biology*, **141** 21-32.

Milligan, C.L. and Wood, C.M. (1987) Regulation of blood oxygen transport and red cell pHi after exhaustive exercise in rainbow trout (*Salmo gairdneri*) and starry flounder (*Platichthys stellatus*). *Journal of Experimental Biology*, **133** 263-282.

Mitchell, G.S., Gleeson, T.T. and Bennett, A.F. (1981) Pulmonary oxygen transport during activity in lizards. *Respiration Physiology*, **43** 365-375.

Mokuda, O., Sakamoto, Y., Kawagoe, R., Ubukata, E. and Shimizu, N. (1992) Epinephrine augments cortisol secretion from isolated perfused adrenal glands of guinea pigs. *American Journal of Physiology*, **262** E806-E809.

Monge, C. and León-Velarde, F. (1991) Physiological adaptation to high altitude: Oxygen transport in mammals and birds. *Physiological Reviews*, **71** 1135-1172.

Motais, R., Garcia-Romeu, F. and Borgese, F. (1987) The control of Na^+/H^+ exchange by molecular oxygen in trout erythrocytes: a possible role of hemoglobin as a transducer. *Journal of General Physiology*, **90** 197-207.

Motais, R., Fievet, B., Garcia-Romeu, F. and Thomas, S. (1989) Na^+-H^+ exchange and pH regulation in red blood cells: role of uncatalyzed H_2CO_3 dehydration. *American Journal of Physiology*, **256** C728-C735.

Nakano, T. and Tomlinson, N. (1967) Catecholamine and carbohydrate concentrations in rainbow trout (*Salmo gairdneri*) in relation to physical disturbance. *Journal of the Fisheries Research Board of Canada*, **24 (8)** 1701-1715.

Neumann, P., Holeton, G.F. and Heisler, N. (1983) Cardiac output and regional blood flow in gills and muscles after exhaustive exercise in rainbow trout (*Salmo gairdneri*). *Journal of Experimental Biology*, **105** 1-14.

Nikinmaa, M. (1992) Membrane transport and control of hemoglobin-oxygen affinity in nucleated erythrocytes. *Physiological Reviews*, **72** 301-321.

Nikinmaa, M. and Huestis, W.H. (1984) Adrenergic swelling of nucleated erythrocytes: cellular mechanisms in a bird, domestic goose, and two teleosts, striped bass and rainbow trout. *Journal of Experimental Biology*, **113** 215-224.

Nikinmaa, M. and Tufts, B.L. (1989) Regulation of acid and ion transfer across the membrane of nucleated erythrocytes. *Canadian Journal of Zoology*, **67** 3039-3045.

Nilsson, S. (1984) *Autonomic Nerve Function in the Vertebrates*. Zoophysiology Series, Springer-Verlag, Berlin, 253 pp.

Nilsson, S. (1997) The autonomic nervous system of the dog and the dogfish: A comparative approach. *Acta Physiologica Scandinavica*, **161** 39-46.

Nilsson, S. and Grove, D.J. (1974) Adrenergic and cholinergic innervation of the spleen of the cod: *Gadus morhua*. *European Journal of Pharmacology*, **28** 135-143.

Nilsson, S., Forster, N.E., Davison, W. and Axelsson, M. (1996) Nervous control of the spleen in the red-blooded Antarctic fish, *Pagothenia borchgrevinki*. *American Journal of Physiology*, **39** R599-R604.

Nonnotte, G., Maxime, V., Truchot, J.-P., Williot, P. and Peyraud, C. (1993) Respiratory responses to progressive ambient hypoxia in the sturgeon, *Acipenser baeri*. *Respiration Physiology*, **91** 71-82.

Olson, K.R. (1998) The cardiovascular system, in *The Physiology of Fishes* (ed. D.H. Evans), CRC Press, Boca Ratan, pp 129-154.

Opdyke, D.F., Carroll, R.G. and Keller, N.E. (1982) Catecholamine release and blood pressure changes induced by exercise in dogfish. *American Journal of Physiology*, **242** R306-R310.

Pagnotta, A., Brooks, L. and Milligan, C.L. (1994) The potential regulatory roles of cortisol in recovery from exhaustive exercise in rainbow trout. *Canadian Journal of Zoology*, **72** 2136-2146.

Perry, S.F. and Bernier, N.J. (1998) The acute adrenergic stress response in fish: Facts and fiction. *Aquaculture*, in press.

Perry, S.F. and Gilmour, K.M. (1996) Consequences of catecholamine release on ventilation and blood oxygen transport during hypoxia and hypercapnia in an elasmobranch (*Squalus acanthias*) and a teleost (*Oncorhynchus mykiss*). *Journal of Experimental Biology*, **199** 2105-2118.

Perry, S.F. and Reid, S.D. (1992a) Relationship between blood O_2 content and catecholamine levels during hypoxia in rainbow trout and American eel. *American Journal of Physiology*, **263** R240-R249.

Perry, S.F. and Reid, S.D. (1992b) The relationship between β-adrenoceptors and adrenergic responsiveness in trout (*Oncorhynchus mykiss*) and eel (*Anguilla rostrata*) erythrocytes. *Journal of Experimental Biology*, **167** 235-250.

Perry, S.F. and Reid, S.D. (1993) β-adrenergic signal transduction in fish: Interactive effects of cortisol and catecholamines. *Fish Physiology and Biochemistry*, **11** 195-203.

Perry, S.F. and Reid, S.G. (1994) The effects of acclimation temperature on the dynamics of catecholamine release during acute hypoxia in the rainbow trout, *Oncorhynchus mykiss*. *Journal of Experimental Biology*, **186** 289-307.

Perry, S.F. and Thomas, S. (1991) The effects of endogenous or exogenous catecholamines on blood respiratory status during acute hypoxia in rainbow trout (*Oncorhynchus mykiss*). *Journal of Comparative Physiology B*, **161** 489-497.

Perry, S.F. and Thomas, S. (1993) Rapid respiratory changes in trout red blood cells during Na^+/H^+ exchange activation. *Journal of Experimental Biology*, **180** 27-37.

Perry, S.F. and Wood, C.M. (1989) Control and coordination of gas transfer in fishes. *Canadian Journal of Zoology*, **67** 2961-2970.

Perry, S.F., Daxboeck, C. and Dobson, G. (1985) The effect of perfusion flow rate and adrenergic stimulation on oxygen transfer in the isolated, saline-perfused head of rainbow trout (*Salmo gairdneri*). *Journal of Experimental Biology*, **116** 251-269.

Perry, S.F., Kinkead, R., Gallaugher, P. and Randall, D.J. (1989) Evidence that hypoxemia promotes catecholamine release during hypercapnic acidosis in rainbow trout (*Salmo gairdneri*). *Respiration Physiology*, **77** 351-364.

Perry, S.F., Fritsche, R., Kinkead, R. and Nilsson, S. (1991) Control of catecholamine release *in vivo* and *in situ* in the Atlantic cod (*Gadus morhua*) during hypoxia. *Journal of Experimental Biology*, **155** 549-566.

Perry, S.F., Kinkead, R. and Fritsche, R. (1992) Are circulating catecholamines involved in the control of breathing by fishes. *Review of Fish Biology and Fisheries*, **2** 65-83.

Perry, S.F., Fritsche, R. and Thomas, S. (1993) Storage and release of catecholamines from the chromaffin tissue of Atlantic hagfish, *Myxine glutinosa*. *Journal of Experimental Biology*, **183** 165-184.

Perry, S.F., Reid, S.G. and Salama, A. (1996) The effects of repeated physical stress on the β-adrenergic response of the rainbow trout red blood cell. *Journal of Experimental Biology*, **199** 549-562.

Pettersson, K. and Johansen, K. (1982) Hypoxic vasoconstriction and the effects of adrenaline on gas exchange efficiency in fish gills. *Journal of Experimental Biology*, **97** 263-272.

Peyraud-Waitzenegger, M. (1979) Simultaneous modifications of ventilation and arterial PO$_2$ by catecholamines in the eel, *Anguilla anguilla* L: participation of α and β effects. *Journal of Comparative Physiology*, **129B** 343-354.

Peyreaud-Waitzenegger, M. and Soulier, P. (1989) Ventilatory and cardiovascular adjustments in the European eel (*Anguilla anguilla*) exposed to short term hypoxia. *Experimental Biology*, **48** 107-122.

Peyraud-Waitzenegger, M., Barthelemy, L. and Peyraud, C. (1980) Cardiovascular and ventilatory effects of catecholamines in unrestrained eels (*Anguilla anguilla* L.). *Journal of Comparative Physiology*, **138B** 367-375.

Pickering, A.D. (1981) Introduction: The concept of biological stress, in *Stress and Fish* (ed. A.D. Pickering), Academic Press, London, pp 1-9.

Piiper, J., Baumgarten, D. and Meyer, M. (1970) Effects of hypoxia upon respiration and circulation in the dogfish *Scyliorhinus stellaris*. *Comparative Biochemistry and Physiology*, **36** 513-520.

Piiper, J., Meyer, M., Worth, H. and Willmer, H. (1977) Respiration and circulation during swimming activity in the dogfish *Scyliorhinus stellaris*. *Respiration Physiology*, **30** 221-239.

Piiper, J., Scheid, P., Perry, S.F. and Hughes, G.M. (1986) Effective and morphometric oxygen-diffusing capacity of the gills of the elasmobranch *Scyliorhinus stellaris*. *Journal of Experimental Biology*, **123** 27-41.

Pizarro, J., Warner, M.M., Ryan, M., Mitchell, G.S. and Bisgard, G.E. (1992) Intracarotid norepinephrine infusions inhibit ventilation in goats. *Respiration Physiology*, **90** 299-310.

Playle, R.C., Munger, R.S. and Wood, C.M. (1990) Effects of catecholamines on gas exchange and ventilation in rainbow trout (*Salmo gairdneri*). *Journal of Experimental Biology*, **152** 353-367.

Podolin, D.A., Munger, P.A. and Mazzeo, R.S. (1991) Plasma catecholamine and lactate responses during graded exercise with varied glycogen conditions. *Journal of Applied Physiology*, **71** 1427-1433.

Pollard, T.M. (1995) Use of cortisol as a stress marker - practical and theoretical problems. *American Journal of Human Biology*, **7** 265-274.

Postlethwaite, E.K. and McDonald, D.G. (1995) Mechanisms of Na$^+$ and Cl$^-$ regulation in freshwater-adapted rainbow trout (*Oncorhynchus mykiss*) during exercise and stress. *Journal of Experimental Biology*, **198** 295-304.

Powell, F.L. (1994) Respiratory gas exchange during exercise. *Advances in Veterinary Science and Comparative Medicine*, **38A** 253-285.

Primmett, D.R.N., Randall, D.J., Mazeaud, M. and Boutilier, R.G. (1986) The role of catecholamines in erythrocyte pH regulation and oxygen transport in rainbow trout (*Salmo gairdneri*) during exercise. *Journal of Experimental Biology*, **122** 139-148.

Randall, D.J. (1982) The control of respiration and circulation in fish during exercise and hypoxia. *Journal of Experimental Biology*, **100** 275-288.

Randall, D.J. and Daxboeck, C. (1982) Cardiovascular changes in the rainbow trout (*Salmo gairdneri* Richardson) during exercise. *Canadian Journal of Zoology*, **60** 1135-1140.

Randall, D.J. and Daxboeck, C. (1984) Oxygen and carbon dioxide transfer across fish gills, in *Fish Physiology* (eds. W.S. Hoar and D.J. Randall), Vol. XA, Academic Press, London, pp 263-314.

Randall, D.J. and Perry, S.F. (1992) Catecholamines, in *Fish Physiology. The Cardiovascular System* (eds. D.J. Randall and W.S. Hoar), Vol. XIIB, Academic Press, New York, pp 255-300.

Rees, A., Harvey, S. and Phillips, J.G. (1985) Transitory corticosterone responses of ducks (*Anas platyrhynchos*). *General and Comparative Endocrinology*, **59** 100-104.

Reid, S.D. and Perry, S.F. (1991) The effects and physiological consequences of raised levels of cortisol on rainbow trout (*Oncorhynchus mykiss*) erythrocyte β-adrenoreceptors. *Journal of Experimental Biology*, **158** 217-240.

Reid, S.D., Lebras, Y. and Perry, S.F. (1993) The *in vitro* effect of hypoxia on the trout erythrocyte β-adrenergic signal transduction system. *Journal of Experimental Biology*, **176** 103-116.

Reid, S., Moon, T.W. and Perry, S.F. (1992) Rainbow trout hepatocyte β-adrenoceptors, catecholamine responsiveness and effects of cortisol. *American Journal of Physiology*, **262** R794-R799.

Reid, S.G. and Perry, S.F. (1995) The effects of chronic hypoxia on red blood cell high affinity β-adrenoceptors in the rainbow trout, *Oncorhynchus mykiss*. *Fish Physiology and Biochemistry*, **14** 519-523.

Reid, S.G., Furimsky, M. and Perry, S.F. (1994) The effects of physical stress or fasting on catecholamine storage and release in the rainbow trout, *Oncorhynchus mykiss*. *Journal of Fish Biology*, **45** 365-378.

Reid, S.G., Vijayan, M.M. and Perry, S.F. (1996) Modulation of catecholamine storage and release by cortisol and ACTH in the rainbow trout, *Oncorhynchus mykiss*. *Journal of Comparative Physiology B*, **165** 665-676.

Reid, S.G., Bernier, N. and Perry, S.F. (1998) The adrenergic stress response in fish: Control of catecholamine storage and release. *Comparative Biochemistry and Physiology C*, **120** 1-27.

Ristori, M.T. and Laurent, P. (1985) Plasma catecholamines and glucose during moderate exercise in the trout: comparisons with bursts of violent activity. *Experimental Biology*, **44** 247-253.

Ristori, M.T. and Laurent, P. (1989) Plasma catecholamines in rainbow trout (*Salmo gairdneri*) during hypoxia. *Experimental Biology*, **48** 285-290.

Roberts, J.L. and Rowell, D.M. (1988) Periodic respiration of gill-breathing fishes. *Canadian Journal of Zoology*, **66** 182-190.

Roosevelt, T.S., Wennhold-Ruhmann, A. and Nelson, D.A. (1972) A protective effect of glucocorticoids in hypoxic stress. *American Journal of Physiology*, **223** 30-33.

Salama, A. and Nikinmaa, M. (1988) The adrenergic responses of carp (*Cyprinus carpio*) red cells: effects of PO_2 and pH. *Journal of Experimental Biology*, **136** 405-416.

Salama, A. and Nikinmaa, M. (1990) Effect of oxygen tension on catecholamine-induced formation of cAMP and on swelling of carp red blood cells. *American Journal of Physiology*, **259** C723-C726.

Samaja, M., Di Prampero, P.E. and Cerretelli, P. (1986) The role of 2,3-DPG in the oxygen transport at altitude. *Respiration and Physiology*, **64** 191-202.

Samaja, M., Mariani, C., Prestini, A. and Cerretelli, P. (1997) Acid-base balance and O_2 transport at high altitude. *Acta Physiologica Scandinavica*, **159** 249-256.

Saunders, D.K. and Fedde, M.R. (1994) Exercise performance of birds. *Advances in Veterinary Science and Comparative Medicine*, **38B** 139-190.

Saunders, R.L. and Sutterlin, A.M. (1970) Cardiac and respiratory responses to hypoxia in the sea raven, *Hemitripterus americanus* and an investigation of possible control mechanisms. *Journal of the Fisheries Research Board of Canada*, **28** 491-503.

Scherrer, D., Lach, E., Landry, Y. and Gies, J.P. (1997) Glucocorticoid modulation of muscarinic and beta-adrenergic receptors in guinea pig lung. *Fundamentals in Clinical Pharmacology*, **11** 111-116.

Shams, H. and Scheid, P. (1987) Respiration and blood gases in the duck exposed to normocapnic and hypercapnic hypoxia. *Respiration Physiology*, **67** 1-12.

Shelton, G. and Boutilier, R.G. (1982) Apnoea in amphibians and reptiles. *Journal of Experimental Biology*, **100** 245-273.

Shelton, G., Jones, D.R. and Milsom, W.K. (1986) Control of breathing in ectothermic vertebrates, in *Handbook of Physiology. Section 3 The Respiratory System. Volume II Control of Breathing* (eds. N.S. Cherniak and J.G. Widdicombe), American Physiological Society, Bethesda, Maryland, pp 857-909.

Sinha, N.P. and Dejours, P. (1980) Ventilation and blood acid-base balance of the crayfish as functions of water oxygenation (40 to 1500 Torr). *Comparative Biochemistry and Physiology*, **65A** 432.

Smith, D.G. (1978) Neural regulation of blood pressure in rainbow trout (*Salmo gairdneri*). *Canadian Journal of Zoology*, **56** 1678-1683.

Smith, J.J. and Kampine, J.P. (1990) *Circulatory Physiology–The Essentials*. Williams and Wilkins, Baltimore, 345 pp.

Soivio, A., Nikinmaa, M. and Westman, K. (1980) The blood oxygen binding properties of hypoxic *Salmo gairdneri*. *Journal of Comparative Physiology*, **136** 83-87.

Sorensen, B. and Weber, R.E. (1995) Effects of oxygenation and the stress hormones adrenaline and cortisol on the viscosity of blood from the trout *Oncorhynchus mykiss*. *Journal of Experimental Biology*, **198** 953-959.

Stevens, E.D. (1968) The effect of exercise on the distribution of blood to various organs in rainbow trout. *Comparative Biochemistry and Physiology*, **25** 615-625.

Stringer, W., Wasserman, K., Casaburi, R., Pörszäz, J., Maehara, K. and French, W. (1994) Lactic acidosis as a facilitator of oxyhemoglobin dissociation during exercise. *Journal of Applied Physiology*, **76** 1462-1467.

Sundin, L.I. (1995) Responses of the branchial circulation to hypoxia in the Atlantic cod, *Gadus morhua*. *American Journal of Physiology*, **37** R771-R778.

Sutton, J.R., Reeves, J.T., Wagner, P.D., Groves, B.M., Cymerman, A., Malconian, M.K., Rock, P.B., Young, P.M., Walter, S.D. and Houston, C.S. (1988) Operation Everest II: oxygen transport during exercise at extreme simulated altitude. *Journal of Applied Physiology*, **64** 1309-1321.

Swenson, E.R. (1990) Kinetics of oxygen and carbon dioxide exchange, in *Advances in Comparative and Environmental Physiology* (ed. R.G. Boutilier), Springer-Verlag, Berlin, pp 163-210.

Swift, D.J. (1981) Changes in selected blood component concentrations of rainbow trout, *Salmo gairdneri* Richardson, exposed to hypoxia or sublethal concentrations of phenol or ammonia. *Journal of Fish Biology*, **19** 45-61.

Swift, D.J. (1982) Changes in selected blood component values of rainbow trout, *Salmo gairdneri* Richardson, following the blocking of the cortisol response with betamethasone and subsequent exposure to phenol or hypoxia. *Journal of Fish Biology*, **21** 269-277.

Takeda, T. (1990) Ventilation, cardiac output and blood respiratory parameters in the carp, *Cyprinus carpio*, during hyperoxia. *Respiration Physiology*, **81** 227-240.

Talbot, C.R. and Stiffler, D.F. (1991) Effects of hypoxia on acid-base balance, blood gases, catecholamines and cutaneous ion exchange in the larval tiger salamander (*Ambystoma tigrinum*). *Journal of Experimental Zoology*, **257** 299-305.

Tang, Y. and Boutilier, R.G. (1988) Correlation between catecholamine release and degree of acidotic stress in rainbow trout, *Salmo gairdneri*. *American Journal of Physiology*, **255** R395-R399.

Taylor, A.C. and Spicer, J.E. (1991) Acid-base disturbances in the haemolymph of the prawns, *Palaemon elegans* (Rathke) and *P. serratus* (Pennant) (Crustacea: decapoda) during exposure to hypoxia. *Comparative Biochemistry and Physiology*, **98A** 445-452.

Taylor, C.R., Karas, R.H., Weibel, E.R. and Hoppeler, H. (1987) Adaptive variation in the mammalian respiratory system in relation to energetic demand: II. Reaching the limits to oxygen flow. *Respiration Physiology*, **69** 7-26.

Taylor, E.W. (1982) Control and co-ordination of ventilation and circulation in crustaceans: Responses to hypoxia and exercise. *Journal of Experimental Biology*, **100** 289-319.

Taylor, E.W. and Barrett, D.J. (1985) Evidence of a respiratory role for the hypoxic bradycardia in the dogfish *Scyliohinus canicula* L. *Comparative Biochemistry and Physiology*, **80A** 99-102.

Taylor, E.W. and Wilson, R.W. (1989) The cardiovascular and respiratory responses to intra-arterial injection of adrenaline in the dogfish *Scyliorhinus canicula* L. *Journal of Physiology*, **418** 133.

Tetens, V. and Christensen, N.J. (1987) Beta-adrenergic control of blood oxygen affinity in acutely hypoxia exposed rainbow trout. *Journal of Comparative Physiology B*, **157** 667-675.

Tetens, V. and Lykkeboe, G. (1981) Blood respiratory properties of rainbow trout, *Salmo gairdneri*: Responses to hypoxia acclimation and anoxic incubation of blood in vitro. *Journal of Comparative Physiology*, **145** 117-125.

Tetens, V. and Lykkeboe, G. (1985) Acute exposure of rainbow trout to mild and deep hypoxia: O_2 affinity and O_2 capacitance of arterial blood. *Respiration Physiology*, **61** 221-235.

Thomas, S. and Hughes, G.M. (1982) A study of the effects of hypoxia on acid-base status of rainbow trout blood using an extracorporeal blood circulation. *Respiration Physiology*, **49** 371-382.

Thomas, S. and Motais, R. (1990) Acid-base balance and oxygen transport during acute hypoxia in fish, in *Animal Nutrition and Transport Processes 2. Transport, Respiration and Excretion: Comparative and Environmental Aspects* (ed. J.-P. Truchot), Karger, Basel, pp 76-91.

Thomas, S. and Perry, S.F. (1992) Control and consequences of adrenergic activation of red blood cell Na^+/H^+ exchange on blood oxygen and carbon dioxide transport in fish. *Journal of Experimental Zoology*, **263** 160-175.

Thomas, S., Poupin, J., Lykkeboe, G. and Johansen, K. (1987) Effects of graded exercise on blood gas tensions and acid-base characteristics of rainbow trout. *Respiration Physiology*, **68** 85-97.

Thomas, S., Fievet, B., Claireaux, G. and Motais, R. (1988) Adaptive respiratory responses of trout to acute hypoxia. I. Effects of water ionic composition on blood acid-base status response and gill morphology. *Respiration Physiology*, **74** 77-90.

Thomas, S., Kinkead, R., Wood, C.M., Walsh, P.J. and Perry, S.F. (1991) Desensitization of adrenaline-induced red blood cell H^+ extrusion *in vitro* after chronic exposure of rainbow trout (*Salmo gairdneri*) to moderate environmental hypoxia. *Journal of Experimental Biology*, **156** 233-248.

Thomas, S., Perry, S.F., Pennec, Y. and Maxime, V. (1992) Metabolic alkalosis and the response of the trout, *Salmo fario*, to acute severe hypoxia. *Respiration Physiology*, **87** 91-104.

Thomas, S., Fritsche, R. and Perry, S.F. (1994) Pre- and post-branchial blood respiratory status during acute hypercapnia or hypoxia in rainbow trout, *Oncorhynchus mykiss*. *Journal of Comparative Physiology B*, **164** 451-458.

Thorarensen, H., Gallaugher, P.E., Kiessling, A.K. and Farrell, A.P. (1993) Intestinal blood flow in swimming Chinook salmon *Oncorhynchus tshawytscha* and the effects of haematocrit on blood flow distribution. *Journal of Experimental Biology*, **179** 115-129.

Truchot, J.-P. (1975) Changements de l'état acid-base du sang en fonction del l'oxygénation de l'eau chez le crabe *Carcinus maenas* (L.). *Journal de Physiologie, Paris*, **70** 583-592.

Truchot, J.-P. (1987) *Comparative Aspects of Extracellular Acid-Base Balance*. Zoophysiology Series, Springer-Verlag, Berlin, 248 pp.

Truchot, J.-P., Toulmond, A. and Dejours, P. (1980) Blood acid-base balance as a function of water oxygenation: a study at two different ambient CO_2 levels in the dogfish, *Scyliorhinus canicula*. *Respiration Physiology*, **41** 13-28.

Tufts, B.L. and Perry, S.F. (1998) Carbon dioxide transport and excretion, in *Fish Physiology. Fish Respiration* (eds. S.F. Perry and B.L. Tufts), Vol. XVII, Academic Press, San Diego, pp 229-281.

Tufts, B.L. and Randall, D.J. (1989) The functional significance of adrenergic pH regulation in fish erythrocytes. *Canadian Journal of Zoology*, **67** 235-238.

Tufts, B.L., Mense, D.C. and Randall, D.J. (1987) The effects of forced activity on circulating catecholamines and pH and water content of erythrocytes in the toad. *Journal of Experimental Biology*, **128** 411-418.

Turner, D.L. (1991) Cardiovascular and respiratory control mechanisms during exercise: An integrated view. *Journal of Experimental Biology*, **160** 309-340.

Val, A.L. (1996) Surviving low oxygen levels: lessons from fishes of the Amazon, in *Physiology and Biochemistry of the Fishes of the Amazon* (eds. A.L. Val, V.M.F. Almeida-Val and D.J. Randall), INPA, Manaus, pp 59-73.

Van Dijk, P.L.M. and Wood, C.M. (1988) The effect of β-adrenergic blockade on the recovery process after strenuous exercise in the rainbow trout, *Salmo gairdneri* Richardson. *Journal of Fish Biology*, **32** 557-570.

Van Raaij, M.T.M., van den Thillart, G.E.E.J.M., Vianen, G.J., Pit, D.S.S., Balm, P.H.M. and Steffens, A.B. (1996) Substrate mobilization and hormonal changes in rainbow trout (*Oncorhynchus mykiss*, L.) and common carp (*Cyprinus carpio*, L.) during deep hypoxia and subsequent recovery. *Journal of Comparative Physiology*, **166** 443-452.

Virtanen, E. and Forsman, L. (1987) Physiological responses to continuous swimming in wild salmon (*Salmo salar* L.) parr and smolt. *Fish Physiology and Biochemistry*, **4** 157-163.

Warner, M.M. and Mitchell, G.S. (1990) Ventilatory responses to hyperkalemia and exercise in normoxic and hypoxic goats. *Respiration Physiology*, **82** 239-250.

Warner, M.M. and Mitchell, G.S. (1991) Role of catecholamines and β-receptors in ventilatory response during hypoxic exercise. *Respiration Physiology*, **85** 41-53.

Wasser, J.S. and Jackson, D.C. (1991) Effects of anoxia and graded acidosis on the levels of circulating catecholamines in turtles. *Respiration Physiology*, **84** 363-377.

Wasser, J.S., Warburton, S.J. and Jackson, D.C. (1991) Extracellular and intracellular acid-base effects of submergence anoxia and nitrogen breathing in turtles. *Respiration Physiology*, **83** 239-252.

Wasserman, K. (1994) Coupling of external to cellular respiration during exercise: the wisdom of the body revisited. *American Journal of Physiology*, **266** E519-E539.

Wasserman, K., Whipp, B.J. and Casaburi, R. (1986) Respiratory control during exercise, in *Handbook of Physiology. Section 3 The Respiratory System. Volume II Control of Breathing* (eds. N.S. Cherniak and J.G. Widdicombe), American Physiological Society, Bethesda, Maryland, pp 595-619.

Weber, R.E. (1995) Hemoglobin adaptations to hypoxia and altitude - the phylogenetic perspective, in *Hypoxia and the Brain* (eds. J.R. Sutton, C.S. Houston and G. Coates), Queen City Printers, Burlington, Vermont, pp 31-44.

Weber, R.E. and Jensen, F.B. (1988) Functional adaptations in hemoglobins from ectothermic vertebrates. *Annual Review of Physiology*, **50** 161-179.

Weber, R.E. and Lykkeboe, G. (1978) Respiratory adaptations in carp blood. Influences of hypoxia, red cell organic phosphates, divalent cations and CO_2 on hemoglobin-oxygen affinity. *Journal of Comparative Physiology*, **128** 127-137.

Weil, J.V. (1986) Ventilatory control at high altitude, in *Handbook of Physiology Section 3 The Respiratory System Volume II Control of Breathing* (eds. N.S. Cherniack and J.G. Widdicombe), American Physiological Society, Bethesda, Maryland, pp 703-727.

Wells, R.M.G. and Weber, R.E. (1990) The spleen in hypoxic and exercised rainbow trout. *Journal of Experimental Biology*, **150** 461-466.

West, J.B. (1982) Respiratory and circulatory control at high altitudes. *Journal of Experimental Biology*, **100** 147-157.

West, J.B. (1989) Physiological responses to severe hypoxia in man. *Canadian Journal of Physiology and Pharmacology*, **67** 173-178.

West, J.B., Hackett, P.H., Maret, K.H., Milledge, J.S., Peters, R.M., Pizzo, C.J. and Winslow, R.M. (1983) Pulmonary gas exchange on the summit of Mount Everest. *Journal of Applied Physiology*, **55** 678-687.

Wheatly, M.G. (1987) Physiological responses of the rock crab *Cancer irroratus* (Say) to environmental hyperoxia. I. Acid-base regulation. *Physiological Zoology*, **60** 398-405.

Wheatly, M.G. (1989) Physiological responses of the crayfish *Pacifastacus leniusculus* to environmental hyperoxia I. Extracellular acid-base and electrolyte status and transbranchial exchange. *Journal of Experimental Biology*, **143** 33-51.

Wheatly, M.G. and Taylor, E.W. (1981) The effect of progressive hypoxia on heart rate, ventilation, respiratory gas exchange and acid-base status in the crayfish *Austropotamobius pallipes*. *Journal of Experimental Biology*, **92** 125-141.

Whipp, B.J. and Ward, S.A. (1982) Cardiopulmonary coupling during exercise. *Journal of Experimental Biology*, **100** 175-193.

Whipp, B.J., Ward, S.A., Lamarra, N., Davis, J.A. and Wasserman, K. (1982) Parameters of ventilatory and gas exchange dynamics during exercise. *Journal of Applied Physiology*, **52** 1506-1513.

Wilkes, P.R.H., Walker, R.L., McDonald, D.G. and Wood, C.M. (1981) Respiratory, ventilatory, acid-base and ionoregulatory physiology of the white sucker *Catostomus commersoni*: The influence of hyperoxia. *Journal of Experimental Biology*, **91** 239-254.

Winslow, R.M., Samaja, M. and West, J.B. (1984) Red cell function at extreme altitude on Mount Everest. *Journal of Applied Physiology*, **56** 109-116.

Withers, P.C., Hillman, S.S. and Kimmel, P.B. (1988a) Effects of activity, hemorrhage, and dehydration on plasma catecholamine levels in the marine toad (*Bufo marinus*). *General and Comparative Endocrinology*, **72** 63-71.

Withers, P.C., Hillman, S.S., Simmons, L.A. and Zygmunt, A.C. (1988b) Cardiovascular adjustments to enforced activity in the anuran amphibian, *Bufo marinus*. *Comparative Biochemistry and Physiology*, **89A** 45-49.

Wood, C.M. (1988) Acid-base and ionic exchange at gills and kidney after exhaustive exercise in the rainbow trout. *Journal of Experimental Biology*, **136** 461-481.

Wood, C.M. (1991a) Acid-base and ion balance, metabolism, and their interactions, after exhaustive exercise in fish. *Journal of Experimental Biology*, **160** 285-308.

Wood, C.M. (1991b) Branchial ion and acid-base transfer in freshwater teleost fish: Environmental hyperoxia as a probe. *Physiological Zoology*, **64** 68-102.

Wood, C.M. (1994) HCO_3^- dehydration by the blood of rainbow trout following exhaustive exercise. *Respiration Physiology*, **98** 305-318.

Wood, C.M. and Jackson, E.B. (1980) Blood acid-base regulation during environmental hyperoxia in the rainbow trout (*Salmo gairdneri*). *Respiration Physiology*, **42** 351-372.

Wood, C.M. and LeMoigne, J. (1991) Intracellular acid-base responses to environmental hyperoxia and normoxic recovery in rainbow trout. *Respiration Physiology*, **86** 91-113.

Wood, C.M. and Munger, R.S. (1994) Carbonic anhydrase injection provides evidence for the role of blood acid-base status in stimulating ventilation after exhaustive exercise in rainbow trout. *Journal of Experimental Biology*, **194** 225-253.

Wood, C.M. and Perry, S.F. (1985) Respiratory, circulatory, and metabolic adjustments to exercise in fish, in *Circulation, Respiration, and Metabolism* (ed. R. Gilles), Springer-Verlag, Berlin, pp 2-22.

Wood, C.M. and Randall, D.J. (1981a) Haemolymph gas transport, acid-base regulation, and anaerobic metabolism during exercise in the land crab (*Cardisoma carnifex*). *Journal of Experimental Zoology*, **218** 23-35.

Wood, C.M. and Randall, D.J. (1981b) Oxygen and carbon dioxide exchange during exercise in the land crab (*Cardisoma carnifex*). *Journal of Experimental Zoology*, **218** 7-22.

Wood, C.M. and Shelton, G. (1980) The reflex control of heart rate and cardiac output in the rainbow trout: Interactive influences of hypoxia, haemorrhage, and systemic vasomotor tone. *Journal of Experimental Biology*, **87** 271-284.

Wood, C.M., Walsh, P.J., Thomas, S. and Perry, S.F. (1990) Control of red blood cell metabolism in rainbow trout (*Oncorhynchus mykiss*) after exhaustive exercise. *Journal of Experimental Biology*, **154** 491-507.

Wood, C.M., Perry, S.F., Walsh, P.J. and Thomas, S. (1994) HCO_3^- dehydration by the blood of an elasmobranch in the absence of a Haldane effect. *Respiration Physiology*, **98** 319-337.

Wood, S.C. and Johansen, K. (1973) Blood oxygen transport and acid-base balance in eels during hypoxia. *American Journal of Physiology*, **225** 849-851.

Wood, S.C., Johansen, K. and Weber, R.E. (1975) Effects of ambient PO_2 on hemoglobin-oxygen affinity and red cell ATP concentrations in a benthic fish, *Pleuronectes platessa*. *Respiration Physiology*, **25** 259-267.

Xu, H.Y. and Olson, K.R. (1993) Significance of circulating catecholamines in regulation of trout splanchnic vascular resistance. *Journal of Experimental Zoology*, **267** 92-96.

Yamamoto, K., Itazawa, Y. and Kobayashi, H. (1980) Supply of erythrocytes into the circulating blood from the spleen of exercised fish. *Comparative Biochemistry and Physiology*, **65A** 5-11.

Yamamoto, K., Itazawa, Y. and Kobayashi, H. (1985) Direct observation of fish spleen by an abdominal window method and its application to exercised and hypoxic yellowtail. *Japanese Journal of Ichthyology*, **31** 427-433.

Young, D.B., Srivastava, T.N., Fitzovich, D.E., Kivlighn, S.D. and Hamaguchi, M. (1992) Potassium and catecholamine concentrations in the immediate post exercise period. *American Journal of Medical Science*, **304** 150-153.

Young, M., Rose, R.S., Sutton, J.R., Green, H.J., Cymerman, A. and Houston, C.S. (1989) Operation Everest II: plasma lipid and hormonal responses during a simulated ascent of Mt. Everest. *Journal of Applied Physiology*, **66** 1430-1435.

Zelnik, P.R. and Goldspink, G. (1981) The effect of exercise on plasma cortisol and blood sugar levels in the rainbow trout, *Salmo gairdneri* Richardson. *Journal of Fish Biology*, **19** 37-43.

3 Impact of stress on animal intermediate metabolism

A.B. Steffens and S.F. de Boer

3.1 Introduction

All living organisms require a continuous supply of energy to cover energy expenditure (EE). Energy expenditure can vary from the situation at rest to that during vigorous exercise. The supply of energy for the tissues in the body is derived from anaerobic glycolysis and aerobic breakdown of the main energy substrates glucose and free fatty acids (FFA). Circulating glucose and FFA are derived from the fairly large stores of glycogen in liver and muscle, and from the large amounts of triglycerides in fat tissues, respectively. Utilization of amino acids derived from excess of dietary amino acids and from hydrolyzed body proteins plays only a minor role and is estimated to cover maximally 4% of EE (Simonson and De Fronzo, 1990). These amino acids are de-aminated mainly in the liver and then converted to glucose and FFA, which are subsequently utilized. Under resting conditions and on a normal diet (i.e. containing 55% carbohydrate energy, 35% fat energy and 10% protein energy) the respiratory quotient (RQ), i.e. the ratio between CO_2 production and O_2 utilization, is 0.85 in the rat (Benthem *et al.*, 1994). This implies that both glucose and FFA contribute approximately 50% to the energy supply since the RQ would have a value of 0.7 or 1.0, respectively, if only FFA or glucose were utilized. During moderate exercise in which EE increases from a basal level of 5.27 watt kg^{-1} to 14.2 watt kg^{-1}, estimated to be about 60% of Vo_{2max}, the RQ decreases to 0.79. This means that relatively more FFA are utilized which results in a contribution to EE of 70% by fat oxidation. The remaining 30% of EE is covered by glucose utilization (Benthem *et al.*, 1994).

It has been found that the blood glucose and plasma FFA concentrations amount to 100 mg dl^{-1} and 5 mg dl^{-1}, respectively, for the resting rat (Benthem *et al.*, 1994). In the exercising rat, blood glucose and plasma FFA concentrations increase to 145 mg dl^{-1} and 20 mg dl^{-1}, respectively. This indicates that the individual amounts of glucose and FFA in the blood circulation of resting rats are sufficient to cover their metabolic needs for about 2 min and 20 s, respectively. During exercise the situation is probably not very different in view of the circulating amounts of substrates, although the contribution of blood glucose to cover metabolic needs is difficult to estimate because glucose originating from muscle glycogenolysis becomes more involved. Contrary to the situation of moderate exercise, severe exercise when Vo_{2max} is approaching 100% leads to nearly only glucose utilization to cover EE. The reasons are: (1) transport of O_2 to the active muscles becomes a limiting factor to guarantee aerobic oxidation of glucose and FFA; (2) excess of acetyl CoA due to increased glycolytic degradation of glucose to pyruvate and acetyl CoA in the cytosol competes with FFA for carnitine. Acetyl CoA reacts with carnitine to form acetylcarnitine, which is transported across the mitochondrial membrane by carnitine acetyltransferase. Because of the excess of acetyl CoA an insufficient amount of carnitine remains to transport FFA as fatty acetylcarnitine across the mitochondrial membrane (McGarry et al., 1977).

From these data it can be concluded that regulation of blood glucose and plasma FFA must be very accurate and matched with EE. This is controlled by the central nervous system and autonomic neural afferents sensing plasma substrate levels and probably also the rate of utilization and size of the reserves. Substrate release during rest and exercise is affected by efferent autonomic neurons, neuroendocrine factors and several hormones. The central nervous system can be considered the main controller where afferent and efferent messages are matched.

Considering the importance of aerobic breakdown of glucose and FFA to cover EE, special attention should be paid to organisms that can sustain hypoxia and even anoxia for longer periods. A good example in this respect is the carp. The question arises as to the regulation of energy supply under hypoxic and anoxic conditions in this animal.

3.2 Regulation of glucose and FFA release in the periphery

Blood glucose levels must be accurately defended because both hypoglycaemia and hyperglycaemia lead to pathological conditions. When blood glucose levels decline below 65 mg dl^{-1} nervous tissue does not function properly because uptake of glucose, the main fuel for nervous tissue, is hampered. Hyperglycaemic blood glucose levels higher than 140 mg dl^{-1} cause glycosylation of cell membrane proteins ultimately leading to dysfunction of numerous membrane processes (Murata et al., 1997). Deviations in plasma FFA levels do not have such serious consequences and are therefore not defended so accurately. However, a chronically elevated level can lead to cell membrane damage (Katz and Messinco, 1981). In principle, glucose and FFA turnover are tightly linked because an increase in blood glucose and plasma insulin levels leads to increased lipogenesis and glycogenesis whereas a decrease in blood glucose and plasma insulin levels results in lipolysis and glycogenolysis.

To prevent hypoglycaemia three lines of defence are effective during food deprivation as well as during exercise. The first line consists of suppressing insulin release from the B-cell and enhancing glucagon release from the A-cell of the islets of Langerhans. Insulin and glucagon released into the pancreatic duodenal vein act on the liver as their first target. Suppression of insulin release inhibits glucose uptake via insulin-dependent glucose transporters ($GLUT_4$) mainly in membranes of adipocytes and resting striated muscle cells. In addition, glycogenesis in the liver is prevented by inactivation of liver glycogen synthase which is converted from the active D form into the inactive I form (Shimazu, 1986). Glucagon converts inactive phosphorylase-b to active phosphorylase-a, causing glycogenolysis. Because the liver contains–contrary to the muscles–the enzyme glucose-6-phosphatase which converts glucose-6-phosphate into glucose, it is able to release glucose into the blood circulation. Further, glucagon is the major stimulus for gluconeogenesis. Thus, glucagon is the main factor to stimulate hepatic glycogenolysis and gluconeogenesis during exercise and starvation, although the decrease in insulin release facilitates this process (Wasserman *et al.*, 1989); in particular, the glucagon insulin ratio seems to be important in this respect (Wasserman *et al.*, 1995). Thus, the pancreatic hormones can be considered to be the main controllers of glucose turnover in the liver which are also the first to come into action.

The sympathetic nervous system can be considered to act as the second line of defence. The sympathetic nervous system consists of two branches: (1) the neural branch innervating e.g. the alimentary tract with related organs like liver and pancreas (both exocrine and endocrine) and the cardiovascular system, (2) the adrenal medullary branch. Activation of both branches of the sympathetic nervous system can be assessed by measuring plasma noradrenaline (NA) and adrenaline (A) concentrations. Here it should be mentioned that during moderate exercise (60% of Vo_{2max}), contrary to data presented in textbooks, the adrenal medulla releases only A and not NA, at least in the rat (Scheurink *et al.*, 1989a). Also, during insulin-induced hypoglycaemia counter-regulation to prevent a further decline in blood glucose concentration is only achieved by release of A and not by release of NA (Vollmer *et al.*, 1992). However, the adrenal medulla releases NA when the rat is subjected to cold stress (Vollmer *et al.*, 1992). When the adrenal medulla does not release NA, circulating NA originates only from the sympathetic nerve endings, mainly from those innervating the cardiovascular system. NA and A stimulate liver glycogenolysis by direct stimulation of α_1-adrenoceptors present in the membrane of liver parenchymal cells and indirectly by prostaglandins released from non-parenchymal cells also after stimulation of α_1-adrenoceptors in the membrane of these cells (Gardemann *et al.*, 1992). Lipolysis in adipocytes, eliciting increased production of FFA, is stimulated by activation of β_3-adrenoceptors in the adipocyte membrane (Zaagsma and Nahorski, 1990). Noradrenaline has a higher affinity for the β_3-adrenoceptors than A. During moderate exercise plasma A and NA levels attain a value of 0.5 and 2.0 ng ml^{-1} plasma, respectively (Figure 3.1) (Scheurink *et al.*, 1989a). Mimicking these exercise-induced plasma concentrations by exogenous infusion of either 20 ng A or 50 ng NA min^{-1} during 15 or 20 min in resting rats leads to conspicuous results regarding blood glucose and plasma FFA levels (Figures 3.2A and 3.2B). Adrenaline infusion caused an increase in blood glucose only and did not affect plasma FFA levels except for a small

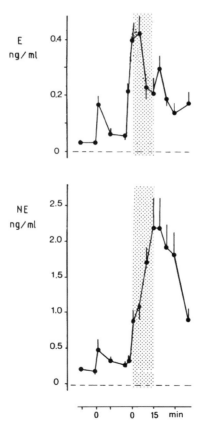

Figure 3.1   Plasma adrenaline (E) and noradrenaline (NE) concentrations before, during and after exercise in rats. Exercise is indicated by the dotted bar (after Scheurink *et al.*, 1989a).

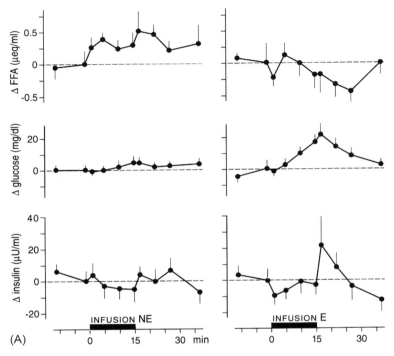

Figure 3.2 (A) Mean changes ± SE of plasma FFA, blood glucose and plasma insulin from preinfusion levels which are average of those of 1 min before infusion start, during intravenous noradrenaline (NE) infusion (left panel) and intravenous E infusion (right panel) at a rate of 20 ng min^{-1} during 15 min. Opposite page: (B) Mean changes ± SE as in (A) during intravenous NE and E infusion at a rate of 50 ng min^{-1} during 20 min.

decline at the infusion end. Infusion of NA resulted in an increase in plasma FFA levels only without an effect on blood glucose concentrations. However, infusion of a higher dose of A (50 ng A min^{-1}) producing a plasma A level similar to that which occurs during stress, also led to an increase in plasma FFA which was accompanied by a large increase in blood glucose concentration (Figure 3.2B). Infusion of 20 ng NA min^{-1} led to only a small increase in plasma FFA levels (Figure 3.2A). From the data of this experiment it can be concluded that during moderate exercise NA and A released into the blood circulation are responsible for lipolysis and glycogenolysis, respectively. In this situation NA can be considered to be a hormone released by the sympathetic nerve endings causing lipolysis in white adipocytes which do not receive direct sympathetic innervation. Noradrenaline does not effect glycogenolysis either in the liver (because NA levels–as occur in the synaptic clefts–are not reached)

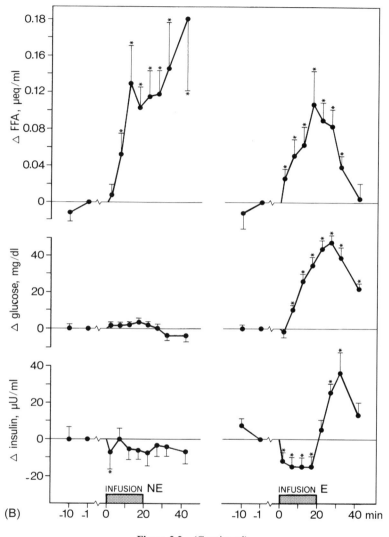

Figure 3.2   (Continued).

or in the muscle cells because glycogenolysis in these cells is mediated by β_2-adrenoceptors for which NA, at least in physiological conditions, has no affinity contrary to A (Gorski and Pietrzyk, 1982).

The contribution of the rich hepatic autonomic nervous innervation in the regulation of liver glucose turnover is still unclear, and this can mainly be attributed to the redundant mechanisms described above. Sympathetic denervation of the liver does not interfere with glucose mobilization during exercise unless glucagon and A release is suppressed underlining the significance of glucagon and A in affecting glucose mobilization (Van Dijk *et al.*, 1994a).

Muscle glycogenolysis due to A-stimulated β_2-adrenoceptors can indirectly contribute to maintenance of blood glucose concentrations during exercise. Muscle glycogenolysis results in diminished uptake of glucose from the circulation by the muscle cells and to increased lactate synthesis (Benthem *et al.*, 1995). In the liver, lactate is converted to glucose by the gluconeogenetic hormones glucagon and adrenaline. These processes might be the main contributors to the increased blood glucose levels during enhanced plasma A levels. In addition, the effects of A and NA on the islets of Langerhans have to be taken into account (Figures 3.2 and 3.3). Both suppress insulin release from the B-cells and enhance glucagon release from the A-cells by an α_2-adrenoceptor mediated mechanism. Adrenaline exerts a slightly stimulating effect on the B-cells by a β_2-adrenoceptor mediated mechanism to guarantee a minimal insulin release during severe sympathetic nervous activity (Benthem *et al.*, 1995). This mechanism prevents complete suppression of glucose uptake by insulin-dependent tissues.

After termination of the catecholaminergic influence a rebound in insulin occurs due to the enhanced blood glucose concentration at that time point. Immediately after termination of their release, the effects of NA and A wane because of their short half-life of 30 s (Ferreira and Vane, 1967). It is evident that the first line of defence (insulin decrease and glucagon increase) and the second line of defence (increased sympathetic activity) are simultaneously active and additional, the more so as glucagon release from the A-cells is stimulated by α-adrenoceptor mechanisms. An outline of all aforementioned processes is depicted in Figure 3.3. Besides the sympathetic nervous system, the parasympathetic nervous system also affects the liver and the islets of Langerhans. Insulin and glucagon release and hepatic glycogenesis are elicited by muscarinic mechanisms (Kaneto *et al.*, 1974, 1975; Shimazu, 1986).

Also, under resting conditions, insulin release from the B-cell is affected by simultaneous activity of the sympathetic and parasympathetic nervous system (Steffens *et al.*, 1991). During stress and exercise the autonomic nervous balance on regulation of hormone release from the islets of Langerhans is shifted into the sympathetic direction.

The third line of defence consists of activation of the hypothalamo–pituitary–adrenal cortex axis (HPA axis) leading to increased corticosterone release (Cryer, 1993). Release of growth hormone also plays a role in glucose counter-regulation (De Feo *et al.*, 1989).

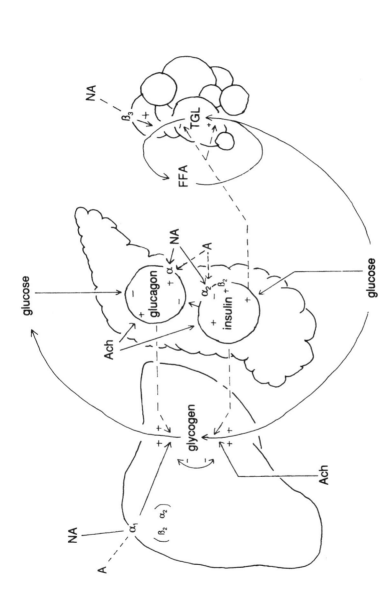

Figure 3.3 Neuronal (—) and hormonal (- - - -) regulation of peripheral energy substrate homeostasis: release of glucose form the liver, secretion of insulin and glucagon from the endocrine pancreas, and release of FFA from white adipose tissue. Ach, acetylcholine; NA, noradrenaline; A, adrenaline; TGL, triglycerides.

3.3   Central nervous control of glucose and FFA release

From the aforementioned data it is evident that maintenance of blood glucose and plasma FFA levels is mainly regulated by peripheral mechanisms only if an animal is at rest and on *ad-libitum* carbohydrate-rich food. Then insulin and glucagon play a major role. However, also in this situation control of insulin and glucagon release by the CNS cannot be excluded. In this respect it is noteworthy that the islets of Langerhans receive a dense sympathetic and parasympathetic innervation. Electrical stimulation of pancreatic vagal nerves leads to increased insulin release (Kaneto *et al.*, 1967). Splanchnic nerve stimulation suppresses insulin release and augments glucagon release (Miller, 1975). Histochemical tracing studies showed that several hypothalamic areas project directly and indirectly on the dorsomotor nucleus of the vagus (DVM) and the intermediolateral column (IML), the motor pool of preganglionic sympathetic nerves in the spinal cord (Luiten *et al.*, 1987). From these motor areas there are direct projections to the islets of Langerhans and the adrenal medulla (Luiten *et al.*, 1987).

There are many reports describing the effects of manipulation of hypothalamic areas on control of blood glucose and plasma FFA levels by interference with the function of the islets of Langerhans, the HPA axis and the autonomic nervous system. An acute lesion in both ventromedial (VMH) and paraventricular (PVN) areas of the hypothalamus causes an immediate increase in activity of the pancreatic parasympathetic nerves with a simultaneous decrease in activity of the pancreatic sympathetic nerves. An acute lesion in the lateral hypothalamic area (LHA) leads to the reverse result (Yoshimatsu *et al.*, 1984). The results of a different experiment clearly show the involvement of the hypothalamus in maintenance of blood glucose and plasma insulin levels. If in a VMH lesioned animal the usually occurring hyperphagia was prevented by strict pair feeding (in quantity and time intervals between meals), nevertheless, with control rats basal plasma insulin levels went up in the weeks after lesioning. Also, meal-stimulated insulin release increased continuously during that period although glucose tolerance was maintained. This is an indication of a slowly deteriorating insulin sensitivity (Balkan *et al.*, 1991).

Infusion of small amounts of NA (an important hypothalamic neurotransmitter) into the VMH leads to increases in blood glucose, plasma FFA and insulin levels whereas infusion of NA into the LHA diminishes plasma FFA levels and enhances plasma insulin levels (Steffens *et al.*, 1984). Infusion of an α-adrenoceptor antagonist into the VMH during exercise in rats leads to exaggerated plasma FFA and attenuated blood glucose levels, whereas infusion of a β-adrenoceptor antagonist causes a drop in blood glucose levels and an attenuated increase in plasma FFA concentrations. Infusion of an α-adrenoceptor antagonist into the LHA during exercise results in an attenuated rise in blood glucose, whereas plasma FFA do not differ from those in the control situation. Infusion of a β-adrenoceptor antagonist into the LHA leads to a drop in blood glucose levels and an attenuated increase in plasma FFA levels during exercise. After termination of exercise blood glucose levels continued to decline after α-adrenoceptor blockade in the VMH as well as in the LHA, whereas an immediate rebound could be observed after β-adrenoceptor blockade of both hypothalamic areas. The drop in blood glucose during exercise after β-adrenoceptor blockade might be attributed to increased glucose uptake which might be due to diminished lipolysis and concomitant attenuated increase in plasma FFA levels causing diminished utilization (Scheurink et al., 1988). Turnover studies of glucose and FFA during exercise have to be performed to corroborate this hypothesis. No differences in plasma insulin levels as compared to exercising control rats could be observed in these experiments. Regarding the neural networks in the hypothalamus involved in glucose and FFA release it can be stated that an extended α-adrenergic network, encompassing the VMH and LHA, affects glucose release during exercise. Free fatty acid release is effectuated by a β-adrenergic network. The exaggerated increase in FFA during exercise with α-adrenergic blockade might be explained as follows.

Increased activity in noradrenergic hypothalamic networks during exercise elicits release of NA from nerve endings in these networks. Presynaptic α2-adreno autoreceptors in these nerve endings inhibit further NA release. If an α-adrenoceptor antagonist is present this inhibition is absent, resulting in an exaggerated NA release (Scheurink et al., 1989a). This excess of NA might lead to enhanced activity in the β-adrenergic network subserving FFA release. Thus hypothalamic noradrenergic networks play an important role in control of blood glucose and plasma FFA levels both during rest and exercise.

Infusion of the neuropeptide NPY into the PVN causes an increase in insulin release and a decrease in sympathetic activity apart from NPY's stimulatory effect on food intake (Van Dijk et al., 1994b). These effects are independent of changes in food intake because food was either not available or the same amount was ingested as in controls.

Most interesting are serotonergic mechanisms in the PVN regarding control of blood glucose and plasma FFA concentrations by interfering with the action of the sympathetic nervous system and the hypothalamo–pituitary–adrenal cortex (HPA) axis. Administration of the serotonin re-uptake blocker norfenfluramine into the PVN in resting rats led to augmented activity of the adrenal medullary branch of the sympathetic nervous system resulting in enhanced plasma A levels and concomitant increase in blood glucose concentrations. The activity of the neural branch of the sympathetic nervous system was unchanged and low as appears from the low plasma NA levels. Also, the plasma FFA levels did not alter. The HPA axis was activated as appears from the increase in plasma corticosterone concentrations. If norfenfluramine was administered in the PVN of exercising rats activation of the neural branch was even attenuated (Scheurink et al., 1993). Postsynaptic 5-HT$_{1A}$ receptors are probably involved because administration of the specific 5-HT$_{1A}$ agonist 8-OH-DPAT into the PVN leads to comparable results (Korte et al., 1991). Thus, the hypothalamus can be considered to be a main integration and outflow area to control blood glucose, plasma FFA via regulation of autonomic nervous activity and peripheral hormone release, e.g. insulin, glucagon and corticosterone.

The way in which the CNS and particularly the hypothalamus is notified to adjust the release of glucose and FFA to exercise stress and food deprivation, is less clear. Information from the periphery (e.g. alimentary tract, liver) and the CNS itself is involved. Changes in glucose concentrations in the portal vein lead to alterations in afferent vagal nerve activity (Niijima, 1989). Neurons in the VMH and LHA are sensitive to changes in insulin glucose and FFA levels in their neighbourhood (Oomura, 1983). These substances can penetrate into the CNS across the blood–brain barrier by carrier systems. The afferent vagal information from the portal vein glucose concentration and also from alimentary tract receptors is carried to the tractus solitarius nucleus (NTS) and from there to several brainstem areas, e.g. noradrenergic areas A$_1$ and A$_6$, dorso motor nucleus of the vagus and the serotonergic raphe nucleus. A$_1$, A$_6$ and raphe nucleus project onto the PVN. Finally, in the case of exercise and stress, activation of the sympathetic nervous system can be achieved by feed forward from higher brain areas (Vissing et al., 1989b).

Insulin and the recently discovered hormone leptin (Zhang et al., 1994) released in relation to the size of the fat mass of an individual, affect metabolism besides their suppressing effect on food intake. Insulin and leptin can cross the blood-brain barrier by means of a saturable carrier system (Banks et al., 1996). Neurons in the arcuate nucleus in the hypothalamus contain many insulin and leptin receptors which inhibit the synthesis of NPY after binding either insulin or leptin (Schwartz et al., 1992, 1996). These NPY-ergic neurons project on the PVN. NPY activity in the PVN decreases metabolism activity via diminished sympathetic tone and increases food intake (Van Dijk et al., 1994b). Leptin also causes activation of the sympathetic nervous system, e.g. sympathetic nerves innervating the thermogenic brown adipose tissue (Haynes et al., 1997). Leptin has also another important effect on the energy balance. It

enhances the release of corticotropin-releasing hormone (CRH) synthesized in neurons of the parvocellular portion of the PVN. Among others,
CRH-containing neurons stimulate neural pathways to the IML leading
to increased sympathetic activity (Haynes *et al.*, 1997) and enhanced
thermogenesis and energy expenditure (Rothwell, 1989; Hwa *et al.*, 1996).
In addition, this system is also intricately involved in stress-induced (fear,
pain, grief, etc.) activation of the HPA axis, leading to elevated levels of
circulating ACTH and glucocorticoids. In many of these processes the
aforementioned 5-HT$_{1A}$ mechanisms contribute to these effects (Korte
et al., 1991; Scheurink *et al.*, 1993). Thus, a reduction in hypothalamic CRH activity has, in essence, the same effect as increased
hypothalamic NPY activity, i.e. a reduced energy expenditure accompanied by increased food intake. However, leptin which is peripherally
secreted, reduced ACTH and glucocorticoid secretion (Ahima *et al.*,
1996), probably by a direct inhibitory effect on the pituitary and adrenal
cortex. The inhibitory effect of peripheral leptin on pituitary-glucocorti-
coid activity intuitively provides a brake to prevent high levels of leptin
being self-perpetuating since glucocorticoids (in addition to peripheral
insulin) are potent stimulants of leptin secretion.

It can be concluded that a number of areas in the hypothalamus are
involved in energy balance and energy expenditure. These areas are
informed about the peripheral energy status by means of the hormones
insulin, leptin and corticosterone and probably also by the metabolic
substrates glucose and FFA. The neurotransmitters noradrenaline,
serotonin and the neuropeptides NPY and CRH play an important role
in the pathways of the CNS. The efferent pathways consist of the
sympathetic nervous system and the HPA axis. Very recently it has been
reported that leptin also increases release of thyroid stimulating hormone
releasing hormone (TRH) causing thyroxin release from the thyroid
gland (Flier and Maratos-Flier, 1998). Thyroxin is one of the most
powerful stimulators of metabolism. By means of these mechanisms stress
interferes with metabolic processes.

3.4   The effects of stress on the control of blood glucose
and plasma FFA concentrations

The term 'stress' is often used but is difficult to define unequivocally.
Originally it was used by Cannon for an overwhelming threat to
homeostasis (Cannon, 1914) but at present it is more used as any
deviation that can alter homeostasis. In that situation the body's stress
effector systems are trying to counteract the disturbing forces in order to
re-establish homeostasis, i.e. the continuous equilibrium of the internal

environment. In this way all information coming from the outside and inside world challenging homeostasis has to be considered as stressors. Outside world and inside world information reach the central nervous system by information from exteroceptors, interoceptors and proprioceptors. The information produced by stressors gathered by the brain results in efferent messages to counteract the deviations produced by the stressors. In this respect the autonomic nervous system and the HPA axis are the main efferent pathways. In this paragraph we will describe the effects of stressors of different severity on the control of blood glucose and plasma FFA concentrations because these are the metabolic substrates to cover energy expenditure which is mostly enhanced because of accompanying increased locomotor activity.

Swimming in water at a temperature of 33°C to prevent cold stress against a countercurrent leads to only a moderate increase in plasma A concentrations (Figure 3.1). However, accurate inspection of Figure 3.1 reveals a dissociation in the increase in plasma NA and A. The basal plasma levels of NA and A are low, $180 \, \text{pg ml}^{-1}$ and $30 \, \text{pg ml}^{-1}$, respectively. Transfer of the rats from the home cage to the waiting platform above the swimming pool leads to an immediate light activation of the adrenal medullary branch as well as the neural branch of the sympathetic nervous system, causing an increase in plasma NA and A concentrations to $500 \, \text{pg ml}^{-1}$ and $180 \, \text{pg ml}^{-1}$, respectively. Then waiting for 20 min on the platform resulted in a decline of plasma NA and A levels to nearly basal levels indicating a waning of sympathetic activity. However, slowly lowering of the platform resulted in a dissociation of the increase in plasma NA and A concentrations. Plasma A increased considerably as soon as the rats got wet paws whereas plasma NA began to increase as soon as the rats started to swim. The dissociation continued during swimming: plasma A decreased whereas plasma NA continued to increase. These results are in agreement with the hypothesis that emotional stress is more related to activation of the adrenal medullary branch and a physical workload more to activation of the neural branch of the sympathetic nervous system (De Boer *et al.*, 1990). The decline in plasma A during swimming is probably due to the light workload (60% $Vo_{2\text{max}}$) in lukewarm water which the rats like. In these experiments the rats were accustomed to the procedure. It is of interest to compare these results with the results obtained in rats subjected to swimming for the first time (Scheurink *et al.*, 1989c). In this situation the experimental set-up is completely new to them which will result in a higher level of emotional stress, mainly anxiety. In Figure 3.4 the plasma NA and A concentrations in rats subjected to swimming for the first time are compared to those in habituated rats. Plasma A attains much higher concentrations in inexperienced animals than in experienced ones whereas the reverse can

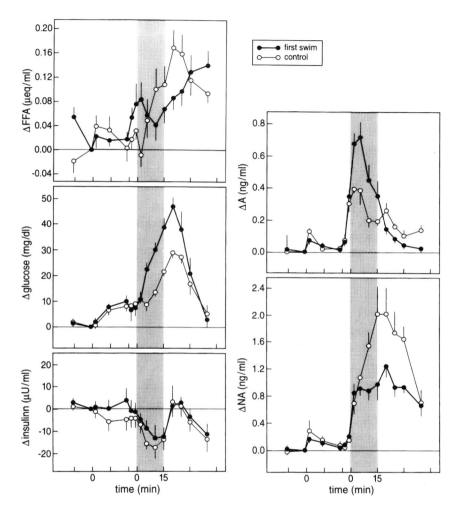

Figure 3.4 Blood glucose, plasma FFA, insulin, adrenaline (A) and noradrenaline (NA) concentrations before, during and after exercise in naive (first swim) and habituated control rats. Exercise is indicated by the dotted bar.

be observed for plasma NA. The exaggerated blood glucose levels and attenuated plasma FFA levels in inexperienced animals can be explained by the altered plasma catecholamine concentrations as described in the second paragraph of this chapter. Blood glucose concentrations are more controlled by A and plasma FFA concentrations more by NA. These observations are corroborated by the results obtained in adrenal medulla ectomized rats subjected to swimming. In these animals A was undetectable both in rest and during exercise whereas the rise in plasma NA concentrations was attenuated during swimming. In these rats even a slight decrease in blood glucose levels could be observed during swimming whereas the increase in FFA was strongly attenuated (Scheurink *et al.*, 1989b).

In another experimental approach rats were subjected to run on a treadmill for 20 min (Vissing *et al.*, 1989a). The workload was 60% of Vo_{2max} which was the same as in the experiments in which rats were subjected to swimming. As can be observed in Table 3.1, the increase in plasma NA concentration is comparable in both exercise conditions. However, plasma A increased continuously during running and reached a level of 6000 pg ml^{-1} at the end of running, i.e. about ten times higher than during swimming. Also, blood glucose levels attained the extreme high value of 180 mg dl^{-1}. Thus, the increase in plasma NA seems to be correlated with the workload which was the same in the swimming and running rat. The emotional stress component is completely different in the running and swimming rat. Rats are good swimmers and they are not subjected to cold stress in the experimental set-up used. In addition emotional stress diminishes during habituation of the animals to the swimming procedure as appears from the diminished A response. Training to run on the treadmill is doubtless very stressful. To run properly on the moving belt for 20 min the rats receive foot shocks and pokes with a fork during the training period if they return to the waiting compartment because of insufficient performance. That they are aware of the possibility of receiving this treatment is apparent from the already high basal plasma A concentration during waiting in the waiting compartment in front of the belt (see Table 3.1). Thus, it can be concluded that changes in plasma NA concentrations are related to workload and changes in plasma A concentrations to emotional stress.

Table 3.1 Plasma NA and A concentrations during swimming and running

	20 min in waiting compartment		10 min after start of exercise	
	Before swimming	Before running	Swimming	Running
NA(pg/ml plasma)	260	410	2400	3000
A(pg/ml plasma)	75	450	250	3600

NA increase caused by swimming: 2140 pg; A increase caused by swimming: 175 pg.
NA increase caused by running: 2590 pg; A increase caused by running: 3150 pg.
NA/A index—swimming: 12, running: 0.8.

Not only does sympathetic activity increase during swimming and running, but the activity of the HPA axis also increases. Both during swimming and running plasma corticosterone concentrations increased to a level of about 50 µg dl^{-1}. However, it has to be taken into consideration that the plasma corticosterone level in the waiting compartment before the running belt was $30\,\mu g\,dl^{-1}$ (Vissing et al., 1989a) and on the waiting platform above the swimming pool $18\,\mu g\,dl^{-1}$ (Scheurink et al., 1990), which is also an indication of increased emotional stress in rats participating in the running experiment.

3.5   Central nervous control of sympathetic and HPA axis activity during stress

As mentioned previously the hypothalamus is one of the most important central nervous areas controlling sympathetic and HPA-axis activity. By means of α- and β-adrenoceptor blockade of several hypothalamic areas, blood glucose and plasma FFA levels can be affected during exercise (Scheurink et al., 1988). Administration of serotonergic agonists into the PVN in resting rats increases the activity of the adrenal medullary branch of the sympathetic nervous system and the HPA axis (Korte et al., 1991; Scheurink et al., 1993). Administration of serotonergic agonists in exercising rats leads to an attenuated activation of the neural branch of the sympathetic nervous system (Scheurink et al., 1993). The dissociation in activation of the neural branch and adrenomedullary branch of the sympathetic nervous system due to either workload or emotional stress can be explained by these data. Emotional stress is accompanied by increased serotonergic activity in the hypothalamus (Shimizu et al., 1989, 1992) and it is quite well tenable that this leads to the observed increase in activity of the adrenal medullary branch of the sympathetic nervous system with concomitant attenuated activation of the neural branch. Taking these data together, it should be expected that administration of serotonergic antagonists into the PVN during exercise would lead to suppressed activity of the adrenal medullary branch of the sympathetic nervous system and the HPA axis and increased activity of the neural branch. However, data in the literature and also the results of experiments performed by ourselves are nearly completely negative. This might be due to insufficient selectivity of the antagonists used because many serotonergic receptor types are present in the PVN, both presynaptically and postsynaptically. Also, other neurotransmitters and neuropeptides might be involved. Alpha adrenoceptor blockade in the PVN during exercise leads to complete suppression of an increase in plasma corticosterone indicating complete suppression of the HPA axis (Scheurink et al., 1990). Beta adrenoceptor blockade in the PVN results in attenuation of activation of the neural branch of the sympathetic nervous system whereas activation of the adrenal medullary branch and HPA axis are completely comparable to the control situation (Scheurink et al., 1990). Increased NPY activity in the PVN leads to suppression of sympathetic activity during food intake (Van Dijk *et al.*, 1994b) and to increased CRH release (Wahlestedt *et al.*, 1987). However, its effects during exercise and emotional stress on metabolism are unknown. Probably also many other neurohumoral factors in the hypothalamus, like insulin and leptin which are involved in regulation of energy intake, affect metabolism during exercise and emotional stress. Future research has to unravel their role in this respect.

Finally, it is worthwhile to pay some attention to the goal of increased activity of especially the adrenal medullary branch of the sympathetic nervous system with concomitant increase in glucose production during emotional stress and especially of the neural branch with concomitant increase in FFA production during exposure to a workload.

If a workload is of moderate intensity 70% of the EE is covered by FFA. Then lipolysis and FFA production can be maintained during long periods because of continuous activation of the neural branch of the sympathetic nervous system. Activity of the adrenal medullary branch has to be low to prevent increased glucose production and utilization because of the relatively small stores. The situation during emotional stress is different. Then glucose is necessary for appropriate functioning of the central nervous system which is completely dependent on glucose to cover its metabolic needs. In addition, often a sudden escape from the source of emotional stress is necessary which includes a workload of high intensity to be covered nearly completely by glucose. Then activation of the adrenal medullary branch of the sympathetic nervous system is useful because of its effects on glucose production.

Finally, it should be borne in mind that activation of the sympathetic nervous system and, to a lesser extent, the HPA axis during stress and exercise also adjust the cardiovascular system to the increased demands. How the demands of metabolism and cardiovascular adjustments are matched at the central nervous level is an intriguing question.

3.6 Metabolic adaptation to hypoxia in fishes

In the preceding paragraphs, the effects of exercise and different emotional stressors on the activity of the sympathetic nervous system and HPA axis in mammals have been described. During prolonged times of stress some animals can survive under hypoxic and even anoxic circumstances. Examples of survivors under hypoxic circumstances are carps and goldfishes. Under these circumstances carbohydrates become the major substrate for covering EE leading to depletion of glycogen stores in all glycogen-containing tissues and to increases in plasma glucose levels (Van den Thillart and Van Raaij, 1995; Van Raaij *et al.*,

1996). Glycogenolysis is, as in the mammal, achieved by catecholamines and glucagon (Janssens and Waterman, 1988). Lipolysis and plasma FFA concentrations are controlled differently during hypoxia. During hypoxia, plasma FFA concentrations decline in spite of an enormous increase in plasma NA levels (Van Raaij *et al.*, 1996). Infusion of NA into the blood circulation of a carp under normoxic conditions also leads to a considerable suppression of plasma FFA levels (Van Raaij *et al.*, 1995). The decrease in plasma FFA concentrations can be due to (1) increased utilization, (2) increased lipogenesis, (3) decreased lipolysis. Increased utilization can be excluded because FFA is oxidized by β-oxidation which is oxygen dependent. Increased lipogenesis can also be excluded because plasma insulin, the main lipogenetic factor, is suppressed during hypoxia and NA infusion (Janssens and Waterman, 1988; Van Raaij *et al.*, 1996). Thus, decreased lipolysis remains as the cause of declining plasma FFA levels in the carp during hypoxia. This reaction is very useful because FFA cannot be utilized and possible damaging reactions of too-high plasma FFA levels are prevented in this way. The cause of decreased lipolysis is under investigation. It can be due to either different receptors in the adipocyte membrane of carps as compared to mammalian adipocytes or to differences in post-receptor processes.

Activation of the HPA axis in fishes is comparable to the HPA activation in mammals (Van Raaij *et al.*, 1996). At present, nearly nothing is known regarding central nervous system control of metabolism in fish.

3.7   Concluding remarks

Emotional stress and physical work profoundly affect glucose and FFA metabolism, mainly via the sympathetic nervous system and, to a lesser extent, via the HPA axis. Emotional stress mainly activates the adrenal medullary branch of the sympathetic nervous system leading to increased A release from the adrenal medulla. Adrenaline elicits a powerful increase in glucose production whereas it scarcely exerts an effect on lipolysis. Physical work mainly activates the neural branch of the sympathetic nervous system resulting in NA release from the sympathetic nerve endings. Circulating NA is a powerful lipolytic substance with minor effects on glucose production. Free fatty acids are the main substrate to cover EE during prolonged moderate physical work whereas glucose is the main substrate to cover EE during explosive activities as can occur during acute emotional stress. This suggests that the nature of stress induces release of the appropriate metabolic substrate (either glucose or FFA) via activation of the appropriate branch of the sympathetic nervous system as indicated by the NA/A index (Table 3.1). Proper adjustments of substrate release occur also under totally different types of stress in different species, e.g. hypoxia (hypoxia tolerance) in fish – e.g. the carp. Because of lack of oxygen, EE is covered by anaerobic glycolysis with simultaneous prevention of lipolysis and FFA utilization, in spite of the fact that activation of the sympathetic nervous system and the HPA axis are similar in mammals. This is effectuated by suppression of lipolysis by NA in the carp. Thus, in mammals and fishes, stress induces a similar activation of the sympatho-adrenomedullary system and HPA axis. However, due to differences at the receptor or post-receptor level, activation or inhibition of lipolysis may occur. It can be concluded that the nature of stress leads to appropriate substrate release to cover metabolic needs existing in that period.

References

Ahima, R.S., Prabakaran, D., Mantzoros, C., Qu, D., Lowell, B., Maratos-Flier, E. and Flier, J.S. (1996) Role of leptin in neuroendocrine response to fasting. *Nature*, **382** 250-252.

Balkan, B., Steffens, A.B., Bruggink, J.E. and Strubbe, J.H. (1991) Hyperinsulinemia and glucose tolerance in obese rats with lesions in the ventromedial hypothalamus: dependence on food intake and route of administration. *Metabolism*, **40** 1092-1100.

Banks, W.A., Kastin, A.J., Huang, W., Jaspan, J.B. and Maness, L.M. (1996) Leptin enters the brain by a saturable system independent of insulin. *Peptides*, **17 (2)** 305-311.

Benthem, L., Bolhuis, J.W., Van der Leest, J., Steffens, A.B., Zock, J.P. and Zijlstra, W.G. (1994) Methods for measurement of energy expenditure and substrate concentrations in swimming rats. *Physiology and Behavior*, **56 (1)** 151-159.

Benthem, L., Van der Leest, J., Steffens, A.B. and Zijlstra, W.G. (1995) Metabolic and hormonal responses to adrenoceptor antagonists in exercising rats. *Metabolism*, **44 (2)** 245-253.

Cannon, W.B. (1914) The emergency function of the adrenal medulla in pain and in the major emotions. *American Journal of Physiology*, **33** 356-372.

Cryer, P.E. (1993) Glucose counterregulation: prevention and correction of hypoglycemia in humans. *American Journal of Physiology*, **264** E149-E155.

De Boer, S.F., De Beun, R., Slangen, J.L. and Van der Gugten, J. (1990) Dynamics of plasma catecholamine and corticosterone concentrations during reinforced and extinguished operant behavior in rats. *Physiology and Behavior*, **47 (4)** 691-698.

De Feo, P.M., Perriello, G., Torlone, E., Ventura, M.M., Santeusanio, F., Brunett, P., Gerich, J.E. and Bolli, G.B. (1989) Demonstration of a role for growth hormone in glucose counterregulation. *American Journal of Physiology*, **256** E835-E843.

Ferreira, S.H. and Vane, J.R. (1967) Half-lifes of peptides and amines in the circulation. *Nature*, **215** 1237-1240.

Flier, J.S. and Maratos-Flier, E. (1998) Obesity and the hypothalamus. Novel peptides for new pathways. *Cell*, **92** 437-440.

Gardemann, A., Püschel, G.P. and Jungermann, K. (1992) Nervous control of liver metabolism and hemodynamics. *European Journal of Biochemistry*, **207** 399-411.

Gorski, J. and Pietrzyk, K. (1982) The effect of beta-adrenergic receptor blockade on intramuscular glycogen mobilization during exercise in the rat. *European Journal of Applied Physiology*, **48** 201-205.

Haynes, W.G., Morgan, D.A., Walsh, S.A., Mark, A.L. and Sivitz, W.I. (1997) Receptor mediated regional sympathetic nerve activation by leptin. *Journal of Clinical Investigation*, **100** 270-278.

Hwa, J.J., Ghibaudi, L., Compton, D., Fawzi, A.B. and Strader, C.D. (1996) Intracerebroventricular injection of leptin increases thermogenesis and mobilizes fat metabolism in ob/ob mice. *Hormone and Metabolic Research*, **28** 659-663.

Janssens, P.A. and Waterman, J. (1988) Hormonal regulation of gluconeogenesis and glycogenolysis in carp (*Cyprinus carpio*) liver pieces cultured in vitro. *Comparative Biochemistry and Physiology*, **91A** 451-455.

Kaneto, A., Kosaka, K. and Nakao, K. (1967) Effects of stimulation of the vagus nerve on insulin secretion. *Endocrinology*, **80** 530-536.

Kaneto, A., Miki, E. and Kosaka, K. (1974) Effects of vagal stimulation on glucagon and insulin secretion. *Endocrinology*, **95** 1005-1010.

Kaneto, A., Miki, E. and Kosaka, K. (1975) Effects of β- and β_2-adrenoceptor stimulants infused intrapancreatically on glucagon and insulin secretion. *Endocrinology*, **97** 1166-1173.

Katz, A.M. and Messinco, F.C. (1981) Lipid-membrane interactions and the pathogenesis of ischemic damage in the myocardium. *Circulation Research*, **48 (1)** 1-16.

Korte, S.M., Van Duin, S., Bouws, G.A.H., Koolhaas, J.M. and Bohus, B. (1991) Involvement of hypothalamic serotonin in activation of the sympathoadrenal medullary system and hypothalamo-pituitary-adrenocortical axis in male Wistar rats. *European Journal of Pharmacology*, **197** 225-228.

Luiten, P.G.M., Ter Horst, G.J. and Steffens, A.B. (1987) The hypothalamus, intrinsic-connections and outflow pathways to the endocrine system in relation to the control of feeding and metabolism. *Progress in Neurobiology*, **28** 1-55.

McGarry, J.D., Mannaerts, G.P. and Foster, D.W. (1977) A possible role for malonyl-CoA in the regulation of hepatic fatty acid oxidation and ketogenesis. *Journal of Clinical Investigation*, **60** 265-270.

Miller, R.E. (1975) Neural inhibition of insulin secretion from the isolated canine pancreas. *American Journal of Physiology*, **229** 144-149.

Murata, T., Nagai, R., Ishibashi, T., Inomuta, H., Ikaed, K. and Horinchi, S. (1997) The relationship between accumulation of advanced glycation end products and expression of vascular endothelial growth factor in human diabetic retinas. *Diabetologia*, **40** 764-769.

Niijima, A. (1989) Nervous regulation of metabolism. *Progress in Neurobiology*, **33** 135-147.

Oomura, Y. (1983) Glucose as a regulator of neural activity, in *Advances in Metabolic disorders*. Vol. 10, *CNS Regulation of Carbohydrate Metabolism* (ed. A. J. Szabo) Academic Press, New York, pp 31-65.

Rothwell, N. (1989) Central effects of CRF on metabolism and energy balance. *Neuroscience Biobehavior Reviews*, **14** 263-271.

Scheurink, A.J.W., Steffens, A.B. and Benthem, L. (1988) Central and peripheral adrenoceptors affect glucose, free fatty acids and insulin in exercising rats. *American Journal of Physiology*, **255** R547-R556.

Scheurink, A.J.W., Steffens, A.B., Bouritius, H., Bruntink, R., Remie, R. and Zaagsma, J. (1989a) Adrenal and sympathetic catecholamines in exercising rats. *American Journal of Physiology*, **256** R155-R160.

Scheurink, A.J.W., Steffens, A.B., Bouritius, H., Bruntink, R., Remie, R. and Zaagsma, J. (1989b) Sympathoadrenal influence on glucose, FFA, and insulin levels in exercising rats. *American Journal of Physiology*, **256** R161-R168.

Scheurink, A.J.W., Steffens, A.B., Dreteler, G.H., Benthem, L. and Bruntink, R. (1989c) Experience affects exercise-induced changes in catecholamines, glucose, and FFA. *American Journal of Physiology*, **256** R169-R173.

Scheurink, A.J.W., Steffens, A.B. and Gaykema, R.P.A. (1990) Paraventricular hypothalamic adrenoceptors and energy metabolism in exercising rats. *American Journal of Physiology*, **259** R478-R484.

Scheurink, A.J.W., Leuvenink, H. and Steffens, A.B. (1993) Metabolic and hormonal responses to hypothalamic administration of norfenfluramine in rats. *Physiology and Behavior*, **53 (5)** 889-898.

Schwartz, M.W., Sipols, A.J., Marts, J.L., Sanacora, G., Shite, J.D., Scheurink, A.J.W., Kahn, S.E., Baskin, D.G., Figlewicz, D.P. and Porte, D. Jr. (1992) Inhibition of hypothalamic neuropeptide Y gene expression by insulin. *Endocrinology*, **130** 3608-3616.

Schwartz, M.W., Baskin, D.G., Bukowski, T.R., Kuijper, J.L., Foster, D., Lasser, G., Prunkard, D.E., Porte, D. Jr., Woods, S.C., Seeley, R.J. and Weigle, D.S. (1996) Specificity of leptin action on elevated blood glucose levels and hypothalamic neuropeptide Y gene expression in ob/ob mice. *Diabetes*, **45** 531-535.

Shimazu, T. (1986) Neuronal control of intermediate metabolism, in *Neuroendocrinology* (eds. S. Lightman and B. Everitt) Blackwell, Oxford, pp 304-330.

Shimizu, N., Oomura, Y. and Aoyagi, K. (1989) Electrochemical analysis of hypothalamic serotonin metabolism accompanied by immobilization stress in rats. *Physiology and Behavior*, **46 (5)** 829-834.

Shimizu, N., Take, S., Hori, T. and Oomura, Y. (1992) *In vivo* measurement of hypothalamic serotonin release by intracerebral microdialysis: significant enhancement by immobilization stress in rats. *Brain Research Bulletin*, **28 (5)** 727-734.

Simonson, D.C. and De Fronzo, R.A. (1990) Indirect calorimetry: Methodological and interpretative problems. *American Journal of Physiology*, **258** E399-E410.

Steffens, A.B., Damsma, G., Van der Gugten, J. and Luiten, P.G.M. (1984) Circulating free fatty acids, insulin, and glucose during chemical stimulation of hypothalamus in rats. *American Journal of Physiology*, **247** E765-E771.

Steffens, A.B., Strubbe, J.H., Balkan, B. and Scheurink, A.J.W. (1991) Neuroendocrine factors regulating blood glucose, plasma FFA, and insulin in the development of obesity. *Brain Research Bulletin*, **27 (3/4)** 505-510.

Van den Thillart, G. and Van Raaij, M. (1995) Endogenous fuels: non invasive vs. invasive approaches, in *Biochemistry and Molecular Biology of Fishes* (eds. P.W. Hochachka and T.P. Mommsen) Elsevier Science, Amsterdam, pp 1-63.

Van Dijk, G., Balkan, B., Lindfeldt, J., Bouws, G., Scheurink, A.J.W., Ahren, B. and Steffens, A.B. (1994a) Contribution of epinephrine, glucagon and hepatic innervation on hepatic glucose mobilization in exercising rats. *Acta Physiologica Scandinavica*, **150** 305-313.

Van Dijk, G., Bottone, A.E., Steffens, A.B. and Strubbe, J.H. (1994b) Hormonal and metabolic effects of paraventricular hypothalamic administration of neuropeptide Y during rest and feeding. *Brain Research*, **660** 96-103.

Van Raaij, M.T.M., Van den Thillart, G.E.E.J.M., Hallemeesch, M., Balm, P.H.M. and Steffens, A.B. (1995) Effect of arterially infused catecholamines and insulin on plasma glucose and free fatty acids in carp. *American Journal of Physiology*, **268** R1163-R1170.

Van Raaij, M.T.M., Van den Thillart, G.E.E.J.M., Vianen, G.J., Pit, D.S.S., Balm, P.H.M. and Steffens, A.B. (1996) Substrate mobilization and hormonal changes in rainbow trout (*Oncorhynchus mykiss*, L.) and common carp (*Cyprinus carpio*, L.) during deep hypoxia and subsequent recovery. *Journal of Comparative Physiology*, **166** 443-452.

Vissing, J., Wallace, J.L., Scheurink, A.J.W., Galbo, H. and Steffens, A.B. (1989a) Ventromedial hypothalamic regulation of hormonal and metabolic responses to exercise. *American Journal of Physiology*, **256** R1019-R1026.

Vissing, J., Iwamoto, G.A., Rybicki, J., Galbo, H. and Mitchell, J.H. (1989b) Mobilization of glucoregulatory hormones and glucose by hypothalamic locomotor centers. *American Journal of Physiology*, **257** E722-E728.

Vollmer, R.R., Baruchin, A., Kolibal-Pegher, S.S., Corey, S.P., Stricker, E.M. and Kaplan, B.B. (1992) Selective activation of norepinephrine- and epinephrine-secreting chromaffin cells in rat adrenal medulla. *American Journal of Physiology*, **263** R716-R721.

Wahlestedt, C., Skagerberg, G., Edman, R., Heilig, M., Sundler, F. and Hakanson, R. (1987) Neuropeptide Y (NPY) in the area of the paraventricular nucleus activates the pituitary-adrenocortical axis in the rat. *Brain Research*, **417** 33-38.

Wasserman, D.H., Spalding, J.H., Lacy, D.B., Coburn, C.A., Goldstein, R.E. and Cherrington, A.D. (1989) Glucagon is a primary controller of hepatic glycogenolysis and gluconeogenesis during muscular work. *American Journal of Physiology*, **257** E108-E117.

Wasserman, D.H., O'Doherty, R.M. and Zinker, B.A. (1995) Role of the endocrine pancreas in control of fuel metabolism by the liver during exercise. *International Journal of Obesity and Related Metabolic Disorders*, **19 Suppl. 4** S22-S30.

Yoshimatsu, H., Niijima, A., Oomura, Y., Yamabe, K. and Katafuchi, T. (1984) Effects of hypothalamic lesion on pancreatic autonomic nerve activity in the rat. *Brain Research*, **303** 147-152.

Zaagsma, J. and Nahorski, S.R. (1990) Is the adipocyte β-adrenoceptor a prototype for the recently cloned atypical β$_3$-adrenoceptor? *Trends in Pharmacological Sciences*, **11** 3-7.

Zhang, Y., Proenca, R., Maffei, M., Barone, M., Leopold, L. and Friedman, J.M. (1994) Positional cloning of the mouse obese gene and its human homologue. *Nature*, **372** 425-432.

4 The impact of stress on animal reproductive activities

Tom G. Pottinger

4.1 Introduction

It is well established that stress affects the reproductive system of vertebrates. Numerous research papers and review articles have presented an increasingly complex picture of the interrelationships between the physiological stress response and the reproductive system of mammals, birds, reptiles, amphibians, and fish. However, there has been no previous attempt to provide a taxonomically inclusive overview of the impact of stress on the reproductive system of vertebrates. It is the intention of this chapter to provide an introduction to the current state of our understanding of the interaction of stress with the reproductive system of vertebrates.

4.1.1 Scope

There is an extensive literature concerning the impact of stress on reproductive processes and it is beyond the scope of this chapter to provide a fully comprehensive catalogue of all relevant work in all vertebrate groups. Therefore, where possible, and to avoid unnecessary repetition, review articles will be cited to provide direct access to specific areas of the field. Where appropriate reviews are unavailable, representative research papers will be highlighted. The intention is to be comprehensive in breadth of coverage but selective in depth. Inevitably, omissions will occur because of limits on space.

4.1.2 The concept of stress

The current concept of physiological stress and the history of research in this field are well documented (see, for example, Chrousos and Gold, 1992; Johnson *et al.*, 1992). A central tenet of the theory which holds that the stress response is an adaptive strategy to cope with a perceived threat to homeostasis is that non-essential activities are curtailed to facilitate a redirection of resources towards survival. This, it is believed, accounts for the fact that physiological and behavioural processes associated with reproduction are, either deliberately, or as an inadvertent consequence of the redirection of resources, 'shut down' when the stress response is activated. In circumstances where the animal is responding to a threat which is successfully overcome or avoided, no long-term problems are manifested within the reproductive system. However, under conditions of chronic stress, or of repeated intermittent exposure to acutely stressful stimuli, adverse effects on reproductive function are observed. It is perhaps worth emphasising that the adverse effects on growth, immunocompetence and reproduction that occur as a consequence of hypothalamic–pituitary–adrenal (HPA) activation should be considered to arise from what is an essentially adaptive response operating under conditions and circumstances with which it did not necessarily evolve to cope.

There has been considerable debate regarding the appropriate terminology to employ when discussing the topic of physiological stress (see for example Pickering, 1981; Levine, 1985; Toates, 1995). For the purposes of this review, the term **stressor** will be employed to denote the destabilising stimulus, the term **stress response** will define the primary neuroendocrine response to the stressor, and exposure to a stressor with subsequent activation of the stress response will be considered to induce a state of **stress** in the animal. The scope of this article is restricted to situations where the activation of the neuroendocrine stress response occurs, and where effects of stress on the reproductive system can be attributed directly to this response. Therefore, changes in the reproductive system related to factors such as exposure to toxic compounds, or the effects of starvation or metabolic imbalance, are excluded from consideration. Although an element of the response of animals to these types of challenge may involve activation of the stress response, the primary cause of reproductive dysfunction may lie elsewhere.

4.1.3 Stress and reproduction

The mechanisms which underlie stress-induced reproductive dysfunction are best understood in mammals but an increasing body of work provides an insight into similar processes in lower vertebrates. However, the imperatives which have driven attempts to understand the mechanisms and effects of stress-induced reproductive dysfunction vary according to the animal groups concerned. Thus, the rodent model has provided much of the basic information on physiological mechanisms associated with the effects of stress on the reproductive system (e.g. Gunin, 1996; Roozendaal et al., 1995); studies on primates have focused, in addition to basic mechanistic studies, on the role of social stress on reproductive modulation (e.g. Sapolsky, 1985; Ziegler et al., 1995); studies on human systems have in many cases been directed towards understanding factors underlying infertility (Negro-Vilar, 1993; Berga, 1995; Harlow et al.,

1996; Xiao and Ferin, 1997) and general reproductive health (Lederman, 1995). Domestic/farm animals have been the focus of studies concerned with understanding the effects of agricultural practices on reproduction and in optimising reproductive performance in captivity (Coubrough, 1985; Liptrap, 1993; Dobson and Smith, 1995), a consideration which has also led to studies on species whose survival may depend on captive breeding programmes (Kreeger et al., 1992). Similar considerations have led to studies on the impact of stress on reproduction in economically important non-mammalian vertebrates such as poultry and fish, both of which are reared intensively (e.g. Campbell et al., 1994; Etches et al., 1984). There is also a significant body of basic research which addresses the fundamental biology of the stress response and its impact on reproduction in birds (e.g. Wilson and Follett, 1976), reptiles (e.g. Lance and Elsey, 1986), amphibians (e.g. Paolucci et al., 1990) and fish (e.g. Pickering et al., 1987).

For clarity, the effects of stress on reproduction will be considered for each major vertebrate group in turn. The main topics considered are: the impact of stress on the reproductive endocrine system, the effects of stress on gamete quality, modifications of reproductive behaviour caused by stress, and the mechanistic basis of such effects. The reciprocal relationship between the pituitary–gonad axis and pituitary–adrenal axis will also be considered where information is available. The assumption is made that the reader is familiar with the principal components of the reproductive system in each of the groups discussed.

4.2 Mammals

The effect of stressors on the reproductive system is most comprehensively understood for the mammals. However, the range of species studied is small and most of the information available can confidently be applied only to the rodent, primate or human.

4.2.1 The mammalian reproductive system

The vertebrate reproductive cycle is a complex system of interacting signals originating from and terminating at both the brain (hypothalamus and pituitary) and gonad (ovary or testes) (Lavy et al., 1991). In mammals, key elements of this system include the pituitary gonadotropins (Ishii, 1991), follicle stimulating hormone (FSH) and luteinising hormone (LH), together with representatives of three classes of steroid hormones secreted by the gonadal tissue: progestogens, oestrogens and androgens (Bourne, 1991; Selcer and Leavitt, 1991). The synthesis and release of the pituitary hormones is controlled by hypothalamic gonadotropin-releasing hormones (GnRH; King and Millar, 1991). Complex feedback loops exist within the hypothalamic–pituitary–gonad (HPG) axis. This assemblage of hormones interact to stimulate growth and development of the reproductive apparatus, promote the appearance of secondary sexual characters, initiate and sustain gametogenesis and coordinate reproductive behaviour to maximise the likelihood of successful fertilisation of the ovum. For more detail see Hadley (1988), Dalkin and Marshall (1997) and contributions within Pang and Schreibman (1991a,b).

4.2.2   Effects of stress on the mammalian reproductive endocrine system

Much of what is known regarding the effects of stress on reproduction in mammals is derived from studies on the laboratory rat. Moberg (1987) points out that the laboratory rat has been subject to many generations of inadvertent selection for reproduction under suboptimal conditions and may therefore not represent an ideal model system for studies of this nature. Nonetheless, the rodent, together with certain primates, remains the primary source of data on stress-induced reproductive dysfunction. There is no satisfactory alternative to the use of laboratory animals of known pedigree under controlled conditions but attempts have been made to employ experimental environments which provide a compromise between the theoretical ideal of free-ranging animals and wholly un-natural confinement (e.g. Monder et al., 1994a).

The effects of stress on the reproductive system of mammals may be manifested in a number of ways including delays in the onset of puberty, behavioural alterations, failure or delay in ovulation, failure of embryo implantation, suppression of spermatogenesis, spontaneous abortion or infant mortality and reduced fecundity (Johnson et al., 1992). However, the effects observed depend upon the duration of the stressful stimulus. While chronic stress results in an overall inhibition of reproductive function, exposure to acute stressors may have a stimulatory or facilitatory effect on aspects of reproduction (see Brann and Mahesh, 1991, for summary).

Studies on the mechanisms underlying reproductive dysfunction under stressful conditions reveal that in most cases these adverse effects are mediated via alterations in the reproductive endocrine system. The interface and interaction between the neuroendocrine components of the stress response and elements of the reproductive system are complex but have proved to be tractable to investigation. A review of the mechanistic basis of the modulation of the HPG axis by stress is provided by Rivier and Rivest (1991).

4.2.3   Hypothalamus: effects of corticosteroids

It is well established that corticosteroids, which are elevated significantly during activation of the stress response, are a primary factor in stress-induced reproductive dysfunction. Numerous sites within the reproductive HPG axis are susceptible to interference by corticosteroids and Moberg (1987) provides a comprehensive account of their effects. However, it is apparent that corticosteroids may exert a facilitatory action within the reproductive system also (see Brann and Mahesh, 1991) and the complexities of the possible interrelationships between the HPG axis and HPA axis are discussed by Nappi and Rivest (1995b). (Two major groups of steroids are produced by the mammalian adrenal cortex: the glucocorticoids, which include cortisol and corticosterone and which have effects on intermediary metabolism, the nervous system, and the immune system, and the mineralocorticoids which include aldosterone and 11-deoxycorticosterone, which have roles in water balance. Whether the primary stress-induced corticosteroid is cortisol or corticosterone is species dependent for mammals. In the context of this article, the generic term corticosteroids will be employed throughout to denote cortisol and corticosterone.)

Interference with reproductive processes during stress is initiated at the highest level of the HPG and HPA cascades. The hypothalamic hormone, gonadotropin-releasing hormone (GnRH; luteinising hormone-releasing hormone, LHRH), is a primary factor controlling the release of LH and FSH from the pituitary and is released in a pulsatile manner (Ferin, 1993). During chronic stress in rats there is a decrease in hypothalamic LHRH content but no loss of sensitivity of the pituitary to exogenous LHRH suggesting that reduction of plasma LH and FSH levels is due to modifications at the hypothalamic level (López-Calderón et al., 1991). Cortisol (C) and the corticosteroid agonist dexamethasone have been shown to suppress release of hypothalamic GnRH in the rhesus monkey (*Macaca mulatta*; Dubey and Plant, 1985) and rat (Rosen et al., 1988) and to alter the pulse frequency of LH release in human females (Saketos et al., 1993). The fact that corticosteroid receptors are present within LHRH neurons (Ahima and Harlan, 1992) provides supporting evidence for a direct effect of corticosteroids on the HPG axis at the level of the hypothalamus during stress. This interpretation is bolstered by the observation that systemic administration of the corticosteroid receptor antagonist RU486 significantly attenuated the acute decline in circulating LH observed in intact male rats subject to immobilisation stress (Briski *et al.*, 1995). These authors also demonstrated that rats pretreated with an intracerebroventricular injection of a corticosteroid receptor agonist RU362 exhibited a greater reduction in plasma LH levels during the first hour of stress than did sham-injected rats. These observations support the hypothesis that corticosteroid receptor-dependent mechanisms are responsible for the inhibition of pituitary LH release during stress.

4.2.4 Hypothalamus: effects of CRH

An early event in the activation of the HPA axis is the secretion of corticotropin-releasing hormone (CRH; also termed corticotropin-releasing factor, CRF) by neurons located within the paraventricular nucleus of the hypothalamus. CRH elicits the release of adrenocorticotropic hormone (ACTH) from the pituitary corticotropes which in turn acts on the adrenal cortex to stimulate the synthesis and release of corticosteroids. Injection of CRH into rhesus monkeys resulted in a decrease in LH and FSH secretion (Olster and Ferin, 1987). The subsequent demonstration that CRH is capable of suppressing LH and FSH secretion even in adrenalectomised rhesus monkeys (Xiao *et al.*, 1989) confirmed that corticosteroids are not the mediator of these CRH-related effects. In contrast with these results from a primate model, systemic administration of CRH in rodents had no effect on pituitary gonadotropin levels (Rivier and Vale, 1984) although infusion of CRH directly into the medial preoptic area of the hypothalamus was successful in causing a decrease in plasma LH levels in rats and in suppressing LHRH release (Rivest *et al.*, 1993), an observation which has been suggested to arise from the differing accessibility of GnRH neurons in rodents and primates to substances entering the peripheral circulation (Ferin, 1993). Thus, the main impact of CRH appears to be interference with the activity of luteinising hormone-releasing hormone (LHRH) neurons A review of the role of CRH in mediating the stress-induced inhibition of LHRH neurons is provided by Rivest and Rivier (1995).

It must be noted that not all species display the same response to CRH infusion. The sheep responds to CRH treatment with an increase in LH secretion (Naylor *et al.*, 1990).

4.2.5 Hypothalamus: effects of opioid peptides

The situation is further complicated by the involvement of opioid peptides in mediating the effects of corticosteroids within the hypothalamus. Naltrexone, an opioid receptor antagonist, attenuates the corticosteroid-induced reduction in plasma LH levels when administered intracranially to rats (Briski and Vogel, 1995) suggesting that corticosteroid receptor-mediated suppression of GnRH activity is brought about in part through mechanisms involving opioid receptors. Administration of naltrexone to rats subjected to restraint stress did not prevent the inhibitory effect of chronic stress on circulating LH and FSH but did increase plasma concentrations of LH in acutely restrained rats (González-Quijano et al., 1991), a result which was interpreted as indicating that endogenous opiates may influence gonadotropin secretion only during acute, not chronic, stress. The role of β-endorphin in mediating the effects of stress on the reproductive system is considered by Herbert (1995).

4.2.6   Effects of cytokines

Further complexity arises when the influence of cytokines on the HPG axis are considered. The cytokine interleukin-1β has been reported to exert an inhibitory effect on plasma LH levels (Bonavera et al., 1993), affecting both frequency and amplitude of pituitary LH release, and on testosterone (T) levels, when administered via an intracerebroventricular route, and is thought to act by influencing neural pathways linking the brain and the testes, resulting in decreased testicular responses to gonadotropic stimuli (Turnbull and Rivier, 1997). The role of interleukin-1 in stress-induced reproductive dysfunction is reviewed by Rivest and Rivier (1995).

- corticosteroids inhibit hypothalamic GnRH release; corticosteroid receptors have been localised within GnRH neurons
- CRH can act at the hypothalamic level to reduce LH and GnRH release
- opioid peptides may be involved in GnRH suppression during stress
- cytokines may interfere with neural pathways linking the brain and gonads during stress

4.2.7   Pituitary: effects of ACTH and corticosteroids

Various stressors have been demonstrated to exert profoundly disruptive effects on pituitary gonadotropin secretion. For example, in female rats subjected to restraint stress on the day of pro-oestrous there is an almost complete suppression of the preovulatory LH surge (Roozendaal et al., 1995). Numerous studies have implicated elements of the HPA axis in such effects and a straightforward picture can be presented of corticosteroids blocking ovulation by inhibiting the preovulatory increase of LH and FSH in the female (Baldwin and Sawyer, 1974; Baldwin, 1979) and having similarly disruptive effects in the male; acute administration of ACTH or dexamethasone caused a reduction in blood T and LH levels in the ram (Juniewicz *et al.*, 1987). In recent years, the mechanisms underlying these effects have become better understood.

Treatment of male rhesus monkeys with ACTH results in a reduced T response to administered GnRH and a reduction in baseline LH levels but has no effect on the LH response to GnRH (Hayashi and Moberg, 1987). Similar effects were observed following treatment with C indicating that ACTH probably exerts its influence via the adrenal gland. The fact that no effects of ACTH on LH secretion could be detected in adrenalectomised rats (Mann *et al.*, 1985) and that adrenalectomy completely abolishes the stress-induced suppression of plasma LH levels in rats (McGivern and Redei, 1994) strongly suggests a primary role for corticosteroids in the effects of stress on the HPG axis. An indication that corticosteroids can act at the pituitary is provided by the observation that dexamethasone administered to male rats caused a significant decline in GnRH-induced gonadotropin secretion (Rosen *et al.*, 1988) and, *in vitro*, corticosterone (CS) inhibits LHRH-stimulated LH secretion from cultured rat pituitary cells (Kamel and Kubajak, 1987). Cortisol also suppresses GnRH-stimulated FSH release from pig pituitary cells *in vitro* and a similar effect was demonstrated for CRH but not for ACTH (Li, 1993). However, neither C nor CS was found to influence the abundance of pituitary GnRH receptors in male rats, suggesting that if corticosteroids do exert an inhibitory effect on pituitary gonadotropin release it must be downstream of the GnRH receptor itself (Suter *et al.*, 1988) possibly by uncoupling GnRH receptors from the LH secretory process or by inhibiting secretion of LH directly. Direct effects of corticosteroids on the pituitary gonadotropes themselves is suggested by the immuno-cytochemical detection of corticosteroid receptors within these cell types (Kononen *et al.*, 1993). However, contradictory evidence exists regarding the sensitivity of the pituitary to corticosteroid influence. Pituitaries removed from rats pretreated with C secreted significantly more LH and FSH *in vitro* in response to GnRH stimulation than pituitaries from control animals (Suter and Orosz, 1989) leading to the suggestion that the inhibitory effects of corticosteroids are exerted at a site other than the pituitary. An extra-pituitary site for interference by corticosteroids in gonadotropin secretion was also suggested by Juniewicz *et al.* (1987) who showed that although dexamethasone treatment of rams suppressed T and LH levels in the blood, pituitary responsiveness to LHRH was unaffected. Further levels of complexity were introduced by Baldwin *et al.* (1991) who suggested that corticosteroid-induced inhibition of pituitary LH release is mediated by antagonism of the positive feedback of oestrogen at the pituitary and that corticosteroids may alter LH subunit biosynthesis via oestrogen-dependent mechanisms. There is also evidence that, *in vitro*, ACTH can reduce LH secretion by interfering directly with GnRH action at the pituitary, either by affecting GnRH receptors, or by disrupting oestradiol (E2)-induced LH synthesis (Matteri *et al.*, 1986; Phogat *et al.*, 1997).

There are conflicting reports regarding the effects of acute and chronic stress on LH levels. Charpenet *et al.* (1981) reported that chronic intermittent immobilisation stress resulted in a significant decline in testicular and plasma levels of T, despite there being no apparent effect on plasma LH levels, while Demura *et al.* (1989) observed significant decreases in plasma LH levels in rats subjected to both acute and chronic stress. A variable response of LH to a variety of stressors differing in severity and duration has been reported (Krulich *et al.*, 1974; Briski and Sylvester, 1988). A recent study (Briski, 1996) has in part addressed the question of the effects of variable glucocorticoid output on the direction and magnitude of LH release during stress and concluded that psychological and physical stressors elicited different patterns of CS release and that the CS response was strongly correlated with the pattern of pituitary LH release. Whether a suppression or transient increase in LH levels was observed appeared to be related to the perceived severity of the stressor.

- ACTH may act on the HPG axis indirectly via the adrenal or directly by interfering with GnRH activity at the pituitary
- corticosteroids reduce the sensitivity of the pituitary to GnRH stimulation, but not via effects on GnRH receptor abundance
- these effects are likely mediated by corticosteroid receptors which are present in pituitary gonadotropes
- there are contradictory data which indicate an extra-pituitary site for the suppressive action of corticosteroids with no direct effects on the pituitary
- there are conflicting reports regarding the effects of acute and chronic stress on pituitary GTH release; suppression or elevation?

4.2.8   Ovary: effects of ACTH and corticosteroids

Cortisol administration disrupts the normal oestrus cycle in rhesus monkeys, blocking the release of LH, oestrogens, and progesterone (Hayashi and Moberg, 1990) effects which are partly mediated at the level of the ovary. Corticosteroids have been shown to disrupt the normal profile of steroid production by granulosa cells *in vitro* (Danišová *et al.*, 1987; Kawate *et al.*, 1993); treatment of pigs with ACTH during the luteal phase of the oestrus cycle, resulting in elevated blood corticosteroid levels, leads to a reduction in the number of viable granulosa cells and altered patterns of steroidogenesis which may in turn compromise subsequent follicle development (Viveiros and Liptrap, 1995). Elevated ACTH levels have been shown to reduce significantly the concentration of follicular LH receptors, cause unusual pathological changes in follicles and corpora lutea, and inhibit ovulation in ewes (López-Díaz and Bosu, 1997). These effects were ascribed to the action of corticosteroids although a direct effect of ACTH was not discounted. However, the effect of corticosteroids may differ according to the stage of the ovarian cycle and degree of differentiation of the cell. In follicular phase granulosa cells, corticosteroids may promote FSH action while opposing LH effects on steroidogenesis during the luteal phase (Michael and Cooke, 1994). Michael and Cooke (1994) discuss the role played by two variants of 11β-hydroxysteroid dehydrogenase in regulating the effects of corticosteroids on gonadal tissue.

4.2.9   Ovary: involvement of CRH

CRH has been detected in ovarian tissue (Mastorakos *et al.*, 1993). The induction of a CRH receptor has been demonstrated to occur in ovarian tissue of rats following exposure to a stressor, and at a specific point during the oestrus cycle (Nappi and Rivest, 1995a). This has been interpreted as indicating that the ovary is more susceptible to interference in stressed animals at specific periods within the ovulatory cycle (Nappi and Rivest, 1995b). The direct suppressive effects of CRH on ovarian steroid synthesis have been demonstrated in human and rat granulosa cells (Calogero *et al.*, 1996; Ghizzoni *et al.*, 1997). CRH caused a significant decrease of *in vitro* production of E2 and progesterone, an effect which was blocked by both the alpha-helical CRH-9-41 antagonist and interleukin-1 receptor antagonist suggesting that CRH exerts a CRH- and IL-1 receptor-mediated inhibitory effect on ovarian steroidogenesis. A recent study (Erden *et al.*, 1998) has demonstrated a potent inhibitory effect of CRH on LH-stimulated androgen production in isolated thecal cells from human ovarian follicles that appears to be mediated through the reduction of P450c17 gene expression. The authors suggest that the ovarian CRH system may function as a regulatory factor controlling androgen biosynthesis in the thecal cell compartment and ensuring an optimal substrate level for oestrogen biosynthesis by granulosa cells. Asakura *et al.* (1997) have defined the cellular distribution of the human ovarian CRH system (CRH, type 1 CRH receptor (CRH-R1), and the high affinity CRH-binding protein (CRH-BP)) and suggest that the CRH-BP may play an important role in modulating the responsiveness of the ovarian CRH system because of its ability to compete with CRH for the CRH receptor.

- corticosteroids inhibit ovulation
- corticosteroids disrupt steroid production by granulosa cells *in vitro*
- elevated blood corticosteroid levels reduce the number of viable granulosa cells and alter patterns of ovarian steroidogenesis
- elevated blood ACTH/corticosteroid levels reduce the abundance of follicular LH receptors
- CRH receptors are present in the ovary and intra-ovarian sources of CRH have been identified
- CRH directly suppresses ovarian steroid synthesis, effects which may be mediated in part by cytokines
- intra-ovarian CRH-BP may modulate the effects of CRH

4.2.10   Testis: effects of corticosteroids

Although as noted above certain types of stressor can cause a reduction in pituitary gonadotropin secretion which may contribute to stress-induced decreases in circulating androgen levels (e.g. Armario and Castellanos, 1984), corticosteroids also act directly on the testes to reduce androgen production either by inhibiting steroidogenesis, or by reducing testicular LH receptor content (Bambino and Hsueh, 1981; Hales and Payne, 1989; Fenske, 1997). For example, exposure to an acute stressor disrupts rat testicular steroidogenesis via a mechanism that is independent of changes in circulating levels of LH and the binding characteristics of LH/hCG receptors. The effects of immobilisation stress on the content of testicular steroids and on the activities of 17α-hydroxylase and 17,20-lyase suggest that stress inhibits the activities of both these enzymes (Orr *et al.*, 1994). The mechanism by which testicular androgen production is modified by stress may depend on the nature of the stressor. In rats subjected to acute immobilisation stress a significant reduction in plasma T and dihydrotestosterone (DHT) levels occurred with no concomitant decline in plasma LH levels, whereas chronic immobilisation stress induced a decline in both plasma androgen and LH levels (Marić *et al.*, 1996). In the former case, the activity of testicular 3β-hydroxysteroid dehydrogenase was decreased and the ability of human chorionic gonadotropin (hCG) to stimulate steroid production by the Leydig cells was reduced. In the latter case, there was no effect on basal or hCG-stimulated steroid production by the Leydig cells, suggesting that the mechanisms by which acute and chronic stressors impact at the level of the testis are different; acute stress impacts primarily at the testicular level (decreasing the activity of certain enzymes), while chronic stress exerts effects at the level of the hypothalamic–pituitary axis. There is some disagreement within the literature regarding the exact nature of the impact of a stressor on blood androgen levels. In the examples cited above, there is a consistent depression of blood androgen levels following exposure to both acute and chronic stressors. In contrast, other studies have reported that exposure to acute stressors causes an elevation of blood androgen levels, while it is chronic stress which results in a depression of circulating levels. Cortisol apparently stimulates, not inhibits, T production in pig Leydig cells (Li, 1991).

The relative abundance of various steroid-metabolising enzymes within the gonadal tissue has been shown to play an important role in determining the impact of elevated corticosteroid levels on gonadal function. The enzyme 11β-hydroxysteroid dehydrogenase, which in the testes primarily oxidises corticosteroids to a functionally inactive form (Gao et al., 1997), is present in the testes of socially subordinate (chronically stressed) rats at significantly lower concentrations than in the testes of dominant or control animals (Monder et al., 1994a) leading to the assumption that T production is more vulnerable to interference by corticosteroids in stressed animals. The effect of corticosteroids on 11β-hydroxysteroid dehydrogenase levels has been shown to be mediated by the corticosteroid receptor (Monder et al., 1994b) and it has also been demonstrated that in unstressed animals physiological levels of corticosteroids exert a tonic negative control directly on Leydig cell steroidogenesis and also induce intracellular 11β-hydroxysteroid dehydrogenase activity, thereby offering some protection against corticosteroid-mediated inhibition of T production under unstressed conditions (Gao et al., 1996).

4.2.11   Testis: effects of CRH

CRH is secreted by the Leydig cells of the testis and acts to oppose the influence of LH. CRH also stimulates β-endorphin secretion from the Leydig cells and β-endorphin in turn opposes the action of FSH in the Sertoli cells. The role of CRH as an anti-reproductive factor in the testis is reviewed by Dufau et al. (1993). However, in the mouse, in contrast to the rat, CRH has been reported to directly *stimulate* T production in Leydig cells (Huang et al., 1995). Mouse Leydig cells express CRH-R1, mediating elevation of T production by CRH agonists through cAMP (Heinrich et al., 1998). Huang et al. (1995) cite a number of differences between rat and mouse Leydig cells related to their activity under conditions of stress which indicate that the lack of effect of CRH is not without precedent.

4.2.12   Testis: effects of opioid peptides

As noted above, acute stressors may reduce blood androgen levels while failing to disrupt LH levels (Orr et al., 1994; Marić et al., 1996). When naloxone and naltrexone-methobromide, an opioid receptor antagonist that does not cross the blood–brain barrier, were administered by unilateral intratesticular injection to rats stressed by immobilisation, both opioid receptor antagonists normalised serum T levels in the immobilised rats and opposed the inhibitory effect of immobilisation stress on 3β-hydroxysteroid dehydrogenase and $P450_{17\alpha,\ lyase}$. Acute immobilisation stress decreased basal and hCG-stimulated androgen production by hemitestis preparation, but naloxone added directly to the incubation medium blocked the decrease. These results were interpreted as suggesting that endogenous opioid peptides, together with corticosteroids, are potentially important modulators of testicular steroidogenesis under stress conditions (Kostić et al., 1997).

- corticosteroids can act directly on the testes to reduce steroidogenesis and alter the abundance of LH receptors
- some reports describe elevated blood androgen levels following an acute stressor
- the effect of stress on testes function may be determined by the duration of the stressor
- the activity of steroid-metabolising enzymes within the Leydig cells is modulated by stress
- CRH of testicular origin may have suppressive or stimulatory effects on testes function, depending on species
- opioid peptides oppose the inhibitory effects of stress on testes function

4.2.13　Direct interaction of corticosteroid and androgen receptors

There has recently been the intriguing suggestion that the ability of the androgen and corticosteroid receptors to influence each other's transcriptional activity may be correlated with their ability to form heterodimers at a common DNA site; thus the opposing physiological effects of the androgen and corticosteroid hormones are due to the direct physical interaction between their receptors at the transcriptional level (Chen et al., 1997).

4.2.14　Effects of social stress on reproduction

Most of the experimental work which has enabled an understanding of the mechanisms underlying stress-induced reproductive dysfunction to develop has been carried out in rodents using standardised stressors, such as restraint or foot shock. There is an implicit assumption that the response to such a stimulus is essentially 'non-specific' and may be used to model the response to 'natural' stressors. Whether this is a fair assumption is open to debate. Perhaps the best understood and most-studied 'natural' stressor is that which arises from social interaction. In several species of mammal the level of understanding of the relationship between social factors, the pituitary–adrenal system and reproductive performance has reached a high degree of sophistication. Two main aspects have been considered. That of the effect of social position on reproductive performance (i.e. dominant versus subordinate) and those instances where less specific social pressures result in population-level effects.

The literature concerning the relationship between social status and reproductive success is reviewed exhaustively by Ellis (1995). The overall conclusion reached by Ellis is that there is overwhelming evidence for a positive link between dominance rank and reproductive success and that this relationship is more pronounced for male animals than females. The corollary of this is that subordinate or subdominant animals are disadvantaged (Blanchard *et al.*, 1993). The manner in which animals can modulate the reproductive performance of conspecifics and in turn be affected by other individuals is discussed by Marchlewska-Koj (1997) in the context of rodent reproduction. The role of activation of the hypothalamic–pituitary–adrenal axis in such effects is also considered. In simple terms, the frequency of aggressive encounters between males results in a state of chronic or intermittent stress in the subordinates, or losers, of such encounters. Similar relationships may be established between adults and juveniles within a population. Dominant male sugar gliders (*Petaurus breviceps*) consistently responded to GnRH administration with a more pronounced elevation of blood T levels than subordinate animals from within the same social group (Bradley and Stoddart, 1997). Social status may also modulate the degree of responsiveness to a stressor, or the extent to which the HPG axis is disturbed. In wild baboons (*Papio anubis*), the stress associated with capture suppressed blood LH and T levels but high ranking males displayed a less pronounced reduction in T and in many cases showed transient increases in T following capture (Sapolsky, 1986). However, it is not clear whether the behaviour of dominant females leads to reproductive suppression in subordinate females. Furthermore, it has been suggested that overall, no simple link exists between activation of the HPA axis, stress, and social status (Zayan, 1991). For example, suppression of ovarian cycling in female cotton-top tamarin monkeys (*Saguinus oedipus*) is not closely linked to stress-induced C secretion and C levels are not closely correlated with reproductive condition (Ziegler *et al.*, 1995); no correlation between blood C levels, dominance status, and the timing of sexual maturation was observed in male rhesus monkeys (Bercovitch and Clarke, 1995) and, in rats, whether or not activation of the HPA has a suppressive action on the HPG may depend upon the presence or absence of stimuli of sexual significance (Lemaire et al., 1997).

- social rank is inversely related to reproductive competence
- the data regarding the endocrine basis for this state, and whether stress status modulates reproductive performance in a social context, are contradictory

4.2.15 Reciprocal relationships between the HPA axis and the HPG axis

Consideration of the effects of stress on the reproductive system is complicated by the fact that the response of animals to stress is itself subject to modification by gonadal steroids. In general terms, oestrogens enhance stress responsiveness and androgens exert a suppressive effect on stress responsiveness. This is manifested in the rat as a sexual dimorphism in the responsiveness of the HPA axis to stress, with females showing greater responsiveness than males (Kant et al., 1983; Aloisi et al., 1994; Spinedi et al., 1994). Gonadectomy was found to have no effect on the plasma ACTH and CS response to stress in male rats but reduced the response in females relative to intact individuals. The administration of oestrogen to ovariectomised female rats and T to orchiectomised male rats restored pre-operative values (Leśniewska et al., 1990). Oestrogen treatment of gonadectomised males results in an enhanced CS response to stress (Handa et al., 1994a). The enhanced HPA response of females to stressors is restricted to the early phase of the oestrus cycle because, it is believed, progesterone inhibits the facilitatory effects of oestrogens on ACTH release (Viau and Meaney, 1991). It has been suggested that the effects of oestrogen and progesterone on the HPA axis in rats are elicited by their relative effects on hippocampal mineralocorticoid receptors which mediate the negative feedback exerted by corticosteroids on the HPA axis; oestrogen promotes a decline in receptor abundance while progesterone opposes this effect (Carey et al., 1995). In contrast, administration of a potent glucocorticoid receptor agonist to oestrogen-treated rats failed to evoke the down-regulation of central (hippocampal) glucocorticoid receptors which was observed in control ovariectomised rats exposed to a stressor. This phenomenon was interpreted as indicating that the receptor had lost the ability to autoregulate and was suggested to contribute to oestrogenic effects on stress responsiveness (Burgess and Handa, 1992). Evidence has also been presented which suggests that the CRH gene is directly susceptible to modulation by oestrogens (Vamvakopoulos and Chrousos, 1993).

In males, gonadectomised individuals display a more pronounced CS response to stress than intact animals or gonadectomised animals receiving

DHT (Handa *et al.*, 1994a; Bingaman *et al.*, 1995). A correlate of this observation is that gonadectomy also increases levels of CRH in the hypothalamus of male rats, an increase which was prevented by DHT replacement (Bingaman *et al.*, 1994). The inhibitory effect of androgens on the HPA response to stress in rats is believed to reside within the medial preoptic area of the brain (Viau and Meaney, 1996) and may involve effects on arginine vasopressin regulation of pituitary ACTH release, rather than effects on CRH (Cover *et al.*, 1991; Viau and Meaney, 1996).

Gonadal steroids have been shown to exert effects on the transcription of brain corticosteroid receptors suggesting possible routes by which the steroids may regulate stress responsiveness. The complex effects of the gonadal steroids on brain corticosteroid receptor expression have been summarised by Turner (1997) who concluded that there remain a number of questions regarding the physiological implications of observations to date.

The functional significance of the sex difference in HPA response to stress has yet to be established. It has been suggested that in males, androgen-induced suppression of responsiveness may be directed at reducing the potentially deleterious effects of stress on reproductive processes in males (Handa *et al.*, 1994b) and in females, enhanced responsiveness to stress may represent a mechanism by which environmental conditions unfavourable to reproduction can inhibit reproductive processes (Viau and Meaney, 1991).

- a sex-dependent dimorphism in stress responsiveness is apparent in some species
- in general, oestrogens enhance and androgens inhibit stress responsiveness
- modulation of negative feedback by corticosteroids, alteration in CRH production and changes in brain corticosteroid receptor abundance may contribute to these effects

4.3   Amphibians and reptiles

The impact of stress on the reproductive system of reptiles and amphibians has been the subject of considerable study. Some of this work is summarised in reviews by Greenberg and Wingfield (1987) and Guillette *et al.* (1995).

4.3.1   *The amphibian and reptile endocrine reproductive system*

The main elements of the endocrine reproductive system of amphibians and reptiles have been summarised in a series of review articles (Norris and Jones, 1987) and, in essence, conform to the vertebrate pattern. As is the case for mammals, two distinct gonadotropins have been identified in at least some amphibians and reptiles and the secretion of these is under the control of GnRH (Licht and Porter, 1987; Ishii, 1991). The gonadotropins regulate steroidogenesis within the gonadal tissue (Chieffi and Pierantoni, 1987) with oestrogens of ovarian origin being responsible for promoting vitellogenesis (Ho, 1987; 1991) and final maturation of the oocytes also being steroid dependent (Nagahama, 1987; Jalabert *et al.*, 1991). The endocrine control of ovulation in reptiles and amphibians is discussed by Jones (1987). The testes produce androgens which promote and maintain secondary sexual characters and sustain spermatogenesis (Lofts, 1987; Callard, 1991). As is the case for other vertebrates, the endocrine system is also implicated in the control of reproductive behaviour in reptiles and amphibians (Moore, 1987; Moore *et al.*, 1994). The amphibian adrenal glands are variable in distribution and structure and comprise of intermingled chromaffin and interrenal tissue which may or may not be organised into a discrete gland (Lofts and Bern, 1972). In reptiles two main structural types occur, one similar to that of birds with a discrete gland containing intermingled interrenal and chromaffin elements, the other where a greater separation of the two cell types occurs (Lofts and Bern, 1972). The major stress-induced corticosteroid in both amphibians and reptiles is CS (Hanke and Kloas, 1995).

4.3.2   Effects of stress on the reproductive endocrine system of amphibians and reptiles

It is well established that exposure to stressful stimuli causes perturbations in the endocrine reproductive system of both reptiles (Lance and Elsey, 1986) and amphibians (Licht *et al.*, 1983). The functional consequences of exposure to stressors are less well documented for reptiles and amphibians than for other vertebrate groups and there is as yet less understanding of the mechanistic basis by which stressors interfere with the reproductive system than for mammals. However, there are more data concerning the effects of stressors on reproductive behaviour in reptiles and amphibians than for the other vertebrate groups.

4.3.3   Hypothalamus: effects of stressors and corticosteroids

Having demonstrated that exposure of the rough skinned newt (*Taricha granulosa*) to a variety of stressors resulted in increased blood CS levels and a reduction in reproductive behaviours (Moore and Miller, 1984), it was subsequently shown that exposure to similar stressors or administration of CS resulted in a decline in blood androgen levels and an increase in hypothalamic immunoreactive LHRH levels (Moore and Zoeller, 1985). The data were interpreted as indicating that stress suppresses circulating androgen levels by inhibiting the release of LHRH.

4.3.4 Pituitary: effects of stressors and corticosteroids

The disturbance associated with capture and captivity caused significant reductions in blood gonadotropin (LH) levels in male bullfrogs (*Rana catesbeiana*) within 2–4 h of capture (Licht *et al.*, 1983). The effects of these procedures on gonadotropin levels in females were reportedly less pronounced. A similar decline in blood FSH levels occurred in male painted turtles (*Chrysemys picta*; Licht *et al.*, 1985) associated with capture and serial sampling.

4.3.5 Ovary: effects of stressors and corticosteroids

As might be expected, stressful procedures such as capture and confinement have been reported to suppress circulating levels of ovarian steroids in female reptiles (*Alligator mississippiensis*; Elsey *et al.*, 1991) and amphibians (*Rana esculenta*; Paolucci *et al.*, 1990; Mosconi *et al.*, 1994). However, there are differing accounts of the rate at which the corticosteroid response to stress occurs in various species and the link between corticosteroid elevation and suppression of gonadal steroids does not appear to be as well established in amphibians and reptiles as is the case for other vertebrates. The elevation of blood CS levels in response to the stress associated with capture and captivity in female *Rana esculenta* did not occur until between 48 and 72 h following the initiation of the stressor (Zerani *et al.*, 1991) while a suppression of blood E2 levels was observed within 6 h of capture. The E2 response was apparently dependent on the reproductive stage of the frog, with animals in the post-reproductive period displaying the most pronounced decline in E2 levels while individuals subjected to stress during or prior to the reproductive period displayed an increase in E2 levels prior to a decline. Gobbetti and Zerani (1996) subsequently confirmed these observations in *R. esculenta*, reporting a much delayed elevation in blood CS levels (72 h post-capture) preceded by an increase in blood E2 levels (6–12 h post capture). A slow rise in blood CS levels was observed in female whistling frogs (*Litoria ewingi*) subjected to captivity with no accompanying variation in E2 or T levels (Coddington and Cree, 1995). These authors suggest that the apparently variable response of female frogs to stressors may arise due to the effect of CS on the HPG axis varying according to stage of reproductive development. Licht *et al.* (1983) also observed that capture and captivity caused less disruption to gonadal steroid levels in female bullfrogs than males.

In contrast, elevation of blood CS levels concomitant with the decline in blood E2 levels was observed in female alligators subject to restraint and serial sampling (Elsey *et al.*, 1991). Nonetheless, a link between reproductive state and the nature of the ovarian response to stress may also be present in reptiles. A rapid elevation of blood E2 levels reportedly occurs in female snapping turtles (*Chelydra serpentina*) immediately following capture (Mahmoud *et al.*, 1989) with the extent of elevation being greater in gravid females than in non-gravid females. Although levels of E2 returned to baseline within 7 days there was no subsequent depression of E2 levels.

Negative effects of the corticosteroid analogue dexamethasone and ACTH have been reported on ovarian growth in the frog (*Rana cyanophlyctis*; Kupwade and Saidapur, 1987) and lizard (*Anolis carolinensis*; Summers, 1995) but a positive correlation between blood CS levels and gonadosomatic index has been observed for the side-blotched lizard (*Uta stansburiana*). In common with the other vertebrate groups for which such a relationship has been reported, it is unclear whether this is related to the metabolic demands of reproduction or is indicative of a role for CS in ovarian function (Wilson and Wingfield, 1992). Similar results are reported for the administration of ACTH to female lizards (*Anolis carolinensis*) in which ACTH treatment inhibited ovarian growth only in small (< 2.6 g) lizards while enhancing ovarian growth in larger individuals (Summers, 1995). The author suggested that this may be indicative of a mechanism by which only females capable of surviving adverse conditions invest resources in gonadal development.

4.3.6   Testis: effects of stressors and corticosteroids

The stress associated with capture and confinement has been shown to have a pronounced suppressive effect on blood androgen levels in male reptiles and amphibians including tuatara (*Sphenodon punctatus*; Cree *et al.*, 1990), alligators (*Alligator mississippiensis*; Lance and Elsey, 1986), frogs (*Rana catesbeiana*; Licht *et al.*, 1983; *Rana esculenta*; Paolucci *et al.*, 1990; Gobbetti and Zerani, 1996) and various lizards (*Podarcis sicula sicula*; Manzo *et al.*, 1994; *Urosaurus ornatus*; Moore *et al.*, 1991). However, exceptions have been reported to this generalisation. In the male snapping turtle capture stress is accompanied by an increase in blood T levels which is followed by a decline below initial levels, the extent of the change varying according to the time of year (Mahmoud *et al.*, 1989). This observation contrasts markedly with the effect of capture and handling on the painted turtle (*Chrysemys picta*) in which blood T levels decline precipitously following capture (Licht *et al.*, 1985) and with a subsequent study on snapping turtles (Mahmoud and Licht, 1997) in which captivity and serial sampling caused a significant decline in blood T levels. Differences in responsiveness of the two sexes may also occur. Unlike the female frog, the effect of capture and captivity on blood levels of gonadal steroids in male *R. esculenta* was independent of reproductive status; capture and captivity consistently elicited an immediate decline in blood T levels (Zerani *et al.*, 1991). Some evidence that the impact of stress on the HPG axis may vary according to stage of development in male reptiles is presented by Mahmoud and Licht (1997) who observed that male snapping turtles captured prior to the onset of the reproductive cycle maintained regressed testes during captivity while the testes of those turtles captured after the onset of reproductive development continued to develop normally.

That CS may have a direct suppressive effect on testicular androgen production in reptiles is suggested by *in vitro* studies in which T production by isolated testis of *Podarcis sicula sicula* was reduced by administration of CS (Manzo *et al.*, 1994). However, in an *in vivo* study in which ACTH was administered to male alligators, the decline in circulating T observed following the onset of serial sampling was similar in both ACTH- and saline-injected animals despite there being higher CS levels in the ACTH-treated group (Mahmoud *et al.*, 1996) suggesting that stress-induced androgen suppression may not be mediated by the adrenal gland.

4.3.7   Effects of stress on vitellogenesis

There are no reports of the impact of stressors on vitellogenesis in amphibians or reptiles.

4.3.8   Effects of stress on reproductive behaviour

Territorial male reptiles display agonistic behaviour when confronted with other males. The 'losers' of such encounters display increased CS levels (Greenberg *et al.*, 1984). Elevated CS levels cause a reduction in aggressive behaviour, as shown by administration of the hormone to male side-blotched lizards, which need not be associated with reduced T levels (DeNardo and Licht, 1993). Similar observations were reported for male copperhead snakes (*Agkistrodon contortix*) following fights. Losing individuals displayed elevated blood CS levels (Schuett *et al.*, 1996), consistent with a subordinate status, and suppression of courtship behaviour (Schuett, 1996) but with no observable difference in blood T levels between dominant and subordinate snakes. These observations are consistent with an earlier report of a negative effect of stress and exogenous CS on courtship behaviour in the rough-skinned newt (Moore and Miller, 1984). However, DeNardo and Licht showed that courtship behaviour in the side-blotched lizard was not suppressed by CS and suggested that it is the relative costs of various behaviours which dictates whether they are susceptible to stress-induced inhibition.

The inhibitory effects of stress or CS administration on reproductive (clasping) behaviour in the male rough-skinned newt can be prevented by treatment of the animal with a blocker of GABA synthesis suggesting that it is GABA which mediates the CS-induced inhibition of sexual behaviour in amphibians (Boyd and Moore, 1990). More recent data suggest that the CS signal is detected not by 'conventional' cytosolic corticosteroid receptors but by receptors situated within neuronal membranes and acting rapidly via a non-genomic mechanism (Rose et al., 1993).

4.3.9 Reciprocal relationships between the HPA axis and the HPG axis in reptiles and amphibians

The CS response of the lizard *Cnemidophorus sexlineatus* to an acute handling stressor displayed a sexual dimorphism. Females display a more pronounced increase in CS levels following handling than males (Grassman and Hess, 1992) and gonadectomy reversed this difference. No satisfactory explanation for these differences has yet been proposed.

- stressful stimuli suppress hypothalamic LHRH release in amphibians and reduce blood GTH and gonadal steroid levels in both male and female reptiles and amphibians
- limited evidence suggests that corticosteroids may suppress testicular androgen production
- overall, the link between corticosteroids and suppression of gonadal function is not well established for reptiles and amphibians
- corticosteroids and/or ACTH may have a repressive effect on ovarian growth in some species of reptiles and amphibians and a positive effect in others
- the observed effects may depend upon the stage of reproductive development reached by the animal
- the effect of stress on the reproductive system of male reptiles and amphibians is less variable than the effects on females
- stress-induced corticosterone elevation has profound effects on reproductive behaviour in reptiles and amphibians, reducing or inhibiting behavioural responses

4.4   Birds

Research into the impact of stress on reproductive function in birds can be segregated into that which addresses the problem in the context of natural populations of free-ranging birds, and that research which is concerned with the impact of stressors on the performance of intensively reared poultry.

4.4.1   The avian reproductive system

The essentials of the avian reproductive endocrine system have been summarised in Mikami *et al.* (1983). A considerable impetus to research in this field is provided by the economic importance of the intensively farmed poultry industry and in particular egg production. Consequently, much is known of the control of ovulation in the hen (*Gallus domesticus*) while other areas are less well represented. Factors controlling ovulation in the hen are discussed by Cunningham (1987). A consideration of the impact of stressors on the avian reproductive system is complicated by the fact that the major avian corticosteroid, CS, appears to play a significant role in timing of ovulation (Cunningham, 1987). Birds possess an adrenal gland located similarly to that in mammals. However, internally, the gland is a mixture of interrenal and chromaffin tissue with no zonation (Lofts and Bern, 1972). The major corticosteroid secreted by the avian adrenal during stress is CS (Sandor, 1972; Hanke and Kloas, 1995).

4.4.2   Effects of stress on the avian reproductive endocrine system

The impact of various stressors on the male avian reproductive system is discussed by Edens (1983). Although much of the work cited in that review has been superseded by more recent studies, Edens highlights chronic exposure to high temperature, a problem encountered during intensive rearing of poultry, as a potent suppressor of male reproductive performance and shows that these effects are probably mediated via activation of the HPA axis. The relationship between heat stress and infertility in both male and female birds continues to be an area of study of importance to commercial exploitation of poultry but the exact mechanisms underlying the effects of temperature are yet to be elucidated (McDaniel *et al.*, 1995). A related area of interest is the impact of environmental stressors (drought, extreme weather) on the reproductive performance of free-living birds (e.g. Cain and Lien, 1985; Astheimer *et al.*, 1995).

4.4.3   Hypothalamus: effects of corticosteroids and stressors

There are few data available which reveal the nature of stress-related effects at the level of the hypothalamus in birds. However, in domestic fowl exposed to thermal stress, circulating levels of LH were significantly reduced. Administration of exogenous LHRH produced similar pituitary LH responses in both stressed and unstressed birds. In combination with the observation that the hypothalamic LHRH content had declined in heat-stressed hens it was concluded that the heat-stress-induced reduction in LH levels reflected a suppression of hypothalamic LHRH release (Donoghue et al., 1989).

4.4.4   Pituitary: effects of ACTH, corticosteroids and stressors

Early data indicated that CS, the major corticosteroid in birds, could influence circulating levels of LH when male tree sparrows (*Spizella arborea*) which had received intracerebral CS implants displayed a reduction in blood LH levels accompanied by a block in testes growth (Wilson and Follett, 1976). However, although the administration of CS caused a reduction in circulating LH levels in the hen it did not affect the release of LH by the pituitary when stimulated by GnRH (Etches et al., 1984) suggesting that CS acts at a site other than the pituitary. In a subsequent study CS has been shown to reduce, though not completely abolish, LHRH-stimulated LH release from enzymatically dispersed Japanese quail (*Coturnix coturnix japonica*) pituitary cells (Connolly and Callard, 1987), a result at odds with the earlier observations of Etches et al. (1984). In contrast with these observations, ACTH administration had no effect on blood LH or FSH levels in castrated male ducks (*Anas platyrhynchos*) despite eliciting elevated blood CS levels (Deviche et al., 1980). To complicate matters further Deviche and Hendrick (1981) subsequently reported that the treatment of male ducks with ACTH, CS, or dexamethasone resulted in an increase in circulating LH levels, a result which was rationalised as possible evidence of seasonal variation in the effects of corticosteroids on the HPG axis.

Environmental stressors appear able to modulate the reproductive system. Hyperthermal challenge reduces circulating levels of LH in domestic hens (Novero et al., 1991) although whether this is mediated via elevated CS levels is unknown. Similarly, blood LH levels in male Lapland longspurs (*Calcarius lapponicus*) captured during a snowstorm showed a clear suppression compared to LH levels in birds captured before or after the storm (Astheimer et al., 1995). In this case, suppression of LH levels was accompanied by an increased CS responsiveness to capture stress.

4.4.5 Ovary: effects of ACTH, corticosteroids and stressors

Both the corticosteroid analogue, dexamethasone, and CS block ovulation in the hen (Etches *et al.*, 1984; Moudgal *et al.*, 1991; Petitte and Etches, 1991) and reduce plasma E2 and progesterone levels (Etches *et al.*, 1984; Petitte and Etches, 1988, 1989) but, *in vitro*, CS was found to have no effect on the ability of granulosa cells to respond to LH suggesting that the CS effect was mediated at the pituitary/hypothalamus. This interpretation of the mechanism was supported by the observation that the administration of pregnant mare's serum GTH to CS-treated hens was able to reverse the CS-induced depression of blood E2 levels (Petitte and Etches, 1989). Administration of CS also caused a reduction in one or both of ovarian or oviductal weight (Etches *et al.*, 1984; Williams *et al.*, 1985; Petitte and Etches, 1989,1991). However, paradoxically, the adrenal gland is necessary for normal ovarian development: adrenalectomy causes ovarian regression in the domestic hen (Etches *et al.*, 1984) and at certain stages of the ovulatory sequence, ACTH or CS are capable of inducing ovulation (Etches and Croze, 1983). The possible role of CS in timing ovulation in the domestic hen is discussed by Cunningham (1987). In bird species other than the domestic fowl adverse effects of corticosteroids have also been observed. In bobwhite quail (*Colinus virginianus*) CS has been shown to significantly reduce or completely block egg laying and to cause a reduction in ovary and oviduct weights (Cain and Lien, 1985), a mechanism proposed to account for drought-induced inhibition of reproductive activity; water restriction is accompanied by elevated levels of blood CS in this species.

Adverse effects on ovarian function have been reported to occur in birds exposed to a variety of 'natural' stressors. Oviposition is delayed in hens exposed to social stress and it has been demonstrated that these delays can be abolished by treatment with the β-adrenergic antagonist propanolol (Crossley, 1983; Reynard and Savory, 1997) indicating that the block may be mediated by adrenergic systems. Isolated granulosa cells from the ovaries of hens exposed to heat stress are unable to respond to LH challenge with an increase in progesterone secretion in contrast to tissue from control birds (Novero *et al.*, 1991), an effect unlikely to be CS-mediated according to the data reported above, and heat-stressed birds also display early oviposition and an extended oviposition interval.

4.4.6 Testis: effects of corticosteroids

Few data are available and those which exist are somewhat contradictory. Administration of ACTH to cockerels caused gonadal regression (Flickinger, 1966) but dietary administration of CS to cockerels was found to elicit an increase in testes weight relative to control birds (Siegel *et al.*, 1989). In male bobwhite quail (*Colinus virginianus*) CS administration was shown to cause significant reductions in both testes weight and sperm production (Cain and Lien, 1985).

4.4.7   *Effects of stress on vitellogenesis*

In domestic hens, food and water deprivation resulted in a decline in circulating vitellogenin levels, accompanied by decreases in blood E2, progesterone, and LH levels (Sekimoto *et al.*, 1990). However, no evidence was presented which suggested involvement of the HPA axis in these effects although the authors speculated that this was the case and water deprivation is known to elevate CS levels in other species (Cain and Lien, 1985).

4.4.8   *Effects of stress and corticosteroids on reproductive behaviour in birds*

The impact of stressful stimuli on reproductive behaviour in poultry is discussed by Ottinger and Mench (1989). These authors report observations on delayed sexual maturation and delays in the onset of mating behaviour in subordinate cockerels (Grosse and Craig, 1960; Flickinger, 1961) but note that more recent studies have failed to provide a definitive link between social status and chronic stress. Corticosterone administered to free-living song sparrows (*Melospiza melodia*) caused a marked reduction in responsiveness to territorial intrusion (Wingfield and Silverin, 1986); however, no effects were observed on blood LH and T levels leading the authors to suggest that, although stressors affect behaviour, gonadal function is protected during episodes of stress to ensure that normal reproductive behaviour can be rapidly resumed after the stressful stimulus has ceased. Corticosterone has also been demonstrated to markedly reduce parental behaviour in the pied flycatcher, *Ficedula hypoleuca* (Silverin, 1986).

4.4.9   *Effects of social stress on reproduction*

Particular interest in the effects of social stress on birds has arisen in relation to the practices employed by the intensive poultry farming industry. It has been reported that birds provided with less cage space produce fewer eggs than those with more available space. Crowding-induced decreases in ovulation rate are postulated to account for the decline in production by crowded birds (Hester and Wilson, 1986) although a reduction in access to food and water may contribute.

4.4.10   Reciprocal relationships between the HPA axis and the HPG axis

In common with other vertebrates, there is evidence that a sexual dimorphism in responsiveness to stressors may exist in birds. However, the apparently straightforward relationship between sex and stress responsiveness reported for mammals and fish does not appear to hold true for birds. A greater responsiveness to capture stress was noted in male white-crowned sparrow, *Zonotrichia leucophrys gambelii*, than females when T levels in males were maximal (Astheimer *et al.*, 1994) and other examples of the same phenomenon are cited by Wingfield *et al.* (1995). There is some consistency between these observations and those of Wang and Edens (1993) who demonstrated that stress-induced CS levels in cockerels were elevated by T treatment and depressed by E2 treatment—the reverse of what has been reported to occur in mammals and fish. Modulation of stress responsiveness in these instances may be a means by which essential reproductive activity is 'protected' from stress-induced inhibition.

Evidence that certain species of birds inhabiting regions subject to severe environmental conditions may display a reduction in stress responsiveness during the breeding season to prevent interference with normal reproductive processes was presented by Wingfield *et al.* (1992) for species resident in a desert region. A study of stress responsiveness in several species of Arctic birds failed to confirm this hypothesis (Wingfield *et al.*, 1995). Rather than being related to the requirements of breeding in a severe environment, modulation of stress responsiveness was more closely related to the degree of parental care displayed. The reasons for this relationship have yet to be established.

- stress and corticosteroids reduce circulating LH levels in birds but it is unclear from the equivocal data whether direct effects occur at the pituitary
- some studies have reported that corticosteroids and ACTH have a stimulatory effect on pituitary LH release, leading to suggestions that reproductive status may be a factor dictating response
- corticosteroids block ovulation and reduce blood levels of gonadal steroids in females but may also trigger ovulation under certain conditions
- corticosteroids cause a reduction in growth of the testes and ovary and reduce sperm production
- corticosteroids inhibit important reproductive behaviour patterns
- no simple relationship between sex and stress responsiveness exists in birds; some species may selectively modulate responsiveness to stressors to avoid interference in reproductive processes

4.5 Fish

Understanding of both the factors controlling reproductive processes in fish, and the impact of stressors on such processes, has increased significantly since the earliest review of the interaction between stress and reproduction in fish (Billard *et al.*, 1981) and this progress is reflected in two recent reviews (Wendelaar Bonga, 1997; Pankhurst and Van Der Kraak, 1997). The extensive literature concerning the effects of pollutants or toxicants on the reproductive system of fish (e.g. Ruby *et al.*, 1993; McMaster *et al.*, 1996; Tam and Zhang, 1996) has not been considered relevant to this chapter because of the uncertainty over the mechanisms underlying such effects. The reader is referred instead to a review of the impact of pollutants on fish reproduction by Kime (1995).

4.5.1 The fish reproductive system

The fish endocrine reproductive system broadly conforms to the vertebrate pattern. However, such a generalisation is complicated by the existence of many species-specific reproductive strategies and the fact that much of what is known regarding reproduction in fish has been established from studies in a limited range of salmonid and cyprinid species. Gonadotropin-releasing hormone (GnRH) of hypothalamic origin exerts a stimulatory signal on the pituitary gonadotropin-producing cells (see review by Peter and Yu, 1997). Two gonadotropins are released by the fish pituitary (GTH I and GTH II) which exert effects at the gonad and promote the synthesis and release of androgens, progestogens and oestrogens. GTH I appears to be analogous to mammalian FSH in that it is primarily implicated in gametogenesis and steroidogenesis while GTH II functions in a fashion similar to mammalian LH and stimulates final maturation of the gametes (see Xiong *et al.*, 1994; Tyler and Sumpter, 1996; Cyr and Eales, 1996 for references). The identity of some piscine gonadal steroids differs from the mammalian model. The major male-specific androgen in teleost fish is 11-ketotestosterone (11KT); T is present in the blood of both male and females in large amounts. The major progestogens are 17α,20β,-dihydroxy-4-pregnen-3-one (17α,20βP) and 17α,20β,21-trihydroxy-4-pregnen-3-one. Oestradiol-17β has a vitellogenic role in fish, stimulating hepatic production of the yolk precursor vitellogenin which is sequestered by the developing oocytes. Detailed reviews of the identity and function of fish reproductive steroids are provided by Kime (1993) and Borg (1994). In contrast to other vertebrates, fish do not possess a discrete adrenal gland, rather the steroid-secreting cells are dispersed around the walls of the posterior cardinal veins within the anterior kidney (Lofts and Bern, 1972). Hence, the adrenal homologue is referred to as the interrenal tissue and the stress response activates the hypothalamic–pituitary–interrenal axis in fish. The principal corticosteroid secreted during stress in fish is C (Hanke and Kloas, 1995).

4.5.2 Effects of stress on the fish reproductive system

Our current understanding of the modulation of fish reproductive processes by stressors is limited by comparison with what is known of the process in mammals. In addition, and in common with other vertebrate groups, the range of experimental animals from which most of the information has been obtained is narrow. However, as the range of species studied expands, it is becoming clear that the basic principles established from earlier work have a wide currency. Nonetheless, too few studies have been conducted to permit the formulation of a definitive consensus on the response of the fish reproductive system to stress.

It is clear from the available data that exposure to stressful stimuli can significantly disrupt the reproductive system of fish. This is manifested, in functional terms, in a number of ways. Repeated random exposure of rainbow trout, *Oncorhynchus mykiss*, to an acute stressor during the 9 months preceding ovulation resulted in a significant delay in ovulation and a reduction in egg size in stressed females, compared to unstressed individuals, and in a reduced sperm count in stressed males. More importantly, the survival of progeny of stressed parents was lower than that of unstressed parents (Campbell *et al.*, 1992). Smaller eggs and a reduction in the survival of progeny were also reported for rainbow trout exposed to two periods of chronic stress during the final stages of the reproductive cycle (Campbell *et al.*, 1994). A more recent study on rainbow trout in which fish were exposed to stressors at different stages of the reproductive cycle also demonstrated stress-induced disruption of reproductive processes but with some differences from the preceding studies. Exposure to stressors either during final maturation or throughout the maturational cycle resulted in earlier ovulation, while exposure to stress during the early stages of vitellogenesis resulted in differences in relative fecundity, smaller eggs and smaller swim-up fry (Contreras-Sánchez *et al.*, 1998). However, no differences in survival between the progeny of stressed and unstressed parents were observed in this latter study. The authors discuss their results in the context of the strategies available to females to cope with unstable environmental conditions during the reproductive period (Contreras-Sánchez *et al.*, 1998). Cod (*Gadus morhua*) which were exposed to a net-handling stressor at regular intervals prior to spawning produced higher numbers of deformed larvae among their offspring than were observed among the progeny of control fish (Wilson *et al.*, 1995). The rapid degeneration of ovarian tissue (atresia) observed in recently captured female snook (*Centropomus undecimalis*) was attributed to the stress associated with capture and transport (Wallace *et al.*, 1993) and high stress-induced C levels in wild-caught walleye (*Stizostedion vitreum*) were suggested to account for the inhibition of final oocyte maturation and ovulation observed in females (Barry *et al.*, 1995). Increased levels of follicular atresia were observed in the ovaries of red gurnard, *Chelidonichthys kumu*, captured from the wild and held in captivity (Clearwater and Pankhurst, 1997). These data clearly indicate that reproductive processes in fish, as in other vertebrates, are susceptible to influence by factors which evoke a stress response.

4.5.3   Hypothalamus

Up to three forms of GnRH have been identified as occurring in the brain of fish species (Peter and Yu, 1997) but to date, nothing is known of the effect of stressors on their regulation.

4.5.4   Pituitary: effects of stressors and corticosteroids

It has been demonstrated that exposure of male brown trout (*Salmo trutta*) to a brief handling/confinement stressor results in a transient elevation of GTH (Pickering *et al.*, 1987). This was interpreted by the authors either as arising from a cessation of negative feedback by gonadal steroids, the levels of which were at the same time depressed, or representing a response akin to that observed in mammalian systems in which a brief or mild stressor elicits an increase in GTH levels. A similar elevation of GTH levels has been reported for acutely stressed salmon (*O. kisutch*; Leatherland *et al.*, 1982). In contrast, chronic or prolonged exposure to stressors results in a suppression of circulating GTH levels in rainbow trout (Zohar, 1980; Bry and Zohar, 1980) and white sucker (*Catostomus commersoni*; Van Der Kraak *et al.*, 1992).

It appears likely that elevated blood C levels play a role in stress-induced GTH suppression in chronically stressed fish; when chronically administered to brown and rainbow trout, C can reduce both pituitary GTH content and circulating GTH levels (Carragher *et al.*, 1989). There is limited evidence for direct effects of C on GTH production. The incubation of pituitaries from male rainbow trout together with C *in vitro* resulted in a reduction of GTH secretion and pituitary GTH content (Carragher and Sumpter, 1990a). However, the concentration of C required to achieve this effect (1000 ng ml^{-1}) was supraphysiological for a salmonid. There has yet to be a demonstration of stress-induced alterations in pituitary sensitivity to GnRH in fish. There was no apparent difference in the GTH response of sturgeon (*Acipenser transmontanus*) to GnRH administered following stressors of varying severity (Faulkner and Moberg, 1997); however, no unstressed absolute control was included in the study, complicating interpretation of the results.

4.5.5 Ovary: effects of stressors and corticosteroids

A positive relationship between circulating corticosteroid levels and reproductive status has been reported for salmonid fish (Pickering and Christie, 1981) but a definite role for C in female reproductive development has yet to be established. Most of the available data indicate that elevated C levels are associated with adverse effects on reproductive status in fish. Confinement of female brown trout resulted in elevated blood C levels accompanied by a reduction in blood T levels but had no effect on E2 levels despite there also being a significant decline in circulating levels of vitellogenin (Campbell *et al.*, 1994). Suppression of circulating levels of T and/or E2 in females have been reported following capture from the wild for a number of species including spotted sea trout (*Cynoscion nebulosis*; Safford and Thomas, 1987), snapper (*Pagrus auratus*; Carragher and Pankhurst, 1991), white sucker (Van Der Kraak *et al.*, 1992), rainbow trout (Pankhurst and Dedual, 1994) and red gurnard (Clearwater and Pankhurst, 1997). Lower levels of plasma E2 and vitellogenin in the blood of wild-caught brown trout, captured and maintained in tanks, than in cultured brown trout were interpreted to arise as a consequence of the associated stress (Norberg *et al.*, 1989).

One of the steroids most closely associated with final maturation of the gametes in female fish, 17α,20βP, appears not to be as susceptible to the influence of stressors as other steroids of ovarian origin. No effects on blood levels of 17α,20βP were observed in white sucker (McMaster *et al.*, 1994) or in rainbow trout (Pankhurst and Dedual, 1994) exposed to stressors which were effective in lowering circulating levels of other gonadal steroids. Levels of 17α,20βP were actually elevated in the blood of female snapper (Carragher and Pankhurst, 1991) following capture and confinement.

Whether these changes in circulating steroid levels are mediated indirectly by modulation of GTH secretion, or by direct action of corticosteroids at the ovary, remains to be resolved. Either explanation may apply to the observation that administration of C to female tilapia (*Oreochromis mossambicus*) reduced both T and E2 levels (Foo and Lam, 1993a). However, chronic administration of C to female brown trout resulted in a reduction in blood levels of T and E2 but had no apparent effects on blood GTH levels (Carragher *et al.*, 1989) suggesting that C may act directly on ovarian tissue. In contrast with this, C administration had no effect on blood E2 levels in immature rainbow trout (Carragher *et al.*, 1989; Pottinger and Pickering, 1990) and the evidence for direct effects of C on fish ovarian tissue *in vitro* is contradictory. Sumpter *et al.* (1987) observed that C reduced the secretion of E2 by cultured rainbow trout ovarian follicles, a finding later confirmed by Carragher and Sumpter (1990b) for both T and E2 production. An attempt to repeat this study resulted in equivocal results, with C successfully suppressing E2 release in ovarian tissue from only a low proportion of fish tested (Pankhurst *et al.*, 1995a). A consistent inhibitory effect of C on E2 production was not observed in ovarian follicles from goldfish (*Carassius auratus*), carp (*Cyprinus carpio*) or snapper when incubated with a range of doses of C (Pankhurst *et al.*, 1995b). Nor could an effect of C be demonstrated on germinal vesicle breakdown in oocytes from walleye *in vitro*, despite clear evidence for an effect of stress on final oocyte maturation and ovulation *in vivo* (Barry *et al.*, 1995).

It has been speculated that the adverse effects on the progeny of fish exposed to stressors during the period prior to ovulation arise from the transfer of maternal C to the developing oocyte. The egg C content at ovulation has been demonstrated to be a direct function of maternal blood C levels during the pre-ovulatory period (Stratholt *et al.*, 1997); however, these authors were unable to demonstrate any relationship between elevated egg C levels and the time to hatch, the synchrony of hatch, growth or survival of fertilised ova.

4.5.6   Testis: effects of stressors and corticosteroids

Chronic confinement stress caused a prolonged reduction in blood T and 11KT levels in male brown trout and levels of both androgens were also reduced by exposure to a brief handling stressor (Pickering *et al.*, 1987). Androgen levels were also reduced in wild-caught male spotted sea trout (Safford and Thomas, 1987), white sucker (McMaster *et al.*, 1994; Jardine *et al.*, 1996) and brown trout (Melotti *et al.*, 1992). The progressive decline in blood T and 11KT levels in male dab (*Limanda limanda*) following capture and confinement was also attributed to stress associated with these procedures (Canario and Scott, 1991). Similarly, blood T and 11KT levels in the electric fish *Gnathonemus petersii* declined rapidly and significantly following transfer from natural to laboratory conditions (Landsman, 1991, 1993). Interestingly, the decline in androgen levels in males occurred simultaneously with alterations in the pattern of electric organ discharge (EOD). The EOD pattern is androgen-dependent and sexually dimorphic and the author concluded that previous failures to observe a sexual dimorphism in the EOD of captive fish arose due to stress-induced suppression of normal EOD behaviour.

The mechanistic basis of stress-related changes in circulating androgen levels has yet to be identified and it is not clear whether effects are mediated directly at the gonad or occur via effects on the brain–hypothalamus–pituitary axis. Administration of exogenous C caused a reduction in blood T levels in tilapia (Foo and Lam, 1993b) but failed to cause a significant reduction in circulating androgen levels in male brown and rainbow trout (Carragher *et al.*, 1989). No *in vitro* studies have been carried out to establish effects of C local to the testis in fish.

4.5.7   *Effects of stress on vitellogenesis*

Vitellogenesis is a critical process in the preparation for spawning, during which yolk proteins are sequestered by the developing oocytes. In fish, the major yolk precursor is vitellogenin, synthesised in the liver under the control of E2 (Tyler and Sumpter, 1996). Stress is known to impact on vitellogenesis in fish. Exposure of female brown trout to a confinement stressor causes a significant decline in circulating levels of vitellogenin, although no effect on E2 levels was observed (Campbell *et al.*, 1994), and lower plasma vitellogenin levels were observed in wild-caught brown trout subject to capture and tank confinement than in brown trout reared under farm conditions (Norberg *et al.*, 1989). It is likely that a reduction in vitellogenin synthesis/sequestration accounts for the smaller egg size noted in stressed female salmonids (Campbell *et al.*, 1992, 1994; Contreras-Sánchez *et al.*, 1998). In some cases, reduced vitellogenin levels have been accompanied by lower E2 levels suggesting a causal relationship between stress, elevated C levels, and reduced hepatic vitellogenin production. However, in other cases C administration has had no effect on blood E2 levels, for example in immature rainbow trout (Carragher *et al.*, 1989; Pottinger and Pickering, 1990). It is possible that C is able to impede vitellogenesis by reducing the sensitivity of the liver to the oestrogenic signal. Cortisol-induced reduction in the abundance of hepatic oestrogen receptors has been demonstrated to occur in rainbow trout (Pottinger and Pickering, 1990; Pottinger *et al.*, 1991)

Cortisol has been shown to stimulate a short-lived vitellogenin mRNA in *Oreochromis aureus* which is rapidly cleared and apparently does not result in elevated blood vitellogenin levels (Ding *et al.*, 1994).

4.5.8   *Effects of social stress on reproduction*

Spawning was inhibited and blood androgen and oestrogen levels were reduced in tilapia (*Tilapia zilli*) maintained in crowded holding tanks (Coward *et al.*, 1998) but these suppressive effects were reversed when fish were transferred to individual aquaria. Similarly, the presence of adult male swordtails (*Corynopoma riisei*) inhibits the maturation of juveniles (Bushmann and Burns, 1994). In both cases, the authors speculate that the inhibition of reproductive processes may have been in part mediated by activation of the HPI axis, although the possibility that pheromonal factors underlie the effect cannot be dismissed. Dominance status has also been demonstrated to be a factor influencing gonadal steroid levels in male rainbow trout. However, data demonstrating that laboratory-held dominant males had higher levels of testosterone and $17\alpha20\beta P$ than subordinates, and that dominant wild male brown trout had higher levels of 11KT than subordinates were interpreted as indicating positive effects of female pheromones or male–male interactions on dominant fish, not as indicating negative effects of stress on the reproductive system of subordinates (Cardwell *et al.*, 1996). However, Fox *et al.* (1997) actually measured blood C levels in the cichlid *Haplochromis burtoni* in a variety of social environments. They found that territorial (dominant) males had lower blood C levels than non-territorial (subordinate) males and that dominant males also possessed significantly larger GnRH-containing neurons within the hypothalamo–proptic area of the brain than subordinates. The potential complexities of the interrelationships between social status, corticosteroid levels and the reproductive system precluded an immediate interpretation of the significance of these observations.

4.5.9   Reciprocal relationships between the HPI axis and the HPG axis in fish

In common with mammals, a reciprocal relationship between the HPI axis and HPG axis has been demonstrated in fish. Early studies on sockeye salmon (*Oncorhynchus nerka*) suggested that the corticosteroid response to stress was affected by the stage of maturity of the fish (Donaldson and Fagerlund, 1970, 1972; Fagerlund, 1970; Fagerlund and Donaldson, 1969) and these observations were later confirmed for brown and rainbow trout; in both species, mature male fish responded to a standardised stressor with a significantly lower elevation of blood C than was the case for sexually immature fish (Sumpter *et al.*, 1987; Pottinger *et al.*, 1995). Plasma ACTH levels during stress were also reduced in mature male fish suggesting that the suppression of responsiveness was mediated at the brain–pituitary level (Pottinger *et al.*, 1995). A subsequent study demonstrated that the effects could be ascribed, at least in part, to modulation of the stress response by gonadal steroids. Administration of testosterone and 11KT to immature brown and rainbow trout resulted in a significantly attenuated blood ACTH and C response to confinement stress compared to control fish. Administration of E2 was found to enhance the elevation of blood ACTH and C during stress relative to control fish (Pottinger *et al.*, 1996). As is the case for mammals, the functional significance of the modulation of the HPI axis by the HPG axis has yet to be established.

- exposure to stressors can delay ovulation, reduce egg size and sperm count, reduce the size and survival of progeny, and can increase the occurrence of developmental abnormalities in progeny and promote ovarian atresia
- exposure to stressors and administration of corticosteroids reduce blood levels of gonadal steroids in male and female fish
- exposure to chronic stressors reduces blood GTH levels
- blood levels of the yolk protein precursor vitellogenin are reduced by stress
- corticosteroids may act directly at the ovary but the evidence is contradictory
- androgens suppress and oestrogens enhance stress responsiveness in fish

4.6 Conclusion

Understanding the extent to which reproductive processes in animals may be disrupted by stressors, and the mechanisms by which such disruption occurs, is of critical importance for a number of reasons. Awareness of the manner in which stress-related reproductive dysfunction impinges on human and veterinary clinical practice, the commercial production of intensively farmed animals, and also plays a role in the modulating the performance of natural populations of animals in both the terrestrial and aquatic environment, has become greater during the past thirty years. However, there is an imbalance in the level of understanding currently applicable to the various vertebrate groups, and the number of different species studied within each group remains limited. It is reasonable to assume that the complexities of the relationship between physiological stress and the reproductive system in mammals will apply to birds, reptiles and amphibians, and fish. Most of the tools required to undertake the necessary studies are available and it is likely that the next ten years will witness a significant improvement in our understanding of how adverse environmental change affects reproduction in all the vertebrate groups.

References

Ahima, R.S. and Harlan, R.E. (1992) Glucocorticoid receptors in LHRH neurons. *Neuroendocrinology*, **56** 845-850.
Aloisi, A.M., Steenbergen, H.L., van De Poll, N.E. and Farabollini, F. (1994) Sex-dependent effects of restraint on nociception and pituitary-adrenal hormones in the rat. *Physiology and Behaviour*, **55** 789-793.

Armario, A. and Castellanos, J.M. (1984). A comparison of corticoadrenal and gonadal responses to acute immobilization stress in rats and mice. *Physiology and Behaviour*, **32** 517-519.

Asakura, H., Zwain, I.H. and Yen, S.S.C. (1997) Expression of genes encoding corticotropin-releasing factor (CRF), type 1 CRF receptor, and CRF-binding protein and localization of the gene products in the human ovary. *Journal of Clinical Endocrinology and Metabolism*, **82** 2720-2725.

Astheimer, L.B., Buttemer, W.A. and Wingfield, J.C. (1994) Gender and seasonal differences in the adrenocortical response to ACTH challenge in an arctic passerine. *Zonotrichia leucophrys gambelii*. *General and Comparative Endocrinology*, **94** 33-43.

Astheimer, L.B., Buttemer, W.A. and Wingfield, J.C. (1995) Seasonal and acute changes in adrenocortical responsiveness in an arctic-breeding bird. *Hormones and Behaviour*, **29** 442-457.

Baldwin, D.M. (1979) The effects of glucocorticoids on estrogen-dependent luteinizing hormonerelease in the ovariectomized ratand on gonadotropin secretion in the intact female rat. *Endocrinology*, **105** 120-128.

Baldwin, D.M. and Sawyer, C.H. (1974) Effects of dexamethasone on LH release and ovulation in the cyclic rat. *Endocrinology*, **94** 1397-1403.

Baldwin, D.M., Srivastava, P.S. and Krummen, L.A. (1991) Differential actions of corticosterone on luteinizing hormone and follicle-stimulating hormone biosynthesis and release in cultured rat anterior pituitary cells: interactions with estradiol. *Biology of Reproduction*, **44** 1040-1050.

Bambino, T.H. and Hsueh, A.J.W. (1981) Direct inhibitory effect of glucocorticoids upon testicular luteinizing hormone receptor and steroidogenesis *in vivo* and *in vitro*. *Endocrinology*, **108** 2142-2148.

Barry, T.P., Malison, J.A., Lapp, A.F. and Procarione, L.S. (1995) Effects of selected hormones and male cohorts on final oocyte maturation, ovulation, and steroid production in walleye (*Stizostedion vitreum*). *Aquaculture*, **138** 331-347.

Bercovitch, F.B. and Clarke, A.S. (1995) Dominance rank, cortisol concentrations, and reproductive maturation in male rhesus macaques. *Physiology and Behaviour*, **58** 215-221.

Berga, S.L. (1995) Stress and amenorrhea. *The Endocrinologist*, **5** 416-421.

Billard, R., Bry, C. and Gillet, C. (1981) Stress, environment and reproduction in teleost fish, in *Stress and Fish* (ed. A.D. Pickering), Academic Press, London, pp 185-208.

Bingaman, E.W., Magnuson, D.J., Gray, T.S. and Handa, R.J. (1994) Androgen inhibits the increases in hypothalamic corticotropin-releasing hormone (CRH) and CRH immunor-eactivity following gonadectomy. *Neuroendocrinology*, **59** 228-234.

Bingaman, E.W., Van De Kar, L.D., Yracheta, J.M., Li, Q. and Gray, T.S. (1995) Castration attenuates prolactin response but potentiates ACTH response to conditioned stress in the rat. *American Journal of Physiology*, **269** R856-R863.

Blanchard, D.C., Sakai, R.R., McEwen, B., Weiss, S.M. and Blanchard, R.J. (1993) Sub-ordination stress: behavioural, brain, and neuroendocrine correlates. *Behavioural Brain Research*, **58** 113-121.

Bonavera, J.J., Kalra, S.P. and Kalra, P.S. (1993) Mode of action of interleukin-1 in suppression of pituitary LH release in castrated male rats. *Brain Research*, **612** 1-8.

Borg, B. (1994) Androgens in teleost fishes. *Comparative Biochemistry and Physiology*, **109C** 219-245.

Bourne, A. (1991) Androgens, in *Vertebrate Endocrinology: Fundamentals and Biomedical Implications, Volume 4, Part B, Reproduction* (eds. P.K.T. Pang and M.P. Schreibman), Academic Press, San Diego, pp 115-147.

Boyd, S.K. and Moore, F.L. (1990) Evidence for GABA involvement in stress-induced inhibition of male amphibian sexual behaviour. *Hormones and Behaviour*, **24** 128-138.

Bradley, A.J. and Stoddart, D.M. (1997) Plasma androgen, social position, and response to GnRH in the marsupial sugar glider *Petaurus breviceps* (Marsupialia: Petauridae). *Journal of Zoology*, **241** 579-587.

Brann, D.W. and Mahesh, V.B. (1991) Role of corticosteroids in female reproduction. *FASEB Journal*, **5** 2691-2698.

Briski, K.P. (1996) Stimulatory vs inhibitory effects of acute stress on plasma-LH — differential-effects of pretreatment with dexamethasone or the steroid-receptor antagonist, RU-486. *Pharmacology Biochemistry and Behavior*, **55** 19-26.

Briski, K.P. and Sylvester, P.W. (1988) Effect of specific acute stressors on luteinizing hormone release in ovariectomized and ovariectomized estrogen-treated female rats. *Neuroendocrinology*, **47** 194-202.

Briski, K.P. and Vogel, K.L. (1995) Role of endogenous opioid peptides in central glucocorticoid receptor (GR)-induced decreases in circulating LH in the male rat. *Neuropeptides*, **28** 175-181.

Briski, K.P., Vogel, K.L. and McIntyre, A.R. (1995) The antiglucocorticoid, RU486, attenuates stress-induced decreases in plasma-luteinizing hormone concentrations in male rats. *Neuroendocrinology*, **61** 638-645.

Bry, C. and Zohar, Y. (1980) Dorsal aorta catheterization in rainbow trout (*Salmo gairdneri*). Glucocorticoid levels, haematological data and resumption of feeding during five days after surgery. *Reproduction, Nutrition, Développement*, **20** 1825-1834.

Burgess, L.H. and Handa, R.J. (1992) Chronic estrogen-induced alterations in adrenocorticotropin and corticosterone secretion, and glucocorticoid receptor-mediated functions in female rats. *Endocrinology*, **131** 1261-1269.

Bushmann, P.J. and Burns, J.R. (1994) Social control of male sexual maturation in the swordtail characin, *Corynopoma riisei. Journal of Fish Biology*, **44** 263-272.

Cain, J.R. and Lien, R.J. (1985) A model for droght inhibition of bobwhite quail (*Colinus virginianus,*) reproductive systems. *Comparative Biochemistry and Physiology*, **82A** 925-930.

Callard, G.V. (1991) Spermatogenesis, in *Vertebrate Endocrinology: Fundamentals and Biomedical Implications, Volume 4, Part A, Reproduction* (eds. P.K.T. Pang and M.P. Schreibman), Academic Press, San Diego, pp 303-341.

Calogero, A.E., Burrello, N., Negri-Cesi, P., Papale, L., Palumbo, M.A., Cianci, A., Sanfilippo, S. and D'Agata, R. (1996) Effects of corticotropin-releasing hormone on ovarian estrogen production *in vitro. Endocrinology*, **137** 4161-4166.

Campbell, P.M., Pottinger, T.G. and Sumpter, J.P. (1992) Stress reduced the quality of gametes produced by rainbow trout. *Biology of Reproduction*, **47** 1140-1150.

Campbell, P.M., Pottinger, T.G. and Sumpter, J.P. (1994) Preliminary evidence that chronic confinement stress reduces the quality of gametes produced by brown and rainbow trout. *Aquaculture*, **120** 151-169.

Canario, A.V.M. and Scott, A.P. (1991) Levels of 17α, 20α-dihydroxy-4-pregnen-3-one, $3\beta,17\alpha,20\alpha$-trihydroxy-5β-pregnane, and other sex steroids in blood plasma of male dab *Limanda limanda* (marine flatfish) injected with human chorionic gonadotropin. *General and Comparative Endocrinology*, **83** 258-264.

Cardwell, J.R., Sorensen, P.W., Van Der Kraak, G.J. and Liley, N.R. (1996) Effect of dominance status on sex hormone levels in laboratory and wild-spawning male trout. *General and Comparative Endocrinology*, **101** 333-341.

Carragher, J.F. and Pankhurst, N.W. (1991) Stress and reproduction in a commercially important marine fish, *Pagrus auratus* (Sparidae), in *Proceedings of the Fourth International Symposium on Reproductive Physiology of Fish, 1991* (eds. A.P. Scott, J.P. Sumpter, D.E. Kime and M.S. Rolfe), FishSymp 91, Sheffield, pp 253-255.

Carragher, J.F. and Sumpter, J.P. (1990a) Corticosteroid physiology in fish, in *Progress in Comparative Endocrinology* (eds. A. Epple, C.G. Scanes and M.H. Stetson), Wiley-Liss, New York, pp 478-492.

Carragher, J.F. and Sumpter, J.P. (1990b) The effect of cortisol on the secretion of sex steroids from cultured ovarian follicles of rainbow trout. *General and Comparative Endocrinology*, **77** 403-407.

Carragher, J.F., Sumpter, J.P., Pottinger, T.G. and Pickering, A.D. (1989) The deleterious effects of cortisol implantation on reproductive steroids in two species of trout, *Salmo trutta* L. and *Salmo gairdneri* Richardson. *General and Comparative Endocrinology*, **76** 310-321.

Carey, M.P., Deterd, C.H., de Koning, J., Helmerhorst, F. and De Kloet, E.R. (1995) The influence of ovarian steroids on hypothalamic-pituitary-adrenal regulation in the female rat. *Journal of Endocrinology*, **144** 311-321.

Charpenet, G., Tache, Y., Forest, M.G., Haour, F., Saez, J.M., Bernier, M., Ducharme, J.R. and Collu, R. (1981) Effects of chronic intermittent immobilization stress on rat testicular androgenic function. *Endocrinology*, **109** 1254-1258.

Chen, S.Y., Wang, J., Yu, G.Q., Liu, W.H. and Pearce, D. (1997) Androgen and glucocorticoid receptor heterodimer formation - A possible mechanism for mutual inhibition of transcriptional activity. *Journal of Biological Chemistry*, **272** 14087-14092.

Chieffi, G. and Pierantoni, R. (1987) Regulation of ovarian steroidogenesis, in *Hormones and Reproduction in Fishes, Amphibians, and Reptiles* (eds. D.O. Norris and R.E. Jones), Plenum Press, New York, pp 117-144.

Chrousos, G.P. and Gold, P.W. (1992) The concepts of stress and stress system disorders. Overview of physical and behavioural homeostasis. *Journal of the American Medical Association*, **267** 1244-1252.

Clearwater, S.J. and Pankhurst, N.W. (1997) The response to capture and confinement stress of plasma cortisol, plasma sex steroids and vitellogenic oocytes in the marine teleost, red gurnard. *Journal of Fish Biology*, **50** 429-441.

Coddington, E.J. and Cree, A. (1995) Effect of acute captivity stress on plasma concentrations of corticosterone and sex steroids in female whistling frogs, *Litoria ewingi. General and Comparative Endocrinology*, **100** 33-38.

Connolly, P.B. and Callard, I.P. (1987) Steroids modulate the release of luteinizing hormone from quail pituitary cells. *General and Comparative Endocrinology*, **68** 466-472.

Contreras-Sánchez, W.M., Schreck, C.B., Fitzpatrick, M.S. and Pereira, C.B. (1998) Effects of stress on the reproductive performance of rainbow trout (*Oncorhynchus mykiss*). *Biology of Reproduction*, **58** 439-447.

Coubrough, R.I. (1985) Stress and fertility. A review. *Onderstepoort Journal of Veterinary Research*, **52** 153-156.

Cover, P.O., Laycock, J.F., Gartside, I.B. and Buckingham, J.C. (1991) A role for vasopressin in the stress-induced inhibition of gonadotropin secretion: studies in the Brattleboro rat. *Journal of Neuroendocrinology*, **3** 413-417.

Coward, K., Bromage, N.R. and Little, D.C. (1998) Inhibition of spawning and associated suppression of sex steroid levels during confinement in the substrate-spawning *Tilapia zilli. Journal of Fish Biology*, **52** 152-165.

Cree, A., Guillette, L.J., Cockrem, J.F. and Joss, J.M.P. (1990) Effects of capture and temperature stresses on plasma steroid concentrations in male tuatara (*Sphenodon punctatus*). *The Journal of Experimental Zoology*, **253** 38-46.

Crossley, J.C. (1983) Prevention of epinephrine and stress-induced egg laying delay by feeding propanolol to the laying hen. *Poultry Science*, **62** 375-378.

Cunningham, F.J. (1987) Ovulation in the hen: neuroendocrine control. *Oxford Review of Reproductive Biology*, **9** 96-136.

Cyr, D.G. and Eales, J.G. (1996) Interrelationships between thyroidal and reproductive endocrine systems in fish. *Reviews in Fish Biology and Fisheries*, **6** 165-200.

Dalkin, A.C. and Marshall, J.C. (1997) Reproduction and fertility, in *Endocrinology: Basic and Clinical Principles* (eds. P.M. Conn and S. Melmed), Humana Press Inc., Totowa, New Jersey, pp 405-418.

Danišová, A., Šebökovà, E. and Kolena, J. (1987) Effect of corticosteroids on estradiol and testosterone secretion by granulosa cells in culture. *Experimental Clinical Endocrinology*, **89** 165-173.

Demura, R., Suzuki, T., Nakamura, S., Komatsu, H., Odagiri, E. and Demura, H. (1989) Effect of immobilization stress on testosterone and inhibin in male rats. *Journal of Andrology*, **10** 210-213.

DeNardo, D.F. and Licht, P. (1993) Effects of corticosterone on social behaviour of male lizards. *Hormones and Behaviour*, **27** 184-199.

Deviche, P., Balthazart, J., Heyns, W. and Hendrick, J.-Cl. (1980) Endocrine effects of castration followed by androgen replacement and ACTH injections in the male domestic duck (*Anas platyrhynchos*). *General and Comparative Endocrinology*, **41** 53-61.

Deviche, P. and Hendrick, J.-Cl. (1981) Participation of glucocorticoids in the regulation of plasma LH levels in the male domestic duck (*Anas platyrhynchos* L.). *Reproduction, Nutrition, Développement*, **21** 1137-1142.

Ding, J.L., Lim, E.H. and Lam, T.J. (1994) Cortisol-induced hepatic vitellogenin messenger RNA in *Oreochromis aureus* (Steindachner). *General and Comparative Endocrinology*, **96** 276-287.

Dobson, H. and Smith, R.F. (1995) Stress and reproduction in farm animals. *Journal of Reproduction and Fertility Supplement*, **49** 451-461.

Donaldson, E.M. and Fagerlund, U.H.M. (1970) Effect of sexual maturation and gonadectomy at sexual maturity on cortisol secretion rate in sockeye salmon (*Oncorhynchus nerka*). *Journal of the Fisheries Research Board of Canada*, **27** 2287-2296.

Donaldson, E.M. and Fagerlund, U.H.M. (1972) Corticosteroid dynamics in Pacific salmon. *General and Comparative Endocrinology*, **Supplement 3** 254-265.

Donoghue, D.J., Krueger, B.F., Hargis, B.M., Miller, A.M. and El Halawani, M. (1989) Thermal stress reduces serum luteinizing hormone and bioassayable hypothalamic content of luteinizing hormone-releasing hormone in hens. *Biology of Reproduction*, **41** 419-424.

Dubey, A.K. and Plant, T.M. (1985) A suppression of gonadotropin secretion by cortisol in castrated male rhesus monkeys (*Macaca mulatta*) mediated by the interruption of hypothalamic gonadotropin-releasing hormone release. *Biology of Reproduction*, **33** 423-431.

Dufau, M.L., Tinajero, J.C. and Fabbri, A. (1993) Corticotropin-releasing factor: an anti-reproductive hormone of the testis. *FASEB Journal*, **7** 299-307.

Edens, F.W. (1983) Effect of environmental stressors on male reproduction. *Poultry Science*, **62** 1676-1689.

Ellis, L. (1995) Dominance and reproductive success among nonhuman animals: a cross-species comparison. *Ethology and Sociobiology*, **16** 257-333.

Elsey, R.M., Lance, V.A., Joanen, T. and McNease, L. (1991) Acute stress suppresses plasma estradiol levels in female alligators (*Alligator mississippiensis*). *Comparative Biochemistry and Physiology*, **100A** 649-651.

Erden, H.F., Zwain, I.H., Asakura, H. and Yen, S.S.C. (1998) Corticotropin-releasing factor inhibits luteinizing hormone-stimulated P450c17 gene expression and androgen production by isolated thecal cells of human ovarian follicles. *Journal of Clinical Endocrinology and Metabolism*, **83** 448-452.

Etches, R.J. and Croze, F. (1983) Plasma concentrations of LH, progesterone, and corticosterone during ACTH- and corticosterone-induced ovualtion in the hen (*Gallus domesticus*). *General and Comparative Endocrinology*, **50** 359-365.

Etches, R.J., Williams, J.B. and Rzasa, J. (1984) Effects of corticosterone and dietary changes in the hen on ovarian function, plasma LH and steroids and the response to exogenous LH-RH. *Journal of Reproduction and Fertility*, **70** 121-130.

Fagerlund, U.H.M. (1970) Response to mammalian ACTH of the interrenal tissue of sockeye salmon (*Oncorhynchus nerka*) at various stages of sexual maturation. *Journal of the Fisheries Research Board of Canada*, **27** 1169-1172.

Fagerlund, U.H.M. and Donaldson, E.M. (1969) The effect of androgens on the distribution and secretion of cortisol in gonadectomized male sockeye salmon (*Oncorhynchus nerka*) *General and Comparative Endocrinology*, **12** 438-448.

Faulkner, I.N. and Moberg, G.P. (1997) Effects of short term management stress on the ability of GnRHa to induce gonadotropin secretion in male white sturgeon, *Acipenser transmontanus. Aquaculture*, **159** 159-168.

Fenske, M. (1997) Role of cortisol in the ACTH-induced suppression of testicular steroidogenesis in guinea pigs. *Journal of Endocrinology*, **154** 407-414.

Ferin, M. (1993) Neuropeptides, the stress response, and the hypothalamo-pituitary-gonadal axis in the female rhesus monkey. *Annals of the New York Academy of Sciences*, **697** 106-116.

Flickinger, G.L. (1961) Effect of grouping on adrenals and gonads of chickens. *General and Comparative Endocrinology*, **1** 332-340.

Flickinger, G.L. (1966) Effect of prolonged ACTH administration on gonads of sexually mature chickens. *Poultry Science*, **45** 753-761.

Foo, T.W. and Lam, T.J. (1993a) Retardation of ovarian growth and depression of serum steroid levels in the tilapia *Oreochromis mossambicus*, by cortisol implantation. *Aquaculture*, **115** 133-143.

Foo, T.W. and Lam, T.J. (1993b) Serum cortisol response to handling stress and the effect of cortisol implantation on testosterone levels in the tilapia, *Oreochromis mossambicus. Aquaculture*, **115** 145-158.

Fox, H.E., White, S.A., Kao, M.H.F. and Fernals, R.D. (1997) Stress and dominance in a social fish. *Journal of Neuroscience*, **17** 6463-6469.

Gao, H.B., Shan, L.X., Monder, C. and Hardy, M.P. (1996) Suppression of endogenous corticosterone levels *in vivo* increases the steroidogenic capacity of purified rat leydig cells *in vitro. Endocrinology*, **137** 1714-1718.

Gao, H.B., Ge, R.S., Lakshmi, V., Marandici, A. and Hardy, M.P. (1997) Hormonal regulation of oxidative and reductive activities of 11beta-hydroxysteroid dehydrogenase in rat Leydig cells. *Endocrinology*, **138** 156-161.

Ghizzoni, L., Mastorakos, G., Vottero, A., Barreca, A., Furlini, M., Cesarone, A., Ferrari, B., Chrousos, G.P. and Bernasconi, S. (1997) Corticotropin-releasing hormone (CRH) inhibits steroid biosynthesis by cultured human granulosa-lutein cells in a CRH and interleukin-1 receptor- mediated fashion. *Endocrinology*, **138** 4806-4811.

Gobbetti, A. and Zerani, M. (1996) Possible mechanism for the first response to short captivity stress in the water frog, *Rana esculenta. Journal of Endocrinology*, **148** 233-239.

González-Quijano, M.I., Ariznavarreta, C., Martín, A.I., Treguerres, J.A.F. and López-Calderón, A. (1991) Naltrexone does not reverse the inhibitory effect of chronic restraint on gonadotropin-secretion in the intact male rat. *Neuroendocrinology*, **54** 447-453.

Grassman, M. and Hess, D.L. (1992) Sex differences in adrenal function in the lizard *Cnemidophorus sexlineatus*: II. Responses to acute stress in the laboratory. *The Journal of Experimental Zoology*, **264** 183-188.

Greenberg, N. and Wingfield, J.C. (1987) Stress and reproduction: reciprocal relationships, in *Hormones and Reproduction in Fishes, Amphibians, and Reptiles* (eds. D.O. Norris and R.E. Jones), Plenum Press, New York, pp 461-503.

Greenberg, N., Chen, T. and Crews, D. (1984) Social status, gonadal state and the adrenal stress response in the lizard, *Anolis carolinensis. Hormones and Behaviour*, **18** 1-11.

Grosse, A.E. and Craig, J.V. (1960) Sexual maturity of males representing twelve strains and six breeds of chickens. *Poultry Science*, **39** 164-172.

Guillette, L.J., Cree, A. and Rooney, A.A. (1995) Biology of stress: interactions with reproduction, immunology and intermediary metabolism, in *Health and Welfare of Captive Reptiles* (eds. C. Warwick, F.L. Frye and J.B. Murphy), Chapman and Hall, London, pp 32-81.

Gunin, A.G. (1996) Effect of chronic stress on estradiol action in the uterus of ovariectomized rats. *European Journal of Obstetrics & Gynecology and Reproductive Biology*, **66** 169-174.

Hadley, M.E. (1988) *Endocrinology*, 2nd edn, Prentice-Hall International, London.

Hales, D.B. and Payne, A.H. (1989) Glucocorticoid mediated repression of P450scc mRNA and *de novo*, synthesis in cultured Leydig cells. *Endocrinology*, **124** 2099-2144.

Handa, R.J., Nunley, K.M., Lorens, S.A., Louie, J.P., McGivern, R.F. and Bollnow, M.R. (1994a) Androgen regulation of adrenocorticotropin and corticosterone secretion in the male rat following novelty and foot shock stressors. *Physiology and Behaviour*, **55** 117-124.

Handa, R.J., Burgess, L.H., Kerr, J.E. and O'Keefe, J.A. (1994b) Gonadal steroid hormone receptors and sex differences in the hypothalamo-pituitary-adrenal axis. *Hormones and Behaviour*, **28** 464-476.

Hanke, W. and Kloas, W. (1995) Comparative aspects of regulation and function of the adrenal complex in different groups of vertebrates. *Hormone and Metabolic Research*, **27** 389-397.

Harlow, C.R., Fahy, U.M., Talbot, W.M., Wardle, P.G. and Hull, M.G.R. (1996) Stress and stress-related hormones during in-vitro fertilization treatment. *Human Reproduction*, **11** 274-279.

Hayashi, K.T. and Moberg, G.P. (1987) Influence of acute stress and the adrenal axis on regulation of LH and testosterone in the male rhesus monkey (*Macaca mulatta*). *American Journal of Primatology*, **12** 263-273.

Hayashi, K.T. and Moberg, G.P. (1990) Influence of the hypothalamic-pituitary-adrenal axis on the menstrual cycle and the pituitary responsiveness to estradiol in the female rhesus monkey (*Macaca mulatta*). *Biology of Reproduction*, **42** 260-265.

Heinrich, N., Meyer, M.R., Furkert, J., Sasse, A., Beyermann, M., Bonigk, W. and Berger, H. (1998) Corticotropin-releasing factor (CRF) agonists stimulate testosterone production in mouse Leydig cells through CRF receptor-1. *Endocrinology*, **139** 651-658.

Herbert, J. (1995) Stress and reproduction: the role of peptides and other chemical messengers in the brain. *Current Science*, **68** 391-400.

Hester, P.Y. and Wilson, E.K. (1986) Performance of white leghorn hens in response to cage density and the introduction of cage mates. *Poultry Science*, **65** 2029-2033.

Ho, S.-M. (1987) Endocrinology of vitellogenesis, in *Hormones and Reproduction in Fishes, Amphibians, and Reptiles* (eds. D.O. Norris and R.E. Jones), Plenum Press, New York, pp 145-169.

Ho, S.-M. (1991) Vitellogenesis, in *Vertebrate Endocrinology: Fundamentals and Biomedical Implications, Volume 4, Part A, Reproduction* (eds. P.K.T. Pang and M.P. Schreibman), Academic Press, San Diego, pp 91-126.

Huang, B.M., Stocco, D.M., Hutson, J.C. and Norman, R.L. (1995) Corticotropin-releasing hormone stimulates steroidogenesis in mouse leydig cells. *Biology of Reproduction*, **53** 620-626.

Ishii, S. (1991) Gonadotropins, in *Vertebrate Endocrinology: Fundamentals and Biomedical Implications, Volume 4, Part B, Reproduction* (eds. P.K.T. Pang and M.P. Schreibman), Academic Press, San Diego, pp 33-66.

Jalabert, B., Fostier, A., Breton, B. and Weil, C. (1991) Oocyte maturation in vertebrates, in *Vertebrate Endocrinology: Fundamentals and Biomedical Implications, Volume 4, Part A, Reproduction* (eds. P.K.T. Pang and M.P. Schreibman), Academic Press, San Diego, pp 23-90.

Jardine, J.J., Van Der Kraak, G.J. and Munkittrick, K.R. (1996) Capture and confinement stress in white sucker exposed to bleached kraft pulp mill effluent. *Ecotoxicology and Environmental Safety*, **33** 287-298.

Johnson, E.O., Kamilaris, T.C., Chrousos, G.P. and Gold, P.W. (1992) Mechanisms of stress: a dynamic overview of hormonal and behavioural homeostasis. *Neuroscience and Biobehavioural Reviews*, **16** 115-130.

Jones, R.E. (1987) Ovulation: insights about the mechanisms based on a comparative approach, in *Hormones and Reproduction in Fishes, Amphibians, and Reptiles* (eds. D.O. Norris and R.E. Jones), Plenum Press, New York, pp 203-240.

Juniewicz, P.E., Johnson, B.H. and Bolt, D.J. (1987) Effect of adrenal steroids on testosterone and luteinizing hormone secretion in the ram. *Journal of Andrology*, **30** 190-196.

Kamel, F. and Kubajak, C.L. (1987) Modulation of gonadotropin secretion by corticosterone: interaction with gonadal steroids and mechanism of action. *Endocrinology*, **121** 561-568.

Kant, G.J., Lenox, R.H., Bunnell, B.N., Mougey, E.H., Pennington, L.L. and Meyerhoff, J.L. (1983) Comparison of stress response in male and female rats: pituitary cyclic AMP and plasma prolactin, growth hormone and corticosterone. *Psychoneuroendocrinology*, **8** 421-428.

Kawate, N., Inaba, T. and Mori, J. (1993) Effects of cortisol on the amounts of estradiol-17β and progesterone secreted and the number of luteinizing hormone receptors in cultured bovine granulosa cells. *Animal Reproduction Science*, **32** 15-25.

Kime, D.E. (1993) "Classical" and "non-classical" reproductive steroids in fish. *Reviews in Fish Biology and Fisheries*, **3** 160-180.

Kime, D.E. (1995) The effects of pollution on reproduction in fish. *Reviews in Fish Biology and Fisheries*, **5** 52-95.

King, J.A. and Millar, R.P. (1991) Gonadotropin-releasing hormones, in *Vertebrate Endocrinology: Fundamentals and Biomedical Implications, Volume 4, Part B, Reproduction* (eds. P.K.T. Pang and M.P. Schreibman), Academic Press, San Diego, pp 1-31.

Kononen, J., Honkaniemi, J., Gustafsson, J.A. and Peltohuikko, M. (1993) Glucocorticoid receptor colocalization with pituitary hormones in the rat pituitary gland. *Molecular and Cellular Endocrinology*, **93** 97-103.

Kostić, T., Andric, S., Kovačević, R. and Marić, D. (1997) The effect of opioid antagonists in local regulation of testicular response to acute stress in adult rats. *Steroids*, **62** 703-708.

Kreeger, T.J., Seal, U.S. and Plotka, E.D. (1992) Influence of hypothalamic-pituitary-adrenocortical hormones on reproductive hormones in gray wolves (*Canis lupus*). *The Journal of Experimental Zoology*, **264** 32-41.

Krulich, L., Hefco, E., Illner, P. and Read, C.B. (1974) The effects of acute stress on the secretion of LH, FSH, prolactin and GH in the normal male rat, with comments on their statistical evaluation. *Neuroendocrinology*, **16** 293-311.

Kupwade, V.A. and Saidapur, S.K. (1987) Effect of dexamethasone and ACTH on oocyte growth and recruitment in the frog *Rana cyanophlyctis* during the prebreeding vitellogenic phase. *General and Comparative Endocrinology*, **65** 394-398.

Lance, V.A. and Elsey, R.M. (1986) Stress-induced suppression of testosterone secretion in male alligators. *The Journal of Experimental Zoology*, **239** 241-246.

Landsman, R.E. (1991) Captivity affects behavioural physiology: plasticity in signaling sexual identity. *Experientia*, **47** 31-38.

Landsman, R.E. (1993) The effects of captivity on the electric organ discharge and plasma hormone levels in *Gnathonemus petersii* (Mormyriformes). *Journal of Comparative Physiology*, **A172** 619-631.

Lavy, G., Whitten, P.L. and Naftolin, F. (1991) Introduction to vertebrate reproductive endocrinology, in *Vertebrate Endocrinology: Fundamentals and Biomedical Implications, Volume 4, Part A, Reproduction* (eds. P.K.T. Pang and M.P. Schreibman), Academic Press, San Diego, pp 2-22.

Leatherland, J.F., Copeland, P., Sumpter, J.P. and Sonstegard, R.A. (1982) Hormonal control of gonadal maturation and development of secondary sexual characteristics in coho salmon, *Oncorhynchus kisutch*, from Lakes Ontario, Erie, and Michigan. *General and Comparative Endocrinology*, **48** 196-204.

Lederman, R.P. (1995) Relationship of anxiety, stress, and psychosocial development to reproductive health. *Behavioural Medicine*, **21** 101-112.

Lemaire, V., Taylor, G.T. and Mormède, P. (1997) Adrenal axis activation by chronic social stress fails to inhibit gonadal function in male rats. *Psychoneuroendocrinology*, **22** 563-573.

Leśniewska, B., Miśkowiak, B., Nowak, M. and Malendowicz, L.K. (1990) Sex differences in adrenocortical structure and function. XXVII. The effect of ether stress on ACTH and corticosterone in intact, gonadectomized, and testosterone- or estradiol-replaced rats. *Research in Experimental Medicine*, **190** 95-103.

Levine, S. (1985) A definition of stress? in *Animal Stress* (ed. G.P. Moberg) American Physiological Society, Bethesda, pp 51-69.

Li, P.S. (1991) Effect of cortisol on testosterone production by immature pig Leydig cells. *Journal of Steroid Biochemistry and Molecular Biology*, **38** 205-212.

Li, P.S. (1993) Actions of corticotropin-releasing factor or cortisol on follicle-stimulating hormone secretion by isolated pig pituitary cells. *Life Sciences*, **53** 141-151.

Licht, P. and Porter, D. (1987) Role of gonadotropin-releasing hormone in regulation of gonadotropin secretion from amphibian and reptilian pituitaries, in *Hormones and Reproduction in Fishes, Amphibians, and Reptiles* (eds. D.O. Norris and R.E. Jones), Plenum Press, New York, pp 62-85.

Licht, P., McCreery, B.R., Barnes, R. and Pang, R. (1983) Seasonal and stress-related changes in plasma gonadotropins, sex steroids and corticosterone in the bullfrog, *Rana catesbeiana*. *General and Comparative Endocrinology*, **50** 124-145.

Licht, P., Breitenbach, G.L. and Congdon, J.D. (1985) Seasonal cycles in testicular activity, gonadotropin, and thyroxine in the painted turtle, *Chrysemys picta*, under natural conditions. *General and Comparative Endocrinology*, **59** 130-139.

Liptrap, R.M. (1993) Stress and reproduction in domestic animals. *Annals New York Academy of Sciences*, **697** 275-284.

Lofts, B. (1987) Testicular function, in *Hormones and Reproduction in Fishes, Amphibians, and Reptiles* (eds. D.O. Norris and R.E. Jones), Plenum Press, New York, pp 283-325.

Lofts, B. and Bern, H.A. (1972) The functional morphology of steroidogenic tissues, in *Steroids in Nonmammalian Vertebrates* (ed. D.R. Idler), Academic Press, London, pp 37-125.

López-Calderón, A., Ariznavaretta, C., Gonzàlez-Quijano, M.I., Tresguerres, J.A.F. and Calderón, M.D. (1991) Stress induced changes in testis function. *Journal of Steroid Biochemistry and Molecular Biology*, **40** 473-479.

López-Díaz, M.C. and Bosu, W.T.K. (1997) Effects of ACTH on luteinizing hormone receptors in ovine follicular wall and corpus luteum. *Reproduction, Nutrition, Development*, **37** 599-612.

Mahmoud, I.Y. and Licht, P. (1997) Seasonal changes in gonadal activity and the effects of stress on reproductive hormones in the common snapping turtle, *Chelydra serpentina*. *General and Comparative Endocrinology*, **107** 359-372.

Mahmoud, I.Y., Guillette, L.J., McAsey, M.E. and Cady, C. (1989) Stress-induced changes in serum testosterone, estradiol-17β and progesterone in the turtle *Chelydra serpentina*. *Comparative Biochemistry and Physiology*, **93A** 423-427.

Mahmoud, I.Y., Vliet, K., Guillette, L.J. and Plude, J.L. (1996) Effect of stress and ACTH$_{1-24}$ on hormonal levels in male alligators, *Alligator mississippiensis*. *Comparative Biochemistry and Physiology*, **115A** 57-62.

Mann, D.R., Evans, D., Edoimioya, F., Kamel, F. and Butterstein, G.M. (1985) A detailed examination of the in vivo and in vitro effects of ACTH on gonadotropin secretion in the adult rat. *Neuroendocrinology*, **40** 297-302.

Manzo, C., Zerani, M., Gobbetti, A., DiFiore, M.M. and Angelini, F. (1994) Is corticosterone involved in the reproductive processes of the male lizard, *Podarcis sicula sicula*? *Hormones and Behaviour*, **28** 117-129.

Marchlewska-Koj, A. (1997) Sociogenic stress and rodent reproduction. *Neuroscience and Biobehavioural Reviews*, **21** 699-703.

Marić, D., Kostić, T. and Kovačević, R. (1996) Effects of acute and chronic immobilisation stress on rat Leydig cell steroidogenesis. *Journal of Steroid Biochemistry and Molecular Biology*, **58** 351-355.

Mastorakos, G., Webster, E.L., Friedman, T.C. and Chrousos, G.P. (1993) Immunoreactive corticotropin-releasing hormone and its binding sites in the rat ovary. *Journal of Clinical Investigation*, **92** 961-968.

Matteri, R.L., Moberg, G.P. and Watson, J.G. (1986) Adrenocorticotropin-induced changes in ovine pituitary gonadotropin secretion *in vitro. Endocrinology*, **118** 2091-2096.

McDaniel, C.D., Bramwell, R.K., Wilson, J.L. and Howarth, B. (1995) Fertility of male and female broiler breeders following exposure to elevated ambient temperatures. *Poultry Science*, **74** 1029-1038.

McGivern, R.F. and Redei, E. (1994) Adrenalectomy reverses stress-induced suppression of luteinizing hormone secretion in long-term ovariectomized rats. *Physiology & Behaviour*, **55** 1147-1150.

McMaster, M.E., Munkittrick, K.R., Luxon, P.L., Van Der Kraak, G.J. (1994) Impact of low-level sampling stress on interpretation of physiological responses of white sucker exposed to effluent from a bleached kraft pulp mill. *Ecotoxicology and Environmental Safety*, **27** 251-264.

McMaster, M.E., Van Der Kraak, G.J. and Munkittrick, K.R. (1996) An epidemiologic evaluation of the biochemical basis for steroid hormonal depressions in fish exposed to industrial wastes. *Journal of Great Lakes Research*, **22** 153-171.

Melotti, P., Roncarti, A., Garella, E., Carnevali, O., Mosconi, G. and Polzonettimagni, A. (1992) Effects of handling and capture stress on plasma glucose, cortisol and androgen levels in brown trout, *Salmo trutta morpha fario. Journal of Applied Ichthyology*, **8** 234-239.

Michael, A.E. and Cooke, B.A. (1994) A working hypothesis for the regulation of steroidogenesis and germ cell development in the gonads by glucorticoids and 11β-hydroxysteroid dehydrogenase (11βHSD). *Molecular and Cellular Endocrinology*, **100** 55-63.

Mikami, S.-I., Homma, K. and Wada, M. (eds.) (1983) *Avian Endocrinology*, Springer-Verlag, Berlin.

Moberg, G.P. (1987) Influence of the adrenal axis upon the gonads. *Oxford Reviews of Reproductive Biology*, **9** 456-496.

Monder, C., Sakai, R.R., Miroff, Y., Blanchard, D.C. and Blanchard, R.J. (1994a) Reciprocal changes in plasma corticosterone and testosterone in stressed male rats maintained in a visible burrow system: evidence for a mediating role of testicular 11β-hydroxysteroid dehydrogenase. *Endocrinology*, **134** 1193-1198.

Monder, C., Miroff, Y., Marandici, A. and Hardy, M.P. (1994b) 11β-hydroxysteroid dehydrogenase alleviates glucocorticoid-mediated inhibition of steroidogenesis in rat Leydig cells. *Endocrinology*, **134** 1199-1204.

Moore, F.L. (1987) Regulation of reproductive behaviours, in *Hormones and Reproduction in Fishes, Amphibians, and Reptiles* (eds. D.O. Norris and R.E. Jones), Plenum Press, New York, pp 506-522.

Moore, F.L. and Miller, L.J. (1984) Stress-induced inhibition of sexual behaviour: corticosterone inhibits courtship behaviours of a male amphibian (*Taricha granulosa*). *Hormones and Behaviour*, **18** 400-410.

Moore, F.L. and Zoeller, R.T. (1985) Stress-induced inhibition of reproduction: evidence of suppressed secretion of LH-RH in an amphibian. *General and Comparative Endocrinology*, **60** 252-258.

Moore, F.L., Lowry, C.A. and Rose, J.D. (1994) Steroid-neuropeptide interactions that control reproductive behaviours in an amphibian. *Psychoneuroendocrinology*, **19** 581-592.

Moore, M.C., Thompson, C.W. and Marler, C.A. (1991) Reciprocal changes in corticosterone and testosterone levels following acute and chronic handling stress in the tree lizard, *Urosaurus ornatus. General and Comparative Endocrinology*, **81** 217-226.

Mosconi, G., Carnevali, O., Facchinetti, F., Neri, I. and Polzonetti-Magni, A. (1994) Opioid peptide modulation of stress-induced plasma steroid changes in the frog *Rana esculenta*. *Hormones and Behaviour*, **28** 130-138.

Moudgal, R.P., Mohan, J. and Panda, J.N. (1991) Corticosterone-mediated depression in reproductive functioning of white leghorn hens: action mechanism. *Indian Journal of Animal Sciences*, **61** 803-807.

Nagahama, Y. (1987) Endocrine control of oocyte maturation, in *Hormones and Reproduction in Fishes, Amphibians, and Reptiles* (eds. D.O. Norris and R.E. Jones), Plenum Press, New York, pp 171-202.

Nappi, R.E. and Rivest, S. (1995a) Stress-induced genetic expression of a selective corticotropin-releasing factor-receptor subtype within the rat ovaries: an effect dependent on the ovulatory cycle. *Biology of Reproduction*, **53** 1417-1428.

Nappi, R.E. and Rivest, S. (1995b) Corticotropin-releasing factor (CRF) and stress-related reproductive failure: the brain as a state of the art or the ovary as a novel clue? *Journal of Endocrinological Investigations*, **18** 872-880.

Naylor, A.M., Porter, D.W.F. and Lincoln, D.W. (1990) Central administration of corticotropin-releasing factor in the sheep—effects on secretion of gonadotropins, prolactin and cortisol. *Journal of Endocrinology*, **124** 117-125.

Negro-Vilar, A. (1993) Stress and other environmental factors affecting fertility in men and women: overview. *Environmental Health Perspectives Supplements*, **101 (Suppl. 2)** 59-64.

Norberg, B., Bjornsson, B.T., Brown, C.L., Wichardt, U.P., Deftos, L.J. and Haux, C. (1989) Changes in plasma vitellogenin, sex steroids, calcitonin, and thyroid hormones related to sexual maturation in female brown trout (*Salmo trutta*). *General and Comparative Endocrinology*, **75** 316-326.

Norris, D.O. and Jones, R.E. (eds.) (1987) *Hormones and Reproduction in Fishes, Amphibians, and Reptiles,*, Plenum Press, New York.

Novero, R.P., Beck, M.M., Gleaves, E.W., Johnson, A.L. and Deshazer, J.A. (1991) Plasma progesterone, luteinizing hormone concentrations and granulosa cell responsiveness in heat-stressed hens. *Poultry Science*, **70** 2335-2339.

Olster, D.H. and Ferin, M. (1987) Corticotropin-releasing hormone inhibits gonadotropin secretion in the ovariectomized rhesus monkey. *Journal of Clinical Endocrinology and Metabolism*, **65** 262-267.

Orr, T.E., Taylor, M.F., Bhattacharyya, A.K., Collins, D.C. and Mann, D.R. (1994) Acute immobilization stress disrupts testicular steroidogenesis in adult male-rats by inhibiting the activities of 17α-hydroxylase and 17, 20-lyase without affecting the binding of LH/hCG receptors. *Journal of Andrology*, **15** 302-308.

Ottinger, M.A. and Mench, J.A. (1989) Reproductive behaviour in poultry—implications for artificial insemination technology. *British Poultry Science*, **30** 431-442.

Pang, P.K.T. and Schreibman, M.P. (1991a) *Vertebrate Endocrinology: Fundamentals and Biomedical Implications, Volume 4, Part A Reproduction*, Academic Press, San Diego.

Pang, P.K.T. and Schreibman, M.P. (1991b) *Vertebrate Endocrinology: Fundamentals and Biomedical Implications, Volume 4, Part B Reproduction*, Academic Press, San Diego.

Pankhurst, N.W. and Dedual, M. (1994) Effects of capture and recovery on plasma levels of cortisol, lactate and gonadal steroids in a natural population of rainbow trout. *Journal of Fish Biology*, **45** 1013-1025.

Pankhurst, N.W. and Van Der Kraak, G. (1997) Effects of stress on reproduction and growth of fish, in *Fish Stress and Health in Aquaculture* (eds. G.K. Iwama, A.D. Pickering, J.P. Sumpter and C.B. Schreck), Cambridge University Press, Cambridge, pp 73-93.

Pankhurst, N.W., van Der Kraak, G. and Peter, R.E. (1995a) A reassessment of the inhibitory effects of cortisol on ovarian steroidogenesis, in *Reproductive Physiology of Fish, 1995* (eds. F.W. Goetz and P. Thomas), Fish Symposium 95 Austin, p 195.

Pankhurst, N.W., Van Der Kraak, G. and Peter, R.E. (1995b) Evidence that the inhibitory effects of stress on reproduction in teleost fish are not mediated by the action of cortisol on ovarian steroidogenesis. *General and Comparative Endocrinology*, **99** 249-257.

Paolucci, M., Esposito, V., Di Fiore, M.M. and Botte, V. (1990) Effects of short postcapture confinement on plasma reproductive hormone and corticosterone profiles in *Rana esculenta* during the sexual cycle. *Bollettino di Zoologia*, **57** 253-259.

Peter, R.E. and Yu, K.L. (1997) Neuroendocrine regulation of ovulation in fishes: basic and applied aspects. *Reviews in Fish Biology and Fisheries*, **7** 173-197.

Petitte, J.N. and Etches, R.J. (1988) The effect of corticosterone on the photoperiodic response of immature hens. *General and Comparative Endocrinology*, **69** 424-430.

Petitte, J.N. and Etches, R.J. (1989) The effect of corticosterone on the response of the ovary to pregnant mare's serum gonadotrophin in sexually immature pullets. *General and Comparative Endocrinology*, **74** 377-384.

Petitte, J.N. and Etches, R.J. (1991) Daily infusion of corticosterone and reproductive function in the domestic hen (*Gallus domesticus*). *General and Comparative Endocrinology*, **83** 397-405.

Phogat, J.B., Smith, R.F. and Dobson, H. (1997) Effect of adrenocorticotrophic hormone on gonadotrophin releasing hormone-induced luteinizing hormone secretion in vitro. *Animal Reproduction Science*, **48** 53-65.

Pickering, A.D. (1981) Introduction: the concept of biological stress, in *Stress and Fish* (ed. A.D. Pickering), Academic Press, London, pp 1-9.

Pickering, A.D. and Christie, P. (1981) Changes in the concentrations of plasma cortisol and thyroxine during sexual maturation of the hatchery-reared brown trout, *Salmo trutta* L. *General and Comparative Endocrinology*, **44** 487-496.

Pickering, A.D., Pottinger, T.G., Carragher, J. and Sumpter, J.P. (1987) The effects of acute and chronic stress on the levels of reproductive hormones in the plasma of mature male brown trout, *Salmo trutta* L. *General and Comparative Endocrinology*, **68** 249-259.

Pottinger, T.G. and Pickering, A.D. (1990) The effect of cortisol administration on hepatic and plasma estradiol-binding capacity in immature female rainbow trout (*Oncorhynchus mykiss*). *General and Comparative Endocrinology*, **80** 264-273.

Pottinger, T.G., Campbell, P.M. and Sumpter, J.P. (1991) Stress-induced disruption of the salmonid liver-gonad axis, in *Proceedings of the Fourth International Symposium on Reproductive Physiology of Fish, 1991* (eds. A.P. Scott, J.P. Sumpter, D.E. Kime and M.S. Rolfe), FishSymp 91, Sheffield, pp 114-116.

Pottinger, T.G., Balm, P.H.M. and Pickering, A.D. (1995) Sexual maturity modifies the responsiveness of the pituitary-interrenal axis to stress in male rainbow trout. *General and Comparative Endocrinology*, **98** 311-320.

Pottinger, T.G., Carrick, T.R., Hughes, S.E. and Balm, P.H.M. (1996) Testosterone, 11-ketotestosterone, and estradiol-17β modify baseline and stress-induced interrenal and corticotropic activity in trout. *General and Comparative Endocrinology*, **104** 284-295.

Reynard, M. and Savory, C.J. (1997) Oviposition delays induced by social stress are reversed by treatment with the β-adrenergic blocking agent propanolol. *Poultry Science*, **76** 1315-1317.

Rivest, S. and Rivier, C. (1995) The role of cortisotropin-releasing factor and interleukin-1 in the regulation of neurons controlling reproductive functions. *Endocrine Reviews*, **16** 177-199.

Rivest, S., Polsky, P.M. and Rivier, C. (1993) CRF alters the infundibular LHRH secretory system from the medial preoptic area of female rats: possible involvement of opioid receptors *Neuroendocrinology*, **57** 236-246.

Rivier, C. and Rivest, S. (1991) Effect of stress on the activity of the hypothalamic-pituitary-gonadal axis: peripheral and central mechanisms. *Biology of Reproduction*, **45** 523-532.

Rivier, C. and Vale, W. (1984) Influence of corticotropin-releasing factor (CRF) on reproductive functions in the rat. *Endocrinology*, **114** 914-919.

Roozendaal, M.M., Swarts, H.J.M., Wiegant, V.M. and Mattheij, J.A.M. (1995) Effect of restraint stress on the preovulatory luteinizing hormone profile and ovulation in the rat. *European Journal of Endocrinology*, **133** 347-353.

Rose, J.D., Moore, F.L. and Orchinik, M. (1993) Rapid neurophysiological effects of corticosterone on medullary neurons: relationship to stress-induced suppression of courtship clasping in an amphibian. *Neuroendocrinology*, **57** 815-824.

Rosen, H., Jameel, M.L. and Barkan, A.L. (1988) Dexamethasone suppresses gonadotropin-releasing hormone (GnRH) secretion and has direct pituitary effects in male rats—differential regulation of GnRH receptor and gonadotropin responses to GnRH. *Endocrinology*, **122** 2873-2880.

Ruby, S.M., Idler, D.R. and So, Y.P. (1993) Plasma vitellogenin, 17β-estradiol, T_3 and T_4 levels in sexually maturing rainbow trout *Oncorhynchus mykiss* following sublethal HCN exposure. *Aquatic Toxicology*, **26** 91-101.

Safford, S.E. and Thomas, P. (1987) Effects of capture and handling on circulating levels of gonadal steroids and cortisol in the spotted seatrout, *Cynoscion nebulosus*, in *Reproductive Physiology of Fish, 1987* (eds. D.R. Idler, L.W. Crim and J.M. Walsh), Memorial University of Newfoundland, St. Johns, p 312.

Saketos, M., Sharma, M. and Santford, N.F. (1993) Suppression of the hypothalamic-pituitary-ovarian axis in normal women by glucocorticoids. *Biology of Reproduction*, **49** 1270-1276.

Sandor, T. (1972) Corticosteroids in Amphibia, Reptilia, and Aves, in *Steroids in Nonmammalian Vertebrates* (ed. D.R. Idler), Academic Press, London, pp 253-328.

Sapolsky, R.M. (1985) Stress-induced suppression of testicular function in the wild baboon: role of glucocorticoids. *Endocrinology*, **116** 2273-2278.

Sapolsky, R.M. (1986) Stress-induced elevation of testosterone concentrations in high ranking baboons: role of catecholamines. *Endocrinology*, **118** 1630-1635.

Schuett, G.W. (1996) Fighting dynamics of male copperheads, *Agkistrodon contortrix* (Serpentes, Viperidae): stress-induced inhibition of sexual behaviour in losers. *Zoo Biology*, **15** 209-221.

Schuett, G.W., Harlow, H.J., Rose, J.D., Van Kirk, E.A. and Murdoch, W.J. (1996) Levels of plasma corticosterone and testosterone in male copperheads (*Agkistrodon contortrix*) following stages fights. *Hormones and Behaviour*, **30** 60-68.

Sekimoto, K., Imai, K., Kato, Y. and Takikawa, H. (1990) Acute decrease in vitellogenin synthesis by deprivation of food and water in laying hens. *Endocrinologia Japonica*, **37** 319-330.

Selcer, K.W. and Leavitt, W.W. (1991) Estrogens and progestins, in *Vertebrate Endocrinology: Fundamentals and Biomedical Implications, Volume 4, Part B, Reproduction* (eds. P.K.T. Pang and M.P. Schreibman), Academic Press, San Diego, pp 67-114.

Siegel, P.B., Gross, W.B. and Dunnington, E.A. (1989) Effects of dietary corticosterone in young leghorn and meat-type cockerels. *British Poultry Science*, **30** 185-192.

Silverin, B. (1986) Corticosterone binding proteins and behavioural effects of high plasma levels of corticosterone during the breeding period in the pied flycatcher. *General and Comparative Endocrinology*, **64** 67-74.

Spinedi, E., Salas, M., Chisari, A., Perone, M., Carino, M. and Gaillard, R.C. (1994) Sex differences in the hypothalamo-pituitary-adrenal axis response to inflammatory and neuroendocrine stressors. *Neuroendocrinology*, **60** 609-617.

Stratholt, M.L., Donaldson, E.M. and Liley, N.R. (1997) Stress induced elevation of plasma cortisol in adult female coho salmon (*Oncorhynchous kisutch*) is reflected in egg cortisol content, but does not appear to affect early development. *Aquaculture*, **158** 141-153.

Summers, C.H. (1995) Regulation of ovarian recrudescence: different effects of corticotropin in small and large female lizards, *Anolis carolinensis*. *The Journal of Experimental Zoology*, **271** 228-234.

Sumpter, J.P., Carragher, J., Pottinger, T.G. and Pickering, A.D. (1987) The interaction of stress and reproduction in trout, in *Reproductive Physiology of Fish, 1987*, (eds. D.R. Idler, L.W. Crim and J.M. Walsh), Memorial University of Newfoundland, St. Johns, pp 299-302.

Suter, D.E., Schwartz, N.B. and Ringstrom, S.J. (1988) Dual role of glucocorticoids in regulation of pituitary content and secretion of gonadotropins. *American Journal of Physiology*, **254** E595-E600.

Suter, D.E. and Orosz, G. (1989) Effect of treatment with cortisol in vivo on secretion of gonadotropins in vitro. *Biology of Reproduction*, **41** 1091-1096.

Tam, W.H. and Zhang, X.M. (1996) The development and maturation of vitellogenic oocytes, plasma steroid hormone levels, and gonadotrope activities in acid-stressed brook trout (*Salvelinus fontinalis*). *Canadian Journal of Zoology*, **74** 587-593.

Toates, F. (1995) *Stress. Conceptual and Biological Aspects*. John Wiley & Sons, Chichester.

Turnbull, A.V. and Rivier, C. (1997) Inhibition of gonadotropin-induced testosterone secretion by the intracerebroventricular injection of interleukin-1β in the male rat. *Endocrinology*, **138** 1008-1013.

Turner, B.B. (1997) Influence of gonadal steroids on brain corticosteroid receptors: a minireview. *Neurochemical Research*, **22** 1375-1385.

Tyler, C.R. and Sumpter, J.P. (1996) Oocyte growth and development in teleosts. *Reviews in Fish Biology and Fisheries*, **6** 287-318.

Vamvakopoulos, N.C. and Chrousos, G.P. (1993) Evidence of direct estrogenic regulation of human corticotropin-releasing hormone gene expression. Potential implications for the sexual dimorphism of the stress response and immune/inflammatory reaction. *Journal of Clinical Investigation*, **92** 1896-1902.

Van Der Kraak, G., Munkittrick, M.E., McMaster, M.E., Portt, C.B. and Chang, J.P. (1992) Exposure to bleached kraft mill effluent disrupts the pituitary-gonadal axis of white sucker at multiple sites. *Toxicology and Applied Pharmacology*, **115** 224-233.

Viau, V. and Meaney, M.J. (1991) Variations in the hypothalamic-pituitary-adrenal response to stress during the estrous cycle in the rat. *Endocrinology*, **129** 2503-2511.

Viau, V. and Meaney, M.J. (1996) The inhibitory effect of testosterone on hypothalamic-pituitary-adrenal responses to stress is mediated by the medial preoptic area. *The Journal of Neuroscience*, **16** 1866-1876.

Viveiros, M.M. and Liptrap, R.M. (1995) Altered ovarian follicle function in ACTH-treated gilts. *Animal Reproduction Science*, **40** 107-119.

Wallace, R.A., Boyle, S.M., Grier, H.J., Selman, K. and Petrino, T.R. (1993) Preliminary observations on oocyte maturation and other aspects of reproductive biology in captive female snook, *Centropomus undecimalis*. *Aquaculture*, **116** 257-273.

Wang, S. and Edens, F.W. (1993) Heat-stress response of broiler cockerels to manipulation of the gonadal steroids testosterone and estradiol. *Comparative Biochemistry and Physiology*, **106B** 629-633.

Wendelaar Bonga, S.E. (1997) The stress response in fish. *Physiological Reviews*, **77** 591-625.

Williams, J.B., Etches, R.J. and Rzasa, J. (1985) Induction of a pause in laying by corticosterone infusion or dietary alterations: effects on the reproductive system, food consumption and body weight. *British Poultry Science*, **26** 25-34.

Wilson, B.S. and Wingfield, J.C. (1992) Correlation between female reproductive condition and plasma corticosterone in the lizard *Uta stansburiana*. *Copeia*, **(3)** 691-697.

Wilson, C.E., Crim, L.W. and Morgan, M.J. (1995) The effects of stress on spawning performance and larval development in the Atlantic cod, *Gadus morhua* L., in *Reproductive Physiology of Fish, 1995* (eds. F.W. Goetz and P. Thomas), Fish Symposium 95 Austin, p 198.

Wilson, F.E. and Follett, B.K. (1976) Corticosterone-induced gonadosuppression in photo-stimulated tree sparrows. *Life Sciences*, **17** 1451-1456.

Wingfield, J.C. and Silverin, B. (1986) Effects of corticosterone on territorial behaviour of free-living male song sparrows *Melospiza Melodia*. *Hormones and Behaviour*, **20** 405-417.

Wingfield, J.C., Vleck, C.M. and Moore, M.C. (1992) Seasonal changes of the adrenocortical response to stress in birds of the Sonoran desert. *The Journal of Experimental Zoology*, **264** 419-428.

Wingfield, J.C., O'Reilly, K.M. and Astheimer, L.B. (1995) Modulation of the adrenocortical responses to acute stress in Arctic birds: a possible ecological basis. *American Zoologist*, **35** 285-294.

Xiao, E. and Ferin, M. (1997) Stress-related disturbances of the menstrual cycle. *Annals of Medicine*, **29** 215-219.

Xiao, E., Luckhaus, J., Niemann, W. and Ferin, M. (1989) Acute inhibition of gonadotropin secretion by corticotropin-releasing hormone in the primate - are the adrenal glands involved. *Endocrinology*, **124** 1632-1637.

Xiong, F., Suzuki, K. and Hew, C.L. (1994) Control of teleost gonadotropin gene expression, in *Fish Physiology Volume XIII, Molecular Endocrinology of Fish* (eds. N.M. Sherwood and C.L. Hew), Academic Press, New York, pp 135-158.

Zayan, R. (1991) The specificity of social stress. *Behavioural Processes*, **25** 81-93.

Zerani, M., Amabili, F., Mosconi, G. and Gobbetti, A. (1991) Effects of captivity stress on plasma steroid levels in the green frog, *Rana esculenta*, during the annual reproductive cycle. *Comparative Biochemistry and Physiology*, **98A** 491-496.

Ziegler, T.E., Scheffler, G. and Snowdon, C.T. (1995) The relationship of cortisol levels to social environment and reproductive functioning in female cotton-top tamarins, *Saguinus oedipus*. *Hormones and Behaviour*, **29** 407-424.

Zohar, Y. (1980) Dorsal aorta catheterization in rainbow trout (*Salmo gairdneri*): Its validity in the study of blood gonadotropin patterns. *Reproduction, Nutrition, Développement*, **20** 1811-1823.

5 Histological and histopathological effects of stress

S.E. Wendelaar Bonga and P.H.M. Balm

5.1 Introduction

Physiological, biochemical and behavioural changes of animals in response to adverse environmental factors (stressors) all have their impact on the structures of cells, tissues and organs within the stressed animals. Gross morphological examination, as well as histological and histopathological methods and techniques at light and electron microscope level, are therefore useful tools for analysis of the mechanisms of action of stressors and of the expressions of the stress response. They are useful for medical or veterinary diagnosis, as well as for the monitoring of stress in human and animal individuals and populations. Histological changes in general are more persistent than the underlying physiological and biochemical changes. As a result, histology offers parameters to evaluate the effects of chronic stressors in particular. Histological methods and techniques are often the only feasible way for post-mortem analysis or for animal samples collected during field studies.

The technical possibilities for this kind of analysis have been increased significantly by improvement of classical microscopes and by the development of new types of reagents and instruments. For instance, routine histological techniques have been extended with more advanced methods such as *in situ* hybridization, and the introduction of the confocal laser scanning microscope and of advanced computer assisted image processing have greatly facilitated the study of living cells and cellular processes *in situ* (Farkas *et al.*, 1993).

In the vertebrates, two types of structural stress parameters can be distinguished. The first type of parameters are associated with the activation of the regulatory systems involved in the stress response. These concern in particular the hypothalamic–pituitary–adrenal (HPA) axis, with corticosteroids as the ultimate endocrine factors, and the hypothalamic–sympathetic–chromaffin cell axis, with adrenaline and noradrenaline as the main messengers. During acute and chronic stress the neurons and endocrine cells of both axes show the (ultra-)structural characteristics of high secretory activity (e.g., Sanchez *et al.*, 1998). The role of the parasympathetic part of the autonomic nervous system, with acetylcholine as the main messenger, has long been ignored in stress research. Although its importance is now well recognized (Koolhaas and Bohus, 1991), the pathological aspects of parasympathetic overstimulation during severe stress have hardly received attention so far, and this is reflected in this review.

The second type of parameters concern the structural correlates of the actions of the regulatory factors produced by both axes, such as adaptive changes in the blood circulation and ventilation and mobilization of energy substrates. These may vary from changes in muscle structure and capillary outgrowth to depletion of liver glycogen stores and the pathological effects associated with chronically high stress hormone levels. The response of a vertebrate to a stressor is principally an adaptive response directed at survival of the individual, with characteristic alterations in heart rate, oxygen consumption, mobilization of energy stores and suppression of energy-demanding activities such as growth and reproduction that are not of immediate importance for successful coping with the stressor (see Chapters 2, 3 and 4 in this volume). However, apparently, the stress response is meant to be acute or of a limited duration, as is reflected by the circumstance that prolonged and unsuccessful attempts to make the necessary behavioural and physiological adjustments to an intense and persistent stressor will harm the organism (e.g. Chrousos and Gold, 1992). The effects can be caused or triggered by persistently high circulating levels of stress hormones and aggravated by external factors such as pathogens, and they may vary from degenerative changes resulting from exhaustion of endocrine tissues, cardiac and vascular abnormalities as negative side-effects of prolonged tachycardia and hypertension or ulceration of the alimentary tract and other infectious diseases, to neuronal and muscular degeneration, and deviant behaviour such as anorexia nervosa and melancholic depression (Chrousos and Gold, 1992).

In this chapter the vertebrate literature on the histological and histopathological aspects of stress will be reviewed. The field is exceptionally broad, however, and we have chosen to discuss only the most prominent aspects, which will be illustrated by a few examples. The literature on this subject is clearly dominated by mammalian studies. The number of reports on fishes scores second, whereas those on birds, reptiles and amphibians range from scarce to very scarce. This is reflected in this review, which will mainly focus on mammals and fish. This offers the opportunity to compare the histology and pathology of stress in vertebrate representatives of two different environments, the land and the water.

5.2   The hypothalamic–hypophyseal–adrenal axis of the vertebrates

The hypothalamic–hypophyseal–adrenal axis (HPA axis) and its homologue in fishes, the hypothalamic–hypophyseal–interrenal axis (HPI axis), play a very prominent role in the stress response of all vertebrates, with

CRH, ACTH and glucocorticoids (cortisol or corticosterone depending on the species) as their main messengers. In mammals the cytology of the axis has been described extensively, under control as well as stressed conditions, and has been summarized in several excellent reviews (e.g. Nussdorfer, 1986). Although the attention paid to the HPA (or HPI) axis in non-mammalian vertebrates can hardly be described as adequate given the richness of species (only a reasonable number of studies on birds and fish are present, see reviews by Chester Jones and Henderson, 1980), the available literature indicates that the molecular structure of the messengers, the cellular organization as well as the functioning of the axis show a high degree of similarity among the vertebrates, and this reflects a surprising phylogenetic conservation of the system up from the early Devonian radiation of the fishes (Wendelaar Bonga, 1997). This stability reflects the great importance of the system as well as its marked functional flexibility in adaptation to a great variety of aquatic as well as terrestrial habitats during vertebrate evolution.

The activity of the neuroendocrine system is altered dramatically by exposure to a stressful stimulus, with some functions activated and others inhibited. In the brain, extensive neuropeptide circuits are involved in the regulation of adaptive responses to stressors, and these have also been implicated in stress associated pathology. Numerous neuropeptides, including neurotensin, substance P, neuropeptide Y, opioid peptides, bombesin-related peptides, and CRH, have been shown to operate in these circuits (see reviews by Chrousos and Gold (1992) and Hayden-Hixson and Nemeroff (1993)). In this review we will limit ourselves to some comments on stress-associated changes in the HPA axis.

A pivotal role is played by the neuroendocrine neurons producing CRH, located in the paraventricular nucleus of the hypothalamus and terminating in the median eminence, where CRH acts as a stimulator of the pituitary cells with corticotropic activity, ACTH cells and the MSH cells. Increased secretory activity of the CRH cells, reflected in histological signs of increased synthesis and a decline of CRH immunoreactivity in the median eminence (with the exception of fishes, which have no median eminence) are common observations in stressed animals. This is associated with activation of the ACTH cells and, in a more stressor-dependent fashion, of the MSH cells, as is shown by hypertrophy and hyperplasia of these cells and extension of their secretory compartments (Sanchez et al., 1998). The inhibition of vegetative functions and reproduction during stress is reflected, at the level of the pituitary gland, by concomitant decreased secretory activity of the cells producing growth hormone and gonadotropins which, during chronic stress, may lead to cellular involution and apoptosis of these cells. Comparable phenomena have been described for all vertebrates. Teleost fishes have an additional type of pars intermedia endocrine cell type, the somatolactin cells, and these cells can also react strongly (although in a stressor-dependent fashion) in stressed animals (Kakizawa *et al.*, 1995).

The mammalian adrenal glands, with two or three cortical layers (the zona glomerulosa, the zona fasciculata and, in many mammals, the zona reticularis) concentrically arranged around the adrenal medulla, are the most diversified from a cytological point of view. During stress, in particular the zona fasciculata, the location of glucocorticoid production, and the medullary cells (site of the adrenergic or chromaffin cells) become activated, and during chronic stress these areas account for most of the increase in size of the adrenal glands. The glucocorticoid cells show the typical characteristics of steroidogenesis: many mitochondria, with vesicular and/or tubular cristae, prominent smooth endoplasmic reticulum (SER) and some profiles of granular endoplasmic reticulum (GER), a few Golgi areas, and variable numbers of lysosome-like bodies and lipid globules. The cells are partially separated by a network of sinusoidal blood spaces. They respond to secretagogues, of which ACTH is the most prominent one, with an increase in steroid production and release, which is reflected by mitochondrial proliferation, increase in SER, and a transient drop in lipid globules. Long-term ACTH stimulation leads to cellular proliferation, and marked increases in the mitochondrial and SER compartments and extension of the sinusoidal spaces. The zona glomerulosa cells, which produce the mineralocorticoid aldosterone, and the zona reticularis cells, which secrete sex steroids, are also stimulated by ACTH, although angiotensin II and gonadotropins, respectively, are the main secretagogues. In the adrenal glands of the lower vertebrates (birds, reptiles, amphibians) no clear zonation is present. The homologues of the cortical and medullary cells are arranged in strands and clusters, which are normally intermingled. In birds and reptiles corticosterone is the main product, in amphibians corticosterone and aldosterone (Nussdorfer, 1986). In the bony fishes the adrenal homologue is located in the head kidneys, where layers of corticosteroid cells, in conjunction with the clusters of medullary chromaffin cells, surround the main blood vessels (for structural deviations of this pattern, see Chester Jones and Henderson (1980). In all these groups the ultrastructure of the cortical and medullary homologues are very similar to those of the cells of the mammalian adrenals and this applies to both control and stressed conditions (Nussdorfer, 1986). In fishes cortisol is the major corticosteroid in teleosts, and corticosterone in chondrichthyans.

5.2.1 *Effects associated with hyper- and hypoactivity of the HPA axis*

Numerous deleterious effects reported during chronic stress have been related to hyperactivity of the HPA axis, in particular the hypersecretion of CRH and glucocorticoids. These include reduction of growth, reproduction, degenerative effects on the brain and other organs, and diseases as a result of the immunosuppressive actions of these hormones (Chrousos and Gold, 1992).

Chronic stress is typically associated with increased energy demand as well as reduced appetite—with anorexia nervosa as an extreme—and this leads to depletion of energy stores, in particular liver glycogens and body fat. Adrenalin is the major glycogenolytic factor during stress, with glucocorticoid in a supportive role. The latter hormones also stimulate gluconeogenesis, to the detriment of body proteins, and, together with CRH, they are central switches for reallocation of energy streams from reproductive activities and body growth towards functions promoting immediate survival. This leads to a reduction of body mass, in particular because of loss of mass of organs such as liver, fat tissue, striated musculature and gonads. For fish this can be easily and reliably expressed in the condition factor (body mass: body length^3), a widely used parameter of the general health condition and reflecting how well these animals cope with their environment (Goede and Barton, 1990). The histological reflection of these processes are involution of liver cells and muscle cells, reduction of cell volume but increased metabolic activity of fat cells, and involution of the hypothalamic–pituitary–gonadal axis and the gonads, as well as accessory sex organs.

5.2.1.1   The reproductive system
Reproductive failure is a classic symptom of stress. The inhibitory effects of stressors on reproduction are conspicuous and have been demonstrated in all vertebrate species examined (see reviews by Gerking, 1980; Moberg, 1985; Greenberg and Wingfield, 1987; Torpy and Chrousos, 1996; Pottinger, this volume). The effects are manifest at the level of the hypothalamo–pituitary–gonadal axis, on the development of secondary sex organs and characters, on sperm and oocyte development, gamete maturation and release, development of embryos and offspring, and on the recruitment rate. The reports show a marked similarity for the major vertebrate groups. Inhibition of the reproductive neuroendocrine control mechanisms has been reported at the level of the brainstem and of the hypothalamic neurons producing gonadotropin-releasing hormones (although this has so far not been studied in fish; Pankhurst and Van der Kraak, 1997), as well as for the two types of pituitary cells that secrete FSH and LH (or, in fish, the homologous hormones gonadotropin I and II), and in the cells secreting the gonadal steroids. The resulting reduction of circulating androgen and oestrogen levels leads to gonadal involution, in particular of the early stages of oogenesis. In males, it results in lower sperm counts, with reduced fertility (McGrady, 1984).

Involution of the female gonads can be very dramatic in non-mammalian vertebrates with meso- and megalecithal eggs. The large amounts of yolk required by the ovaries during the vitellogenetic period are produced in the liver and transported as vitellogenins, proteins rich in calcium and phosphate, via the blood to the oocytes. This process is easily disrupted by stressors and this is reflected by involution of liver cells and by reduction of growth or atresia of the maturing oocytes, which can affect most of the gonadal tissue in animals such as amphibians, reptiles or fish that produce large numbers of eggs simultaneously (Figure 5.1). Oocyte

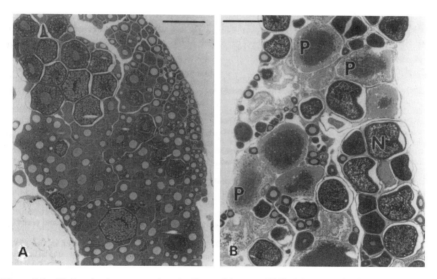

Figure 5.1 Fathead minnow ovaries. A, Control (water pH 8). Many previtellogenic and some vitellogenic oocytes (left upper corner) are present. B, Water pH 6. A few normal oocytes, vitellogenic oocytes and many preovulatory corpora atretica (P) are present. This premature degeneration is typical for stressed fish. Scale bars represent 50 μm. Reproduced with permission from McCormick *et al.* (1989).

atresia begins by erosion of the zona pellucida, and this is followed by swelling and loss of stainability of oocyte yolk material and, finally, disintegration and intra-ovarian resorption (e.g. McCormick *et al.*, 1989). Gamete release is delayed or blocked completely. For reptiles (Mahmoud and Licht, 1997) and fish (Pankhurst and Van der Kraak, 1997) it has been shown that the degree of inhibition by stressors depends on the stage in the gonadal cycle: gonadal growth is blocked more easily at the start of gametogenesis than during subsequent stages. In fish, mature, postvitellogenic follicles appear to be relatively resistant to stress and will continue to undergo final maturation, although spawning may be delayed and the size and numbers of the ova are reduced (Pankhurst and Van der Kraak, 1997). The effects of stress on reproduction are at least partially mediated by endocrine messengers of the HPA axis, with CRH in a prominent role at least in mammals (Chrousos and Gold, 1992). Although high glucocorticoid levels may also be active in this respect, there are also several reports on, for example, reptiles and fish, showing that these steroids have little or no effect (Manzo *et al.*, 1994; Pankhurst *et al.*, 1995) or are even stimulatory, as has been shown for the final maturation of oocytes in fish (Pankhurst and Van der Kraak, 1997).

5.2.1.2   *The gastrointestinal system*

The gastrointestinal system is another organ system that may be affected during stress, which may be mediated by the autonomic nervous system as well as the HPA axis (Archer, 1984). Acute stressors may promote gastric muscular activity and gastrointestinal secretion, peristaltic intestinal motility, and faecal excretion (Buéno and Gué, 1988; Garrick *et al.*, 1988; Lambert and Peacock, 1989). Chronic stress can lead to loss of appetite. The resulting structural effects include intracellular storage of secretory products in the exocrine and endocrine cells of the system and, after prolonged and severe reduction of food intake, cellular involution and loss of all its epithelial cell types, which results in a decrease of the absorptive and secretory capacity. However, such changes are characteristic for low food intake or starvation in general. Typical for chronic stress, however, are the occurrence of pathological changes in the gastric and intestinal mucosa, in particular mucosal erosion and atrophy, hyper- and parakeratosis, and ulceration. Gastric and intestinal ulcers have long been interpreted as mainly resulting from hypersecretion of gastric juices, but now the important contribution of pathogenic organisms has been well established, with pathogens such as *Helicobacter pylori* in humans *Helicobacter pylori* or *Ascaris suum* in pigs (Vaira *et al.*, 1988; O'Brian, 1986) or *Aeromonas* species in reptiles, amphibians and fish as causative agents (Gorden *et al.*, 1979; Goede and Barton, 1990). The mucosa may become corrugated by hyperkeratosis and parakeratosis, and this is followed by mucosal erosion and ulceration. In domestic pigs such phenomena increased from 8% in controls to over 40% in animals after transport and mixing of groups (Hessing *et al.*, 1992). Whereas there are numerous studies on gastric and duodenal pathology as a result of stressors in mammals (e.g. reviews by Weiss, 1977 and Pfeiffer, 1992), for the non-mammalian vertebrates reports on the gastrointestinal tract are scarce. In chickens stressed by elevated temperature for two weeks, reduced food intake and growth rate were associated with decreased villus height and wet and dry mass per unit length of jejunum (Mitchell and Carlisle, 1992). Chickens stressed by water immersion showed erosion of the gizzard epithelium, reduced body weight and reduced antibody titres (Dzaja *et al.*, 1996). In stressed fish reduction of mucous cells (possibly by depletion) and atrophy of the gastric and intestinal mucosae have been described (Peters, 1982; Szakolczai, 1997). Conflict for social dominance in subordinate eels causes serious damage to the stomach. The gastric epithelium shows decreased folding and clear signs of necrosis and erosion, whereas the mucous cells degenerate after depletion of the mucus and the gastric glands atrophy and become partially replaced by connective tissue (Peters, 1982). Detachment of the columnar epithelial cells from the basal membrane as well as epithelial necrosis and inflammation of the lamina propria have been reported several days after capture and transport of the fish (Szakolczai, 1997).

High circulating glucocorticoid levels have long been considered as important mediators of gastrointestinal pathology. They have been reported to raise gastric hydrochloric acid secretion rates and to promote inflammation by reducing immunoresistance. In the gastrointestinal tract of salmonids after anadromous migration to their spawning grounds, when very high cortisol levels prevail, gastric atrophy has been reported and these could be induced in the gastric epithelium by injection of cortisol in Sockeye salmon (McBride and Van Overbeeke, 1971). There are also conflicting reports, however, and it was shown that high corticosterone levels in rats reduced, and reduction of corticosterone secretion increased, the formation and size of gastric erosions (Filaretova *et al.*, 1998)

5.2.1.3 *The skin*
The skin is the largest body organ exposed to the environment and deserves specific attention in this chapter because the skin, in addition to containing many sensory organs and cells—including sensory elements of the immune system—is able to detect potentially threatening or noxious signals, and is a protective barrier that can respond to adverse stimuli, by specific and non-specific actions that are part of the general stress response. These can be mediated by endocrine, or paracrine activity, and be expressed by alterations in, for example, pigmentation, exocrine secretion, keratinization, immune functions, or production of proteins such as heat- or coldshock proteins or metallothioneins. In this section we will concentrate on some actions related to the main hormones involved in the stress response. With respect to these hormones it is of interest that at least the mammalian skin is a target for the hormones of the HPA axis such as CRH, ACTH, MSH and β-endorphin, and also an active site of production of these messengers (Slominski *et al.*, 1993, 1996). Since it has also been reported that keratinocytes produce different cytokines known to modulate the activity of the HPA axis at different levels (Milstone and

Edelson, 1988; Chrousos and Gold, 1992), it has been proposed that the equivalent of the HPA axis is operating in the skin in order to restore peripheral homeostasis during stress (Slominski and Mihm, 1996).

In the highly keratinized skin of terrestrial vertebrates, stress is mainly reflected in increased ageing such as greying and loss of hair in humans and other primates, loss of brilliance of sex coloration of skin, feathers and scales in mammals, birds and reptiles and increased incidence of skin inflammation by pathogens in all vertebrate groups. Skin conditions evoked or exacerbated by stressors including atopic dermatitis, eczema, psoriasis and urticaria are common in humans (Theoharides *et al.*, 1998). The sensitivity of the oral skin to stress was recently confirmed by Cekic-Arambasin *et al.* (1997), who studied a group of patients with recurrent oral aphthous ulceration, before and during the Croatian War. They noticed a significant increase in aphthal recurrence during war time. Patients with a persistent form of this disease have been shown to score significantly higher on an anxiety and depression scale and had higher saliva cortisol levels than patients with a form of the disease responding to therapy (McCartan *et al.*, 1996).

Skin lesions including dermatitis as a result of infestation with viruses, bacteria and ectoparasites have also been reported for birds, reptiles, amphibians and fish (Goldberg and Holshuh, 1993; Klontz, 1995). The pathological phenomena described for the skin of stressed fish include protozoan, bacterial and viral infections, and loss of tissue integrity, in particular between the rays of caudal and pectoral fins, which has been interpreted as necrosis resulting from ischaemia (Klontz, 1995). However, in the typical aquatic vertebrates the poorly or non-keratinized skin has a much more direct relationship with the ambient medium than the thick and keratinized skin of the terrestrial animals, and this is reflected in a higher complexity of cellular composition and functions in the former animals. The transparency of the epidermis of aquatic amphibians and fish offers the possibility of colour display that can be changed by nervous or endocrine innervation in seconds, minutes or days. This is affected by dermal iridophores or chromatophores containing moveable pigment granules. Such processes are responsible for the darkening reported for some fish species during stress (Klontz, 1995) or the melanin patterns in the skin of *Tilapia zillii*, which vary rapidly during social behaviour, including stressful encounters (Hulscher-Emeis, 1992). When stressed, neontetras can change the spectral peak reflected from their light-sensitive iridophores toward longer wavelengths (Nagaishi and Oshima, 1998).

The mucous layer secreted by the mucous cells of the skin epidermis in amphibians and fish has an important protective function in these animals, and this is reflected by marked changes in response to stressors. The mucous cells show increased release activity, which may lead to depletion of their contents and a transient reduction in secretion unless the products of newly differentiated cells become available. In amphibians, a variety of substances, including toxic agents and antibiotic peptides, are released into the mucous layer in response to stressors (Marschal *et al.*, 1992). In fish, the upper layers of the normal epidermal cells (the filament cells) start to release the contents—in which enzymes such as peroxidase have been demonstrated—of small secretory granules produced by these cells into the mucous layer. Also kairomones and pheromones have been reported to be released by fish during stress. Other changes in the skin of stressed fish concern the higher turnover of the epidermal cells, as indicated by increased rates of mitosis, apoptosis and necrosis, the enlargement of intercellular spaces in the epidermis, the infiltration in these spaces of different types of leukocytes, and the extension of the capillary network underlying the epidermis. These changes, with the exception of pavement cell necrosis and leukocyte infiltration, were also observed in the skin of fish after stress-free administration of cortisol (Iger *et al.*, 1994, 1995; Wendelaar Bonga, 1997). In stressed fish, the epidermis covering the primary filaments of the gills shows a marked increase of necrosis and apoptosis of chloride cells, the main ion-transporting cells of the integument (Peters and Hong, 1985; Wendelaar Bonga, 1997).

5.2.1.4   The brain
The brain, in particular the hippocampus, is an important target of steroid hormones, including glucocorticoids, which can easily enter the brain and act on many neurons, in particular those located in the central circuits that lead to their secretion (De Kloet and Voorhuis, 1992). Brain damage has been widely observed in chronically stressed mammals. For instance, victims of prolonged torture have been shown to develop psychiatric disorders as well as cerebral cortical atrophy (Jensen *et al.*, 1982), whereas degeneration and loss of hippocampal neurons has been reported in socially subordinate African vervet monkeys originally caught in the wild and that had been abused by cage mates and died with multiple gastric ulcers and adrenal cortical hyperplasia (Figure 5.2; Uno *et al.*, 1989). It was also observed in three shrews with a low position in the social hierarchy (Fuchs *et al.*, 1995) and in rats exposed to sustained restraint or water immersion (Mizoguchi *et al.*, 1992). The effects reported vary from the reversible decrease of apical dendritic branch points and the length of apical dendrites, to shrinkage of cell bodies, swollen mitochondria, and irreversible loss of neurons, resulting in permanent reduction of hippocampal volume and impaired cognitive ability (Uno *et al.*, 1989; Woolley *et al.*, 1990). In general, neuronal damage and atrophy is concentrated in the same brain areas that contain

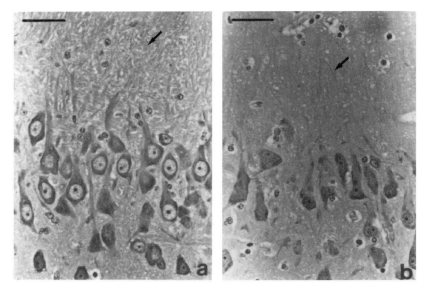

Figure 5.2   Pyramidal neurons in hippocampal CA3 region of vervet monkeys. a, Non-stressed control showing large pyramidal neurons with well-developed dendritic processes and dense mossy fibre endings in zona lucidum (arrow). b, Socially subordinate monkey stressed by social harassment and attack from peers, showing a depletion of neurons with shrunken cell bodies and strophic dendritic processes (arrow). Scale bars, 50 μm. Reproduced with permission from Uno *et al.* (1989).

the highest density of glucocorticoid receptors, most notably the pyramidal neurons of the hippocampal CA regions and of the dentate gyrus, and to a lesser extent the frontal cortex. A direct link has been demonstrated between neuronal degeneration and exposure to high glucocorticoid levels: the same type of brain damage observed in stressed mammals could be produced in rats by experimentally increased circulating glucocorticoid levels, and be prevented in stressed rats by treatment with cyanoketone, a blocker of glucocorticoid synthesis (Magarinos and McEwen, 1995). Exposure of rats for 12 h per day for 3 months to experimentally enhanced levels of corticosterone resulted in a 20% reduction of pyramidal neurons of the hippocampal CA3 area (Sapolsky, 1996). Similar results have been reported for vervet monkeys after implantation of cortisol in the vicinity of the hippocampus (Sapolsky *et al.*, 1990). Administration of the glucocorticoid analogue dexamethasone to pregnant rhesus monkeys induced degeneration and depletion of hippocampal pyramidal and dentate granular neurons in the brain of the foetuses (Figure 5.3; Uno *et al.*, 1990). Moreover, patients suffering from Cushing's syndrome were reported to have a decreased

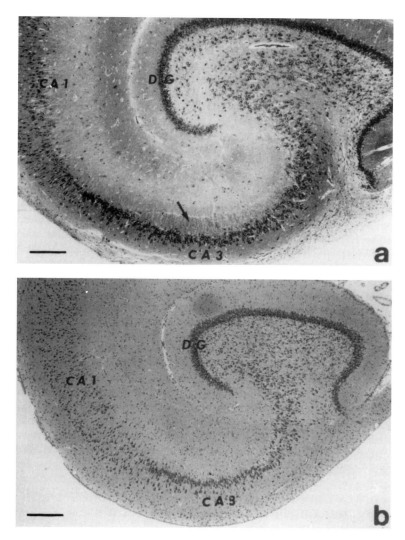

Figure 5.3 Hippocampal gyrus of foetal rhesus monkeys near term (162 days of gestation): a, Vehicle-treated control showing well-developed dentate gyrus (DG) and CA regions with well-arranged CA3 pyramidal neurons forming zona lucidum (arrow); b, Dexamethasone-treated ($4\times1.25\,mg\,kg^{-1}$, at 132 and 133 days of gestation) monkey, showing overall reduction of hippocampal gyrus with poorly developed neurons and regional structures. Scale bars 400 μm. Reproduced with permission from Uno *et al.* (1990).

hippocampal volume to an extent that correlated positively with glucocorticoid levels (Starkman *et al.*, 1992).

Several authors have emphasized the similarities between the sustained effects of stress or experimentally elevated glucocorticoid levels with the symptoms of ageing of the hippocampus. This can partially be explained by the increased sensitivity of the hippocampal neurons to the neurotoxic action of glucocorticoids (Fuxe *et al.*, 1996) and partially by the gradual rise in circulating glucocorticoid levels during ageing, as shown for instance in ageing rats (Sapolsky, 1992). In addition, the ageing brain may also reflect the cumulated effects of stressful experiences during life. Ageing effects on the hippocampus can be reduced by prolonged treatment of rats with the glucocorticoid-receptor blocker RU 486 (Talmi *et al.*, 1993, 1996).

Glucocorticoids have also been reported to increase the sensitivity of hippocampal neurons to the damaging effects of high levels of excitatory amino acids in the brain, and to increase the impact of ischaemia or hypoglycaemia on the hippocampus (Tombaugh *et al.*, 1992; Stein-Behrens *et al.*, 1994; McEwen, 1992).

The mechanism underlying the degenerative actions of glucocorticoids has only partially been elucidated. Clear signs of apoptosis seem to be absent (Masters *et al.*, 1989) and cell death by necrosis seems to be the major mechanism (Sapolsky, 1996). The damage to the cells may be mediated by an increase of the cytosolic calcium ion concentration and by oxygen radical formation, which then ends in damage to membrane lipids, enzymes and cytoskeletal proteins (Stein-Behrens *et al.*, 1994; Sapolsky, 1996).

Not only high glucocorticoid levels, but also chronic hyposecretion of glucocorticoids can induce neuronal degeneration, although this effect seems to be limited to the dentate gyrus of the hippocampus. Increased apoptosis of the granulated neurons in the dentate gyrus has been reported after long-term adrenalectomy to rats, and this effect can be prevented by corticosterone administration (Sloviter *et al.*, 1989).

No studies are known to us on brain damage by high glucocorticoid levels in non-mammalian vertebrates.

5.3 The autonomic nervous system

The sympathetic and parasympathetic branches of the autonomic nerves system and the adrenal medulla alter heart rate, vascular resistance, contractions of the smooth muscles of the digestive system and the secretory activity of several exocrine glands. During stress the release of large amounts of catecholamines from the adrenal medulla and nerve terminals can dramatically increase heart rate, blood pressure and ventilation rate, as well as mobilize glucose from hepatic stores, thus facilitating energy production for the stress response. Since the pioneering studies of Cannon (1929) that resulted in his 'fight or flight' concept, the activation of the sympathetic branch of the autonomic nervous system and the adrenal medulla has been known as an integral part of the response of vertebrates to acute threat.

5.3.1   The cardiovascular system

The massive release of adrenaline, mainly from the adrenal medulla, and noradrenaline from the medulla as well as the overflow from sympathetic nerves, stimulates cardiac output by accelerating heart rate, and raises blood pressure by vasoconstriction of the splanchnic, renal and cutaneous blood vessels. Emotional stress is well known as a contributing factor for the development of degenerative changes of the cardiovascular system in mammals. These changes involve the structure and metabolism of the muscular and endothelial tissues as well as reduction in myocardial capacity, haemodynamic disturbances and, eventually, heart failure. Coronary heart disease, with myocardial infarction as one of the most common forms, is a well-known risk of stress, although stress is only one of the risk factors producing this disorder in humans, with ageing, cigarette smoking, high cholesterol levels, hypertension, obesity and diabetes mellitus as other important causal factors (see reviews by Glass, 1977; Moberg, 1985; Bohus and Koolhaas, 1993).

The damage to the blood vessels is concentrated in the intima (the inner elastin layer of the vessels), the underlying periarterial muscle layer, and the covering endothelium. The most prominent effects are thickening of the smooth muscle coat by proliferation of the myocytes and penetration of these cells in the intima, and hardening and loss of elasticity of the vessel wall by rupture of the elastin fibres and replacement by more fibrous material. The endothelial cell layers undergo changes that facilitate the aggregation of blood platelets which may become incorporated into arterial plaques and these may contribute to the narrowing and hardening of the vessel wall. Damage to the cardiac muscles is reflected in altered, usually reduced, enzymatic activity, in particular of mitochondrial enzymes such as dehydrogenases, oxidases and esterases, disorganization and fragmentation of myofilament bundles, focal necrosis, increased incidence of apoptosis, with signs of lysis of myofilaments, swelling of mitochondria and tubular and sarcoplasmic systems and disruption of mitochondrial cristae. Inflammatory cells may invade the affected vascular wall, where macrophages are scavenging the damaged tissue components.

Under acute stress, arterial changes can occur rapidly, as has been demonstrated for instance in a study on pigs stressed by electrostimulation of the legs, where most of the degenerative changes mentioned above became already visible within 16–48 h after the restraint stress (Jönsson and Johansson, 1974) and in rats exposed for 4 h to −20°C (Lopes *et al.*, 1992). Also chronic exposure to stressors, in particular adverse psychogenic factors, can lead to cardiac and vascular pathology, and irreversible cardiac dysfunction. Atherosclerotic changes have been described for instance in the aorta and coronary arteries of rats kept in a colony with serious social disorder (Henry and Stephens, 1977), cynomolgus monkeys (Manuck *et al.*, 1983) and pigs after social isolation (Ratcliffe *et al.*, 1969). Focal myocardial necrosis and fibrosis has been reported for many species and different stressors, e.g. rats undergoing chronic social stress (Henry and Stephens, 1977), in crowded rabbits (Weber and Van der Walt, 1975), or after restraint in hamsters (Tapp *et al.*, 1989). For pigs exposed to stressful situations, a high incidence of subepicardial and subendocardial haemorrhages in the heart muscle was reported (Hessing, 1993).

The impact of stressors on the cardiovascular system is determined by different factors of which the degree of hypertension produced by the stressors seems to be the most important. In mammals, chronic hypertension originating from stressors (secondary hypertension) has the same structural cardiovascular aetiology as inherited (primary or essential) hypertension, and the extent of cardiovascular lesions is in general directly related to the height of blood pressure (Folkow, 1982; Trevi *et al.*, 1995). Apparently, heart and vessels cannot withstand prolonged, elevated blood pressure, or even brief periods of very high pressure, without substantial structural damage. The effects are at least for an important part mediated by the hypertensive effects of catecholamines, which result from enhanced cardiac output and raised systemic resistance. There is a surprising similarity between the cardio-myopathy caused by such acute stressors and the damage produced by the administration of high doses of catecholamines, as was already shown for rats more than twenty five years ago (Ferrans *et al.*, 1972). Heart failure, through for instance ventricular fibrillation, as well as athero-sclerosis are well-known effects of sustained overactivity of the sympathetic medullary system (Bohus and Koolhaas, 1993). The atherosclerosis resulting from chronic social stress in rats correlated well with the development of irreversible hypertension (Henry *et al.*, 1975). Similarly, Carlsten *et al.* (1994) showed that experimentally induced restraint stress in pigs caused myocardial cell necrosis to an extent directly related to the increase in plasma adrenaline and noradrenaline levels.

The mechanisms involved in the origin of cardiovascular damage during stress are complex, and there is probably more than one causal factor. Several studies have shown that β-adrenoceptor blockers can prevent the structural damage produced by acute stressors or adminis-tration of catecholamines. For instance, pretreatment of pigs with the β-blocker propanolol prevented the myocardial necrosis normally following a restraint stress protocol in these animals, even though the catecholamine levels were higher than in control treated pigs (Häggendahl *et al.*, 1982). The subcellular alterations in the myocardium of rats caused by cold stress could also be prevented by propanolol (Lopes *et al.*, 1992). Interestingly, treatments with some chemicals without β-blocking activity have produced similar results. Pretreatments of pigs with zinc, selenium and α-tocopherol, which effectively reduce cytotoxic free radical levels during stress, reduce the degree of myocardial necrosis following restraint stress, despite the presence of high catecholamine levels (Häggendahl *et al.*, 1987; Carlsten *et al.*, 1994). These results suggest that heart lesions resulting from stress may be caused by β-adrenoceptor-mediated production of cytotoxic free radicals. Oxidative stress is now considered to play a significant role in the development of endothelial dysfunction and disturbance of cardiac structure and function. Other factors proposed to explain myocardial damage during stress include hypoxia of the myocytes caused by overcharging of the heart by catecholamines. Lopes *et al.* (1997) have shown recently that the disruptive subcellular alterations in the myocardium of rats by cold stress can be reduced dramatically by amiodarone, a drug known to decrease myocardial oxygen consumption. Several pathogens, in particular *Chlamydia pneumoniae*, cytomegalovirus and herpes simplex virus, have been demonstrated in human atherosclerotic lesions, and infection with these agents has been suggested to increase the risk of atherosclerosis (Chiu *et al.*, 1997). Experimental infection of rabbits with *C. pneumoniae* was shown to produce atherosclerotic-like changes in the aortas of these animals (Fong *et al.*, 1997; Laitinen *et al.*, 1997). It is highly possible that the immunosuppression during stress promotes this type of arterial infection, and that these pathogens are a contributing factor to the initiation and development of atherosclerosis.

Oxidative damage to the endothelium as for instance caused by inflammation has been identified as a major factor mediating cardiovascular disturbances (Rösen *et al.*, 1995), and drugs effective in inhibiting inflammatory cytokines, nitric oxide (NO) or endothelin are also effective in reducing cardiovascular damage and promoting recovery (e.g. Colucci, 1997). Nitric oxide is a vasorelaxing agent released by many cell types including endothelial cells in response to vasodilating substances such as acetylcholine. It is also produced during inflammation by macrophages and neutrophils when stimulated by cytokines or endotoxins, in particular where it acts at high concentration, as a cytotoxic agent. Prolonged overexcitation or vascular injury can also lead to production of excessive amounts of NO during stress, where chronic hypertension is associated with extensive splanchnic vasodilatation (Pizcueta *et al.*, 1992).

The actions of NO, by interacting with superoxide anion, can lead to the production of hydroxyl radicals known to produce cell damage and injury, including vascular wall necrosis, vascular disruption and oedema (Hogg *et al.*, 1992; Whittle, 1995).

Myocardial remodelling and hypertrophy is a common phenomenon during chronic stress, as an adaptive mechanism to increased haemodynamic load and the resulting damage to cardiovascular structure and function. Typically this leads to an increase in cell size and not cell proliferation, and is accompanied by a transient increase in apoptosis of myocytes, and changes in quantity and composition of the extracellular matrix. Many factors such as cytokines, growth factors and hormones, including catecholamines, are involved in this process (Teerlink *et al.*, 1994; Li *et al.*, 1997).

The relationship between stress and atherosclerosis has also been established for lower vertebrates, from birds to fish. The histopathology is similar to that of mammals (Figure 5.4). It has been established for instance in chickens of both sexes when kept in mixed sex groups (Ratcliffe and Snyder, 1967). Socially stressed roosters had a greater incidence and severity of aortic atherogenesis than non-stressed birds (Wong *et al.*, 1992). Coronary atherosclerosis in fish has first been described in salmonids during and after anadromous migration towards their spawning grounds. The condition was characterized by highly vacuolated, although intact, endothelial cells, thinning and interruption of the inner elastic layers, proliferation of smooth muscle cells of the muscular media layer and penetration of these cells into the intima, and disruption and thinning of the media itself. These phenomena have been ascribed to the severe physiological stress during migration and spawning in combination with the high plasma sex steroid levels in steelhead trout (McKenzie *et al.*, 1978) and with migration in the presence of high circulating levels of apo-β peptide containing low-density lipoproteins in Chinook salmon (Eaton *et al.*, 1984). Similar observations have been reported in studies on steelhead trout and Coho salmon from water containing toxic metals and organic pollutants (House and Benditt, 1981; Muller, 1983). A causal or mediating role of haemodynamic factors has been suggested by Saunders *et al.* (1992) who explained the frequent incidence of atherosclerotic lesions in salmonids with the mechanical stress produced in the coronary artery by the distension of the bulbus arteriosus following contraction of the ventricle. This hypothesis was investigated by García-Garrido *et al.* (1993), who found that the incidence of this type of lesions in dogfish was significantly correlated with areas of high mechanical stress such as arterial bifurcations or high pulsatile flow, as well as with total body length and age, and haemodynamic forces were considered important causal factors.

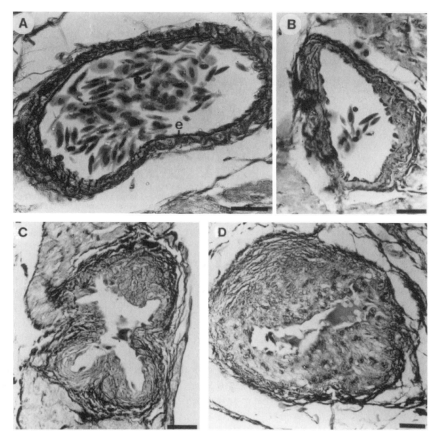

Figure 5.4 Sections of coronary intramyocardial ventricular branches in dogfish (*Scyliorhinus canicula*). A, Normal artery with intact inner elastic layer (e); B–D, Increasing grades of lesion severity. Note breakage and disappearance of the inner elastic layer and thickening of the intimal layer and reduction of the lumen. Scale bars, 30 μm. Reproduced with permission from García-Garrido *et al.* (1993).

5.3.2 The gills of fish

A specific type of histopathological alteration in fish, that may be ascribed to stress-related increase in blood pressure, is the so-called 'epithelial lifting' in the gills. This is the swelling of the respiratory filaments of the gills as a result of the dissociation of the skin epithelium of the underlying basal lamina and associated connective tissue and endothelium lining the blood spaces. This swelling has been reported for fish exposed to a large variety of water pollutants, including heavy metals and organic toxicants (Mallatt, 1985) as well as during stress caused by transport, confinement or handling of fish (Wendelaar Bonga, 1997). It has been interpreted as osmotic swelling after damage of the epithelium by toxic agents. However, epithelial lifting occurs not only in freshwater fish, which are experiencing an osmotic gradient across the integument that might favour osmotic swelling of the intercellular space (inside: ±325 mOsm; water: 1–5 mOsm), but also in seawater fish. These fish are facing an osmotic gradient in the reverse direction (inside: ±335 mOsm l^{-1}) water: ±1000 mOsm l^{-1}). In our opinion epithelial lifting is not a toxic and/or osmotic effect, but a phenomenon caused by the high blood pressure in stressed fish. Many water pollutants are known to produce a stress response in fish (see review by Wendelaar Bonga, 1997). Moreover, we have also observed epithelial lifting in salmon and trout that were stressed by transport or by handling and netting (Wendelaar Bonga, unpublished) or in rainbow trout infected with sea lice on the skin outside the branchial area. Sea lice infection is very stressful for trout (Nolan *et al.*, 1997). Epithelial lifting could furthermore be produced in a so-called 'isolated head' preparation in which the vascular circulation was maintained by a peristaltic pump with an iso-osmotic Ringer fluid replacing the blood. High hydrostatic pressure of the fluid and addition to the fluid of adrenaline to open the branchial sphincters of the vessels to the lamellae lead to the same type of epithelial lifting as produced in severely stressed fish *in vivo* (our unpublished observations).

A second phenomenon typical for aquatic vertebrates is the increase of the permeability to water, ions and even macromolecules of the integument, in particular the branchial epithelia (Mazeaud *et al.*, 1977; McDonald and Milligan, 1997). This leads to increased osmotic uptake of water and passive outward diffusion of ions in freshwater fish, and of osmotic water loss and inflow of ions in seawater fish. These passive movements need active compensation by the fish, and this is reflected histologically in increased differentiation of chloride cells in the epithelium of the branchial filaments, and for instance in salmonid species, migration of these cells to the branchial lamellae. The increased permeability may also facilitate the penetration of antigens from the water into the epithelium of skin and gills (Nakanishi and Ototake, 1997), and this forms an explanation for the migration of leukocytes (in particular lymphocytes and macrophages) from the cutaneous blood vessels into the intercellular spaces of these epithelia, where they can be found singly or in clusters, sometimes in very high numbers. The increased permeability of the integument to water, ions and other substances in stressed fish is most likely caused by high circulating catecholamines. Adrenaline is known to increase the osmotic permeability to water and ions of the gills (McDonald and Milligan, 1997).

5.4 Individual differences in the stress response

The mode of response to a stressor is dependent on extrinsic and intrinsic (genetic) factors, which determine the perception of the stressor by an individual, and its preferred strategy to cope with stressors. Observations on different vertebrate populations, varying from mammals including humans (Glass, 1977; Koolhaas et al., 1997) to birds (Verbeek, 1998) and fish (Van Raaij et al., 1996) have revealed individual variations in behaviour towards a stressor, with active (or pro-active) and passive (or reactive) behaviour as the two main categories. Both behaviour patterns (coping strategies) have their own functional significance and both can be equally successful depending on the social or environmental conditions. The individual differences in behaviour are also reflected at the neuroendocrine level, with sympathetic reactivity towards stressors more pronounced in animals with an active, more aggressive coping style, and reactivity of the HPA axis and parasympathetic nervous system dominating in individuals with a passive coping style. The coping styles are further reflected in the pathology of the stressed individuals, with active copers having a higher sensitivity to pathologies related to overstimulation of the sympathetic system such as cardiovascular disorders, and passive copers with those related to high glucocorticoid levels such as neuronal degeneration in the hippocampus, and infections such as gastrointestinal and epidermal ulcerations (Koolhaas and Van Oortmerssen, 1988). For instance, the incidence of atherosclerotic lesions in male rats after chronic social stress correlated positively not only with the development of hypertension but also with social dominance (Henry et al., 1975), which is characterized by an active coping style and high circulating catecholamine levels during stress (Bohus and Koolhaas, 1993). In a study on domestic pigs exposed to stressful situations, 65.6% of the animals with an active behavioural response showed subepicardial and subendocardial haemorrhages in the heart muscle, and 34.4% of the animals with a passive behavioural response. Only the latter showed adrenocortical hypertrophy (Hessing et al., 1994). Thus, as a result of these individual differences in the stress response of the vertebrates, one may always expect a high degree of individual variation for every stress parameter investigated.

Other factors contributing to individual variation are individual experiences, sex, or life stage. Of great importance are the morphogenetic effects of perinatal stress experiences on the development of the stress response. It has now been well established that the intensity of the response to a standard stressor can be modified substantially by the experience of early emotional and physical stressors. The consequences resulting from strong neonatal stressful stimuli may persist throughout life by altered stress responsiveness effected by modified neuroendocrine secretion patterns, and structurally reflected by signs of different cellular activity such as changed mRNA levels and glucocorticoid receptor densities in the brain. For instance, rats exposed to infantile stimulation or handling, maternal separation, physical trauma, or endotoxin administration, show increased HPA responsiveness to stressors during later life (Meaney *et al.*, 1996). Such changes can also be induced by experimental manipulation of CRH/AVP or cortisol levels (Meaney *et al.*, 1996; De Kloet *et al.*, 1996; McEwen, 1997). These hormones, when applied perinatally, are able to modify persistently the responses of the neuroendocrine system to stressors. Sex hormones not only mediate gender differences in the impact of stressors, but can also greatly modify the impact of stressors of an individual, for instance by modulating hormone receptor densities and hormone secretion rates, for instance of CRH, ACTH and cortisol. Such effects have been reported for all vertebrate groups (Greenberg and Wingfield, 1987; Pottinger *et al.*, 1996). Recently Barry *et al.* (1997) has presented evidence indicating that the rapid degeneration of many tissues and organs of Pacific salmon, resulting in massive mortality of the animals, is mediated by the actions of extremely high cortisol levels in concert with high 17α, 20β-dihydroxy-4-pregnen-3-one levels, which stimulate cortisol synthesis and inhibit cortisol metabolizing enzymes.

Thus, genetic factors as well as life stage and individual experiences are important determinants of the intensity of the stress response and of the type of lesions associated with this response. As a result of the individual variation in the stress response within a population, one may always expect a high degree of individual variation for every stress parameter investigated, including the histological and histopathological parameters.

References

Archer, J. (1984) *Animals under Stress*. Arnold, London.

Barry, T.P., Riebe, D.J., Parrish, J.J. and Malison, J.A. (1997) Effects of 17 alpha, 20 beta-dihydroxy-4-pregnen-3-one on cortisol production by rainbow trout interrenal tissue *in vitro*. *General and Comparative Endocrinology*, **107** 172-181.

Bohus, B. and Koolhaas, J. (1993) Stress and the cardiovascular system: Central and peripheral physiological mechanisms, in *Stress from Synapse to Syndrome* (eds. S.C. Stanford and P. Salmon), Academic Press, London.

Buéno, L. and Gué, M. (1988) Evidence for the involvement of corticotropin-releasing factor in the gastrointestinal disturbances induced by acoustic and cold stress in mice. *Brain Research*, **441** 1-4.

Cannon, W.B. (1929) *Bodily Changes in Pain, Hunger, Fear and Rage*. Appleton Century Crofts, New York.

Carlsten, J., Bjurström, S., Häggendal, J. and Jönsson, L. (1994) Reduction of heart lesions after experimental restraint stress: a study in stress-susceptible pigs. *Journal of Veterinary Medicine*, **A41** 722-730.

Cekic-Arambasin, A., Maler, G., Topic, B. and Mravak-Stipetic, M. (1997) The effect of stress on the occurrence of oral recurrent aphthous ulceration. *Acta Stomatologica Croatica*, **31** 35-41.

Chester Jones, I. and Henderson, I.W. (eds.) (1980) *General, Comparative and Clinical Endocrinology of the Adrenal Cortex*, Academic Press, London.

Chiu, B., Viira, E., Tucker, W. and Fong, I.W. (1997) Chlamydia pneumoniae, cytomegalovirus, and herpes simplex virus in atherosclerosis of the carotid artery. *Circulation*, **96** 2144-2148.

Chrousos, P. and Gold, P.W. (1992) The concepts of stress and stress system disorders. *Journal of the American Medical Association*, **267** 1244-1252.

Colucci, W.S. (1997) Molecular and cellular mechanisms of myocardial failure. *American Journal of Cardiology*, **80** 15L-25L.

De Kloet, E.R. and Voorhuis, Th.A.M. (1992) Neuropeptides, steroid hormones, stress and reproduction. *Journal of Controlled Release*, **21** 105-116.

De Kloet, E.R., Rots, N.Y. and Cools, A.R. (1996) Brain corticosteroid hormone dialogue: slow and persistent. *Cellular and Molecular Neurobiology*, **16** 345-356.

Dzaja, P., Grabarevic, Z., Peric, J., Mazija, H., Prukner-Radovcic, E., Bratulic, M., Zubcic, D. and Ragland, W.L.III (1996) Effects of histamine application and water-immersion stress on gizzard erosion and fattening of broiler chicks. *Avian Pathology*, **25** 359-367.

Eaton, R.P., McConnell, T., Hnath, J.G., Black, W. and Swartz, R.E. (1984) Coronary myointimal hyperplasia in freshwater Lake Michigan salmon (genus *Oncorhynchus*). Evidence for lipoprotein-related atherosclerosis. *American Journal of Pathology*, **116** 311-318.

Farkas, D.L., Baxter, G. and DeBiasio, R.L. (1993) Multimode light microscopy and the dynamics of molecules, cells, and tissues. *Annual Review of Physiology*, **55** 785-817.

Ferrans, V.J., Hibbs, R.G., Ciprinao, P.R. and Buma, L.M. (1972) Histochemical and electron microscopic studies of norepinephrine-induced myocardial necrosis in rats, in *Myocardiology, Recent advances in studies on cardiac structure and metabolism* (eds. E. Bajusz and G. Rona), University Park Press, Baltimore, pp 495-525.

Filaretova, L.P., Filaretov, A.A. and Makara, G.B. (1998) Corticosterone increase inhibits stress-induced gastric erosions in rats. *American Journal of Physiology*, **37** G1024-G1030.

Folkow, B. (1982) Physiological aspects of primary hypertension. *Physiological Reviews*, **62** 347-504.

Fong, I.W., Chiu, B., Viira, E., Fong, M.W., Jang, D. and Mahony, J. (1997) Rabbit model for *Chlamydia pneumoniae* infection. *Journal of Clinical Microbiology*, **35** 48-52.

Fuchs, E., Uno, H. and Flugge, G. (1995) Chronic psychosocial stress induces morphological alterations in hippocampal pyramidal neurons of the tree shrew. *Brain Research*, **673** 275-282.

Fuxe, K., Diaz, R., Cintra, A., Bhatnagar, M., Tinner, B., Gustafsson, J.A., Ogren, S.O. and Agnati, L.F. (1996) On the role of glucocorticoid receptors in brain plasticity. *Cellular and Molecular Neurobiology*, **16** 239-258.

Garcia-Garrido, L., Muñoz-Chápuli, R. and de Andrés, V. (1993) Coronary arteriosclerosis in dogfish (*Scyliorhinus canicula*). An assessment of some potential risk factors. *Arteriosclerosis and Thrombosis*, **13** 876-885.

Garrick, T., Veiseh, A., Sierra, A., Weiner, H. and Taché, Y. (1988) Corticotropin-releasing factor acts centrally to suppress stimulated gastric contractility in the rat. *Regulatory Peptides*, **21** 173-181.

Gerking, S.D. (1980) Fish reproduction and stress, in *Environmental Physiology of Fishes* (ed. Ali Ma), Plenum Press, New York, pp 569-587.

Glass, D.C. (1977) Stress, behavior patterns, and coronary disease. *American Scientist*, **65** 177-182.

Goede, R.W. and Barton, B.A. (1990) Organismic indices and an autopsy-based assessment as indicators of health and condition of fish. *American Fisheries Society Symposium*, **8** 93-108.

Goldberg, S.R. and Holshuh, H.J. (1993) Histopathology in a captive yarrow's spiny lizard, *Sceloporus jarrovii (Phrynosomatidae)*, attributed to the mite *Hirstiella sp. Pterygosomatidae. Transactions of the American Microscopical Society*, **112** 234-237.

Gorden, R.W., Hazen, T.C., Esch, G.W. and Fliermans, C.B. (1979) Isolation of *Aeromonas hydrophila* from the American alligator, *Alligator mississippiensis. Journal of Wildlife Diseases*, **15** 239-243.

Greenberg, N. and Wingfield, J. (1987) Stress and Reproduction: reciprocal relationships, in *Hormones and Reproduction in Fishes, Amphibians and Reptiles* (eds. D.O. Norris and R.E. Jones) Plenum Press, New York, pp 461-503.

Häggendahl, J., Johansson, G., Jönsson, L. and Thorén-Tolling, K. (1982) Effect of propranolol on myocardial cell necroses and blood levels in pigs subjected to stress. *Acta Pharmacologica et Toxicologica*, **50** 58-66.

Häggendahl, J., Jönsson, L., Johansson, G., Bjurström, S., Carlsten, J. and Thorén-Tolling, K. (1987) Catecholamine-induced free radicals in myocardial cell necrosis on experimental stress in pigs. *Acta Physiologica Scandinavica*, **131** 447-452.

Hayden-Hixson, D.M. and Nemeroff, C.B. (1993) Roles of neuropeptides in responding and adaptation to stress, in *Stress from Synapse to Syndrome* (eds. S.C. Stanford and P. Salmon), Academic Press, New York and San Diego, pp 355-391.

Henry, J.P. and Stephens, P.M. (1977) *Stress, Health and the Social Environment: A sociobiological Approach to Medicine*. Springer, Berlin.

Henry, J.P., Stephens, P.M. and Santisteban, A. (1975) A model of psychosocial hypertension showing reversibility and progression of cardiovascular complications. *Circulation Research*, **36** 156-164

Hessing, M. (1993) *Individual behavioural characteristics in pigs and their consequences for pig husbandry*. Thesis, University of Wageningen.

Hessing, M.J.C., Geudeke, M.J., Scheepens, C.J.M., Tielen, M.J.M., Schouten, W.G.P. and Wiepkema, P.R. (1992) Mucosal lesions in the pars oesophagea in pigs: prevalence and influence of stress. *Tijdschrift voor Diergeneeskunde*, **117** 445-450.

Hessing, M.J.C., Hagelsø, A.M., Van Beek, J.A.M., Wiepkema, P.R. and Schouten, W.G.P. (1994) Individual behavioral and physiological strategies in pigs. *Physiology and Behavior*, **55** 39-45.

Hogg, N., Darley-Usmar, V.M., Wilson, T. and Moncada, S. (1992) Production of hydroxyl radicals from the simultaneous generation of superoxide and nitric oxide. *Biochemical Journal*, **281** 419-424.

House, E.W. and Benditt, E.P. (1981) The ultrastructure of spontaneous coronary arterial lesions in steelhead trout (*Salmo gairdneri*). *American Journal of Pathology*, **104** 250-257.

Hulscher-Emeis, T.M. (1992) The variable colour patterns of *Tilapia zillii (Cichlidae)*: Integrating ethology, chromatophore regulation and the physiology of stress. *Netherlands Journal of Zoology*, **42** 525-560.

Iger, Y., Lock, R.A.C., Jenner, H.A. and Wendelaar Bonga, S.E. (1994) Cellular responses in the skin of carp (*Cyprinus carpio*) exposed to copper. *Aquatic Toxicology*, **29** 49-64.

Iger, Y., Balm, P.H.M., Jenner, H.A. and Wendelaar Bonga, S.E. (1995) Cortisol induces stress-related changes in the skin of rainbow trout (*Oncorhynchus mykiss*). *General and Comparative Endocrinology*, **97** 188-198.

Jensen, T.S., Genefke, I.K., Hyldebrandt, N., Pedersen, H., Petersen, H.D. and Weile, B. (1982) Cerebral atrophy in young torture victims. *New England Journal of Medicine*, **307** 1341.

Jönsson, L. and Johansson, G. (1974) Cardiac muscle cell damage induced by restraint stress. *Virchows Archiv B Cell Pathology*, **17** 1-12.

Kakizawa, S., Kaneko, T., Hasegawa, S. and Hirano, T. (1995) Effects of feeding, fasting, background adaptation, acute stress, and exhaustive exercise on the plasma somatolactin concentrations in rainbow trout. *General and Comparative Endocrinology*, **98** 137-146.

Klontz, G.W. (1995) Care of fish in biological research. *Journal of Animal Science*, **73** 3485-3492.

Koolhaas, J.M. and Bohus, B (1991) Coping strategies and cardiovascular risk: a study of rats and mice, in *Behavioral Observations in Cardiovascular Research* (eds. A. Appels, J. Broen and J. Koolhaas), Swets and Zeitlinger, Amsterdam, pp 45-58.

Koolhaas, J.M. and Van Oortmerssen, G.A. (1988) Individual differences in disease susceptibility as a possible factor in the population dynamics of rats and mice. *Netherlands Journal of Zoology*, **38** 111-122.

Koolhaas, J.M., de Boer, S.F. and Bohus, B. (1997) Motivational systems or motivational states: behavioural and physiological evidence. *Applied Animal Behaviour Science*, **53** 131-143.

Laitinen, K., Laurila, A., Pyhala, L., Leinonen, M. and Saikku, P. (1997) *Chlamydia pneumoniae* infection induces inflammatory changes in the aortas of rabbits. *Infection and Immunity*, **65** 4832-4835.

Lambert, K.G. and Peacock, L.J. (1989) Feeding regime affects activity-stress ulcer production. *Physiology and Behaviour*, **46** 743-746.

Li, Q., Li, B., Wang, X., Leri, A., Jana, K.P., Liu, Y., Kajstura, J., Baserga, R. and Anversa, P. (1997) Overexpression of insulin-like growth factor-1 in mice protects from myocyte death after infarction, attenuating ventricular dilation, wall stress, and cardiac hypertrophy. *Journal of Clinical Investigation*, **100** 1991-1999.

Lopes, A.C., Borrotchin, L., Sasso, W.S. and DiDio, L.J.A. (1992) Action of propranolol on the atrial cardiomyocytes of rats submitted to cold stress. *Journal of Submicroscopical Cytology and Pathology*, **24** 187-191.

Lopes, A.C., Mora, O., Sasso, W.S. and DiDio, L.J.A. (1997) Propranolol-like action of amiodarone. An electronmicroscopic study in rats under cold stress. *Journal of Submicroscopical and Cytological Pathology*, **29** 253-256.

Magarinos, A. and McEwen, B. (1995) Stress-induced atrophy of apical dendrites of hippocampal CA3c neurons: Comparison of stressors. *Neuroscience*, **69** 83-87.

Mahmoud, I.Y. and Licht, P. (1997) Seasonal changes in gonadal activity and the effects of stress on reproductive hormones in the common snapping turtle, *Chelydra serpentina*. *General and Comparative Endocrinology*, **107** 359-372.

Mallatt, J. (1985) Fish gill structural changes induced by toxicants and other irritants: a statistical review. *Canadian Journal of Fisheries and Aquatic Sciences*, **42** 630-648.

Manuck, S.B., Kaplan, J.R. and Clarkson, T.B. (1983) Behaviorally induced heart rate reactivity and atherosclerosis in cynomoyglus monkeys. *Psychosomatic Medicine*, **45** 95-108.

Manzo, C., Zerani, M., Gobbetti, A., Di Fiore, M.M. and Angelini, F. (1994) Is corticosterone involved in the reproductive processes of the male lizard, *Podarcis sicula sicula*? *Hormones and Behavior*, **28** 117-129.

Marschal, P., Herrmann, J., Leffler, H., Baroondes, S.H. and Cooper, D.N.W. (1992) Sequence and specificity of a soluble lactose-binding lectin from *Xenopus laevis* skin. *Journal of Biological Chemistry*, **267** 12942-12949.

Masters, J.N., Finch, C.E. and Sapolsky, R.M. (1989) Glucocorticoid endangerment of hippocampal neurons does not involve deoxyribonucleic acid cleavage. *Endocrinology*, **124** 3083-3088.

Mazeaud, M.M., Mazeaud, F. and Donaldson, E.M. (1977) Primary and secondary effects of stress in fish: some new data with a general review. *Transactions of the American Fisheries Society*, **106** 201-212.

McBride, J.R. and Van Overbeeke, A.P. (1971) Effects of androgens, estrogens, and cortisol on the skin, stomach, liver, pancreas and kidney in gonadectomized adult Sockeye salmon (*Oncorhynchus nerka*). *Journal of Fisheries Research Board of Canada*, **28** 485-490.

McCartan, B.E., Lamey, P.J. and Wallace, A.M. (1996) Salivary cortisol and anxiety in recurrent aphthous stomatitis. *Journal of Oral Pathology and Medicine*, **25** 357-359.

McCormick, J.H., Stokes, G.S and Hermanutz, R.O. (1989) Oocyte atresia and reproductive success in fathead minnows (Pimephales promelas) exposed to acidified hardwater environments. *Archives of Environmental Contamination and Toxicology*, **18** 207-214.

McDonald, G. and Milligan, L. (1997) Ionic, osmotic and acid-base regulation in stress, in *Fish Stress and Health in Aquaculture* (eds. G.K. Iwama, A.D. Pickering, J.P. Sumpter and C.B. Schreck), Cambridge University Press, Cambridge, pp 119-144.

McEwen, B. (1992) Reexamination of the glucocorticoid hypothesis of stress and aging. *Progress in Brain Research*, **93** 365-393.

McEwen, B.S. (1997) Hormones as regulators of brain development: life-long effects related to health and disease. *Acta Paediatrica Supplement*, **422** 41-44.

McGrady, A.V. (1984) Effects of psychological stress on male reproduction: a review. *Archives of Andrology*, **13** 1-7.

McKenzie, J.E., House, E.W., McWilliam, J.G. and Johnson, D.W. (1978) Coronary degeneration in sexually mature rainbow and steelhead trout, *Salmo gairdneri*. *Atherosclerosis*, **29** 431-437.

Meaney, M.J., Diorio, J., Francis, D., Widdowson, J., LaPlante, P., Caldji, C., Sharma, S., Seckl, J.R. and Plotsky, P.M. (1996) Early environmental regulation of forebrain glucocorticoid receptor gene expression: Implications for adrenocortical responses to stress. *Developmental Neuroscience*, **18** 49-72.

Milstone, L.M. and Edelson, R.L. (1988) *Endocrine, Metabolic, and Immunologic Functions of Keratinocytes*. New York Academy of Sciences, New York.

Mitchell, M.A. and Carlisle, A.J. (1992) The effects of chronic exposure to elevated environmental temperature on intestinal morphology and nutrient absorption in the domestic fowl (*Gallus domesticus*). *Comparative Biochemistry and Physiology*, **A 101** 137-142.

Mizoguchi, K., Kunishita, T., Chui, D. and Tabira, T. (1992) Stress induces neuronal death in the hippocampus of castrated rats. *Neuroscience Letters*, **138** 157-160.

Moberg, G.P. (1985) Influence of stress on reproduction: measure of well-being, in *Animal Stress* (ed. G.P. Moberg), American Physiological Society, Bethesda MD, pp 245-267.

Muller, R. (1983) Coronary arteriosclerosis and thyroid hyperplasia in spawning coho salmon (*Oncorhynchus kisutch*) from lake Ontario. *Acta Zoologica Pathologica Antwerpen*, **77** 3-12.

Nagaishi, H. and Oshima, N. (1998) Neural control of motile activity of light-sensitive iridophores in the neon tetra. *Pigment Cell Research*, **2** 485-492.

Nakanishi, T. and Ototake, M. (1997) Antigen uptake and immune responses after immersion vaccination. *Developments of Biological Standardization*, **90** 59-68.

Nolan, D.T., Ruane, N.M., Rotllant, J., Wendelaar Bonga, S.E. and Balm, P.H.M. (1997) Modulation of the stress response in rainbow trout (*Oncorhynchus mykiss* Walbaum) by infestation with ectoparasitic lice. The Society for Experimental Biology Annual Meeting, Canterbury.

Nussdorfer, G.G. (1986) Cytophysiology of the adrenal cortex. *International Review of Cytology*, **98** 1-405.

O'Brian, J.J. (1986) Gastric Ulcers, in *Diseases of Swine* chapter 4 (ed. A.D. Leman), Iowa State University Press, USA.

Pankhurst, N.W. and Van der Kraak, G. (1997) Effects of stress on reproduction and growth of fish, in *Fish Stress and Health in Aquaculture* (eds. G.K. Iwama, A.D. Pickering, J.P. Sumpter, and C.B. Schreck), Cambridge University Press, Cambridge, pp 73-93.

Pankhurst, N.W., Van der Kraak, G. and Peter, R.E. (1995) Evidence that the inhibitory effects of stress on reproduction in teleost fish are not mediated by the action of cortisol on ovarian steroidogenesis. *General and Comparative Endocrinology*, **99** 249-257.

Peters, G. (1982) The effect of stress on the stomach of the European eel, *Anguilla anguilla*. *Journal of Fish Biology*, **21** 497-512.

Peters, G. and Hong, L.Q. (1985) Gill structure and blood electrolyte levels of European eels under stress, in *Fish and Shellfish Pathology* (ed. A.E. Ellis), Academic, London, pp 183-196.

Pfeiffer, C.J. (1992) A review of spontaneous ulcer disease in domestic animals: chickens, cattle, horses, and swine. *Acta Physiologica Hungarica*, **80** 149-158.

Pizcueta, J.M., Pique, J.M., Bosch, J., Whittle, B.J.R. and Moncada, S. (1992) Effects of inhibiting nitric oxide biosynthesis on the systemic and splanchnic circulation of rats with portal hypertension. *British Journal of Pharmacology*, **105** 184-190.

Pottinger, T.G., Carrick, T.R., Hughes, S.E. and Balm, P.H.M. (1996) Testosterone, 11-ketotestosterone, and estradiol-17-beta modify baseline and stress-induced interrenal and corticotropic activity in trout. *General and Comparative Endocrinology*, **104** 284-295.

Ratcliffe, H.L. and Snyder, R.L. (1967) Arteriosclerotic stenosis of the intramural arteries of chickens: further evidence of a relation to social factors. *British Journal of Experimental Pathology*, **48** 357-365.

Ratcliffe, H.L., Luginbuhl, H., Schnarr, W.R. and Chacko, K. (1969) Coronary arteriosclerosis in swine: evidence of a relation to behaviour. *Journal of Comparative Physiology and Psychology*, **68** 385-392.

Rösen, P., Ballhausen, T., Bloch, W. and Addicks, K. (1995) Endothelial relaxation is disturbed by oxidative stress in the diabetic rat heart: influence of tocopherol as antioxidant. *Diabetologia*, **38** 1157-1168.

Sanchez, M.M., Aguado, F., Sanchez-Toscano, F. and Saphier, D. (1998) Neuroendocrine and immunocytochemical demonstrations of decreased hypothalamo-pituitary-adrenal axis responsiveness to restraint stress after long-term social isolation. *Endocrinology*, **139** 579-587.

Sapolsky, R. (1992) Do glucocorticoid concentrations rise with age in the rat? *Neurobiology and Aging*, **13** 171-176.

Sapolsky, R.M. (1996) Stress, glucocorticoids, and damage to the nervous system: the current state of confusion. *Stress*, **1** 1-19.

Sapolsky, R., Uno, H., Rebert, C. and Finch, C. (1990) Hippocampal damage associated with prolonged glucocorticoid exposure in primates. *Journal of Neuroscience*, **10** 2897-2904.

Saunders, R.L., Farrell, A.P. and Knox, D.E. (1992) Progression of coronary arterial lesions in Atlantic salmon (*Salmo salar*) as a function of growth rate. *Canadian Journal of Fisheries and Aquatic Sciences*, **69** 878-884.

Slominski, A. and Mihm, M.C. (1996) Potential mechanism of skin response to stress. *International Journal of Dermatology*, **35** 849-851.

Slominski, A., Paus, R. and Wortsman, J. (1993) On the potential role of proopiomelanocortin in skin physiology and pathology. *Molecular and Cellular Endocrinology*, **93** C1-C6.

Slominski, A., Ermak, G. and Mihm, M. (1996) ACTH receptor CYP11A1, CYP17, and CYP21A2 genes are expressed in skin. *Journal of Clinical Endocrinology and Metabolism*, **81** 2746-2749.

Sloviter, R.S., Valiquette, G., Abrams, G.M., Ronk, E.C., Sollas, A.I., Paul, L.A. and Neubort, S.L. (1989) Selective loss of hippocampal granule cells in the mature rat brain after adrenalectomy. *Science*, **243** 535-538.

Starkman, M., Gebarski, S., Berent, S. and Schteingart, C. (1992) Hippocampal formation volume, memory dysfunction, and cortisol levels in patients with Cushing's syndrome. *Biological Psychiatry*, **32** 756-762.

Stein-Behrens, B., Mattson, M., Chang, I., Yeh, M. and Sapolsky, R. (1994) Stress exacerbates neuron loss and cytoskeletal pathology in the hippocampus. *Journal of Neuroscience*, **14** 5373-5380.

Szakolczai, J. (1997) Histopathological changes induced by environmental stress in common carp, Japanese coloured carp, European eel, and African catfish. *Acta Veterinaria Hungarica*, **45** 1-10.

Talmi, M., Carlier, E. and Soumireu-Mourat, B. (1993) Similar effects of aging and corticosterone treatment on mouse hippocampal function. *Neurobiology and Aging*, **14** 239-245.

Talmi, M., Carlier, E., Bengelloun, W. and Soumireu-Mourat, B. (1996) Chronic RU 486 treatment reduces age-related alterations of mouse hippocampal function. *Neurobiology and Aging*, **17** 9-17.

Tapp, W.N., Natelson, B.H. and Creighton, D. (1989) Alprazolam reduces stress-induced mortality in cardiomyopathic hamsters. *Pharmacology and Biochemistry of Behaviour*, **32** 331-336.

Teerlink, J.R., Pfeffer, J.M. and Pfeffer, M.A. (1994) Progressive ventricular remodelling in response to diffuse isoproterenol-induced myocardial necrosis in rats. *Circulation Research*, **75** 105-113.

Theoharides, T.C., Singh, L.K., Boucher, W., Pang, X., Letourneau, R., Webseter, E. and Chrousos, G. (1998) Corticotropin-releasing hormone induces skin mast cell degranulation and increased vascular permeability, a possible explanation for its proinflammatory effects. *Endocrinology*, **139** 403-413.

Tombaugh, G., Yang, S., Swanson, R. and Sapolsky, R. (1992) Glucocorticoids exacerbate hypoxic and hypoglycemic hippocampal injury in vitro: Biochemical correlates and a role of astrocytes. *Journal of Neurochemistry*, **59** 137-145.

Torpy, D.J. and Chrousos, G.P. (1996) The three-way interactions between the hypothalamic-pituitary-adrenal and gonadal axes and the immune system. *Baillieres Clinical Rheumatology*, **10** 181-198.

Trevi, G., Sheiban, I. and Gorni, R. (1995) Myocardial hypertrophy and arterial hypertension. *Giornale Italiano Di Cardiologia*, **25** 1331-1338.

Uno, H., Tarara, R., Else, J., Suleman, M. and Sapolsky, R. (1989) Hippocampal damage associated with prolonged and fatal stress in primates. *Journal of Neuroscience*, **9** 1705-1712.

Uno, H., Lohmiller, L., Thieme, C., Kemnitz, J.W., Engle, M.J., Roecker, E.B. and Farrell, P.M. (1990) Brain damage induced by prenatal exposure to dexamethasone in fetal rhesus macaques. *Developmental Brain Research*, **53** 157-167.

Vaira, D., Holton, J., Londei, M., Bertrand, J., Salmon, P.R., D'Anastasio, C., Dowsett, J.F., Bertoni, F., Grauenfels, P. and Gandolfi, L. (1988) *Campylobacter (Helicobacter) pylori* in abattoir workers: is it a zoonosis? *The Lancet*, 725-726.

Van Raaij, M.T.M., Pit, D.S.S., Balm, P.H.M., Steffens, A.B. and Van den Thillart, G.E.E.J.M. (1996) Behavioural strategy and the physiological stress response in rainbow trout exposed to severe hypoxia. *Hormones and Behaviour*, **30** 85-92.

Verbeek, M. (1998) *Bold or cautious. Behavioural characteristics and dominance in great tits.* Thesis, University of Wageningen.

Weber, H.W. and Van der Walt, J.J. (1975) Cardiomyopathy in crowded rabbits. *Recent Advances in Studies on Cardiovascular Structure and Metabolism*, **6** 441-447.

Weiss, J.M. (1977) Psychosocial and behavioral influences on gastrointestinal lesions in animal models, in *Psychopathology: Experimental Models* (eds. J.D. Maser and M.E.P. Seligman), Freeman, San Francisco, pp 232-269.

Wendelaar Bonga, S.E. (1997) The stress response in fish. *Physiological Reviews*, **77** (3) 591-625.

Whittle, J.R. (1995) Nitric oxide in physiology and pathology. *Histochemical Journal*, **27** 727-737.

Wong, H.Y., Cheng, K.K. and Nightingale, T.E. (1992) Social stress and atherosclerosis in roosters. *Comparative Biochemistry and Physiology*, **A101** 625-629.

Woolley, C., Gould, E. and McEwen, B. (1990) Exposure to excess glucocorticoids alters dendritic morphology of adult hippocampal pyramidal neurons. *Brain Research*, **531** 225-231.

6 Stress-induced immune–endocrine interaction

Alec G. Maule and Scott P. VanderKooi

6.1 Introduction

Our current understanding of the physiological responses to stress has grown from early work by Cannon *et al.* (1927), who defined the fight-or-flight response to a perceived threat, and the concept of homeostasis as the physiological processes by which organisms can maintain a relatively stable internal environment. Selye (1936, 1976) formulated the General Adaptation Syndrome (GAS) to describe the general, non-specific physiological responses that allow an organism to fight or take flight. Central to Selye's GAS is that the central nervous system acts instantaneously to divert the body's bioenergetic resources away from non-protective functions, such as reproduction (see Chapter 4, this volume) or growth (see Chapter 3, this volume) to those activities that will help the organism deal with the threat, such as changing behavior (see Chapter 1, this volume) or respiration (see Chapter 2, this volume). Among Selye's (1936) earliest observations in stressed animals were enlarged adrenal glands and atrophy of the thymus, spleen and lymph nodes (Bleeding ulcers completed his 'triad of the alarm reaction'). The heuristic value of the GAS was questioned when it was discovered that one of the primary hormones regulating physiological systems during stress, glucocorticoids (GC), was also immunosuppressive (Munck *et al.*, 1984; Munck and Guyre, 1991).

Early concerns about the immunological effects of stress were based on studies that described the suppressive effects of GC (Munck *et al.*, 1984). However, several studies have shown enhancement of immune functioning and disease resistance following stress (Gisler *et al.*, 1971; Okimura and Nigo, 1986) and that other stress-induced hormones (e.g. growth hormone, prolactin, endogenous opioids) are immune enhancers (see review: Kelley and Dantzer, 1991). Concerns about the ambiguity of immunosuppression by GC have lessened through an understanding of endocrine–immune interactions (Blalock and Smith, 1985; Blalock, 1994; Besedovsky and Del Rey, 1996), the characterization of immune cells as 'sensory organs' (Blalock, 1984) or a 'mobile immune-brain' (Ottaviani *et al.*, 1997), and the phylogenetic universality of some of these interrelations (Ottaviani and Franceschi, 1996). We agree with Ottaviani and Franceschi (1996) that the stress response is adaptive and that 'Stress can be seen as the most important and complex body reaction to ensure survival. Thus, contrary to common sense, stress must be considered a fundamentally **positive** type of adaptive reaction.'

In this chapter our main objective is to present a phylogenetic examination of the physiological affects of stress on the immune system and disease resistance. To accomplish this we will first define the conditions of stress to be considered in this review. We will also provide a brief summary of the hypothalamic–pituitary–adrenal (HPA) axis and associated hormones, which are the main effectors for translating a stress into physiological action (stress response), and we will describe a generalized immune response. Second, we will describe the ways in which stress-induced changes in neuroendocrine and endocrine hormones affect immune functioning and disease resistance. To avoid confusion, we will use the inclusive term 'endocrine', when referring to hormones of any origin. Our third task will be to summarize the action of immune molecules—immune cytokines and immune-derived endocrine 'mimics'— that have regulatory effects on the endocrine system. Recently many excellent reviews describing endocrine–immune interactions have been published; rather than repeat the summaries of those authors, we will highlight the significant conclusions as they relate to stress and immunity and frequently refer the reader to those reviews. Finally, we will examine the literature on stress-induced immune regulation from invertebrates through mammals; we will concentrate our efforts in describing what is known about the effects of stress on the immune systems of fish — our area of expertise — but we will include information on invertebrates, amphibians and birds. Most of the work in the area of immune-endocrine interactions used mammalian models; we will describe much of that literature in the first three sections of this chapter.

6.2   Scope of the chapter

6.2.1   Stress

We define stress as an external or internal stimulus which disrupts the internal physiology of the organism. In virtually all vertebrates, the primary physiological responses to stress (stress responses) are initiated by activation of the sympathetic nervous system and the HPA axis. A wide range of stimuli can activate these systems; among these stimuli are cognitive stresses including direct physical injury and psychological, or perceived stresses. We will not consider direct physical injury because the injury itself can have physiological consequences that will confound examination of the purely endogenous responses to the stress. One can easily see the need to exclude physical injury when considering stress-induced immune modification because of the confounding effects of an immune response to the injury itself. This definition does not exclude experimental stresses that involve physical contact, such as restraint or crowding, when no tissue damage occurs. We will, however, also consider non-cognitive stimuli (Ottaviani and Franceschi, 1996) such as pathogenic microorganisms or immunologically relevant antigens. The need for this distinction is clear when one considers immune cells as sensory organs that communicate the status of the internal environment to the endocrine system (Blalock, 1984; Besedovsky and Del Rey, 1996).

A recent review by Chrousos and Gold (1992) dealt primarily with the effects of stress-associated disease in humans. We agree with their opening statement about the uniqueness of the human condition: 'Although human societies have become more complex and in many ways more demanding, our physiological mechanisms for coping with adversity have not evolved appreciably over the past several thousand years. Hence, it seems that our physiological responses to social pressures, information overload, and rapid change resemble those set in motion during physical danger and outright threats to survival. Whether these (stress-associated) illnesses have always been with us in abundance or are a more prominent part of the landscape of modern life—which may provide us with a greater variety of adverse situations—is conjecture.' Studies of emotional stress in humans often rely on a subjective measure of stress rather than a specific measure of physiological change. In order to avoid the problem of adequately defining emotional stress (Leonard and Song, 1996) we will not consider studies of human emotional stress that do not include a physiological measure of stress.

6.2.2 *Endocrine response to stress*

Information about a cognitive stress is communicated from the sensory organs to the brain and, hence, to target tissues throughout the body, by two primary groups of biochemical effectors. One group consists of catecholamines that can be secreted from neurons of the sympathetic nervous system and act as neurotransmitters. Catecholamines can also be secreted by the chromaffin cells of the adrenal medulla and act as endocrine hormones (Figure 6.1). Bioactivity of the catecholamines (epinephrine and norepinephrine) is transmitted to target cells by α- and β-adrenergic receptors in the plasma membranes of those cells (Norris, 1996). The second group of effectors are steroid and peptide hormones that originate in cells of the HPA axis (Figure 6.1). Upon activation by a stressful stimulus, the hypothalamus secretes one or more releasing hormones, including corticotropin-releasing hormone (CRH). These

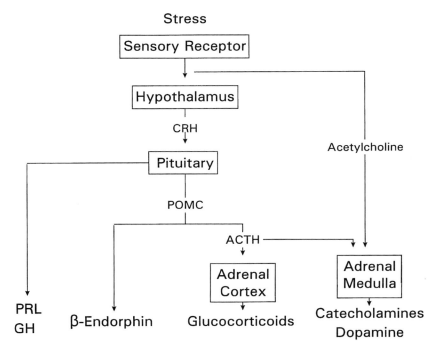

Figure 6.1 Activation of the hypothalamic–pituitary–adrenal (HPA) axis by stress, resulting in the secretion of hormones including corticotropin releasing hormone (CRH), prolactin (PRL), growth hormone (GH), and proopiomelanocortin (POMC) which is cleaved to produce adrenocorticotropic hormone (ACTH) and β-endorphin (β-END).

releasing hormones act primarily on the pituitary gland to stimulate the release of several hormones that ultimately have profound effects on physiological functioning. Relative to the stress response, the most significant of these pituitary secretions is proopiomelanocortin (POMC). Upon enzymatic cleavage, POMC-derived peptides include adrenocorticotropic hormone (ACTH) and β-endorphin. Adrenocorticotropic hormone completes activation of the HPA axis by stimulating cells of the adrenal glands to secrete glucocorticoids and catecholamines.

There are two general receptor-mediated mechanisms through which hormones can affect changes in target cell functioning (Norris, 1996). The first is by activating a plasma membrane receptor which in turn activates a cascade of biochemical reactions leading to the release of a 'second messenger', which, in the case of protein kinase, catalyzes the phosphorylation of another protein that has biological activity within the cell. Peptide hormones usually act through these membrane-associated second messengers (Hadden *et al.*, 1991). Steroid hormones usually have biological action via the second type of receptor. Because they are lipid soluble, steroids perfuse into target cells where they activate specific receptors. The activated receptor then binds to the DNA at sites known as hormone response elements. This binding either enhances or suppresses transcription of a specific gene and the resulting change in translation of a protein alters cellular functioning (Bamberger *et al.*, 1996). We will address the mechanisms of glucocorticoid steroid action in greater detail in section 6.3.4. Virtually all of the endocrine hormones mentioned in this brief synopsis are well conserved throughout the animal kingdom (Ottaviani and Franceschi, 1997) and act through specific receptors in plasma membrane, cytosol or nucleus of target cells, including cells of the immune system. The timing of these responses following an acute stress ranges from less than seconds for sympathetic noradrenergic nerve firing, to several hours required for plasma glucocorticoids to return to close to normal levels after stress.

6.2.3   The immune system

The function of the immune system is to defend the organism from microorganisms (e.g. pathogenic bacteria or virus), inorganic substances (e.g. splinter in a paw), or the organism's own cells gone awry (e.g. tumor cells). Responses of the immune system can be classified as innate or adaptive. Innate immunity includes humoral factors such as lysozyme, complement and acute phase proteins, and cellular components such as phagocytic cells. The ability of these factors and cells to non-specifically attack invading organisms make them an early line of defense.

The first step in an adaptive immune response is to determine that the offending substance does not belong to 'self', or that it is 'altered-self' in the case of tumor cells. After proper identification, the immune system has a complex array of cellular and humoral responses with which to rid the body of the threat and prepare a more rapid and aggressive response should the same threat be encountered in the future (i.e. a secondary or memory response). The cells of the immune system are composed primarily of phagocytes (e.g. monocyte/macrophages, neutrophils) and lymphocytes. There are three classes of lymphocytes—B-cells, T-cells and natural killer (NK) cells. When stimulated by a physicochemically specific antigen, B-cells proliferate and mature into plasma cells which secrete antibodies that bind specifically to that antigen. Similarly, T-cells exhibit antigen specificity and can be classed as T-helper (T_H)-cells, T-suppressor (T_S)-cells, and cytotoxic T-cells. Virtually all of these cells also secrete immune cytokines that communicate information to other cells of the immune system and, as we shall see, to cells of the endocrine system as well.

Figure 6.2 portrays an adaptive, specific immune response to a bacterial pathogen; the letters in the following description correspond to those in the figure. The initial cellular contact with the bacteria is from a phagocytic cell, in this example a macrophage—indicating that the response is occurring in tissue as opposed to the circulation (A). After phagocytizing and lysing the cell, the macrophage affixes bacterial antigens to its own cell membrane and becomes an antigen-presenting cell (B). By presenting the bacterial antigen along with 'self' antigen (i.e. major histocompatibility complex antigens), the macrophage can activate T-cells that have specific receptors for both self and non-self antigens. The macrophage also secretes several cytokines that prepare surrounding tissue, attract and activate lymphocytes and communicate with other physiological systems. Foremost among these are interleukin-1 (IL-1), IL-6, and tumor necrosis factor (TNF). The activated T-cells proliferate and differentiate into T_H-cells that activate B-cells (C), which in turn proliferate and differentiate into antibody-secreting plasma cells (D). Activated T_H-cells also secrete cytokines, the most important being IL-2, which further stimulates T-cells and B-cells. In addition, the T-cells secrete interferon-γ (INF-γ) which activates macrophages. Some of the activated T_H-cells and B-cells become long-lived, memory cells available for rapid responses should they come in contact with same antigen in the future (E). Down-regulation of the immune response is accomplished primarily by eliminating the antigens that activated the system and through the action of T_S-cells, but we now know that the endocrine system has a role in immune regulation, especially during stress. Unlike the endocrine response to an acute stress that can be completed in hours if not minutes, the initial phases of the immune response (phagocytosis) may take hours and the peak antibody response in mammals may take four days or more (Janeway and Travers, 1994). As we shall see, many of the effects of the endocrine stress response have enhancing or suppressing effects on the immune system depending on the temporal relation of stress (or hormone treatment) to immune challenge.

6.3 Endocrine effects on the immune system

Glucocorticoids are the most studied, and perhaps the best understood, of the stress-induced, immunomodulating hormones. Glucocorticoids, their receptors and biological actions will be addressed in depth in subsequent sections. However, the substances leading to GC release from the adrenal cortex also have effects on immune functioning and we will start by summarizing briefly what is know of the effects of these

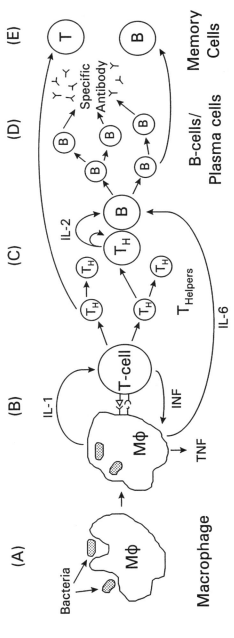

Figure 6.2 A generalized immune response to a bacterial pathogen, including the release of cytokines: tumor necrosis factor (TNF), interleukins (IL-1, -2, -6), and interferon (INF). Letters in parentheses correspond to letters in the text describing the immune response (section 6.2.3).

hormones. Figure 6.3 presents an overview of the key endocrine hormone effects on immune cell functioning.

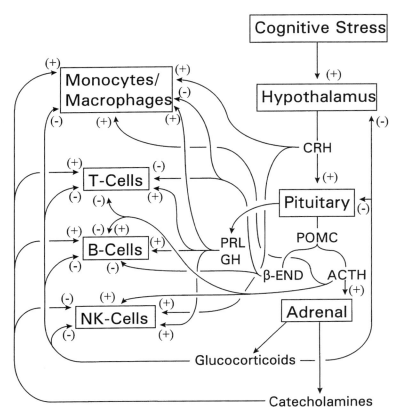

Figure 6.3 Actions of hormones from the hypothalamic–pituitary–adrenal (HPA) axis on the immune system following activation by stress. Although not all studies agree, indications of immune suppression (−) or immune enhancement (+) are based on the predominate conclusions of research reviewed in text. Please refer to Figure 6.1 for definitions of abbreviations.

6.3.1 CRH and POMC

In contrast to GC, the immunomodulating roles of CRH and the POMC-derived ACTH and β-endorphin are not well understood. Receptors for CRH have been identified in mouse spleen in an area rich with macrophages (Webster and de Souza, 1988). Irwin and Jones (1991) report that central nervous system administration of CRH caused a decrease in splenic NK-cell cytotoxicity. However, the mechanism of action is probably by indirect effects of the neurohormone as no effect was seen with subcutaneous CRH administration or when NK-cells were exposed to CRH *in vitro*. Moreover, when catecholamine release was blocked, CRH administration had no effect on NK-cell activity. Direct *in vitro* stimulation of human peripheral blood lymphocytes with CRH resulted in measurable POMC-derived peptides in the cell culture medium (Smith *et al.*, 1986), further supporting the view that CRH has no direct role in immune regulation.

POMC-derived ACTH and β-endorphin have direct effects on the immune system; however, they can suppress or enhance depending on the experimental conditions. Low concentrations of ACTH enhanced, but high concentrations inhibited, secretion of IgM from a mouse B-cell line (Bost *et al.*, 1990). Similarly, the full ACTH molecule (39 amino acids) suppressed antibody and INF-γ production, while steroidogenic ACTH fragments had no effect (Johnson *et al.*, 1982, 1984). That ACTH has a direct role in immune functioning is evident by the presence of specific ACTH receptors on T-cells and B-cells (Clarke and Bost, 1989) and the ability of the hormone to activate second messengers in lymphocytes (Johnson *et al.*, 1988). Smith *et al.* (1992) reported that some of the immunosuppressive effects of ACTH may be from its proteolytic cleavage to melanocyte stimulating hormone (α-MSH).

Studies with β-endorphin and other endogenous opioids have also had mixed results. Shavit *et al.* (1984) reported that stress-induced suppression of NK-cell activity was blocked by the opioid antagonist naloxone; Mandler *et al.* (1986), however, found enhanced NK-cell activity when cells were treated with β-endorphin *in vitro*. Johnson *et al.* (1982) found that *in vitro* antibody responses requiring T-cell activation (T-dependent) were inhibited by much lower concentrations of β-endorphin than were antibody responses that did not require T-cells (T-independent), suggesting that T-cells are more sensitive to β-endorphin than are B-cells. As with ACTH, opioid receptors have been identified in lymphocytes (Wybran *et al.*, 1979) and it is likely that differences in bioactivity are the result of cell-specific differences in receptor numbers or affinity, or the presence of modified ligand fragments (Williamson *et al.*, 1987). Stefano *et al.* (1995) reported that *in vitro* pre-treatment with morphine enhanced, while simultaneous treatment suppressed, the ability of LPS to stimulate immune cells from humans and invertebrates. There is also evidence that the parasite *Schistosoma mansoni* secretes POMC-derived peptides to avoid its host's immune system through immune suppression (Duvaux-Miret *et al.*, 1992). Several chapters in Plotnikoff *et al.* (1991) and Ader *et al.* (1991) are dedicated to the topic of opioid–immune system interaction.

6.3.2   Prolactin and growth hormone

Prolactin and growth hormone (GH) are pituitary peptides that may be the antithesis of GC, in that they are immune enhancing. Recent reviews by Bernton *et al.* (1991), Kelley (1991) and Kelley and Dantzer (1991) describe the actions of GH and PRL as being permissive, and antagonistic to the immunosuppression by GC. Most of what is known about GH and PRL comes from studies with hypophysectomized or hormone-deficient animals in which GH and/or PRL treatment restores normal immune functioning. Receptors for both hormones have been identified on human mononuclear cells, thymocytes and lymphocytes (Kiess and Butenandt, 1985; Russell *et al.*, 1985); however, cells from the thymus (i.e. T-cells) have almost twice as many PRL receptors as cells from the bone marrow (i.e. B-cells) (Dardenne *et al.*, 1994). Bernton *et al.* (1991) describe a series of experiments with mice in which blocking PRL secretion *in vivo* was immunosuppressive and resulted in increased mortality in a pathogen challenge; exogenous PRL treatment reversed these effects. Madden and Felten (1995) describe a mechanism of immune enhancement in which PRL works in concert with IL-2, possibly in the role of second messenger (Blalock, 1994), to induce T-cell proliferation. Interestingly, PRL also induces IL-2 receptors in lymphocytes (Mukherjee *et al.*, 1990). Growth hormone has been identified as an important growth factor in lymphocyte proliferation; however, this GH may be immune-derived and acting in an autocrine or paracrine manner (Weigent *et al.*, 1991). Growth hormone can also activate killing mechanisms in macrophages (Edwards *et al.*, 1988).

6.3.3   Catecholamines

The catecholamines—epinephrine (EPI) and norepinephrine (NE)—can reach target tissues as neurotransmitters or via secretion from the adrenal medulla as endocrine hormones. Virtually all organs of the immune system—thymus, bone marrow, spleen, lymph nodes, gut-associated lymphoid tissue—receive sympathetic noradrenergic innervation (Felten and Felten, 1991). Moreover, T-cells, B-cells, macrophages and neutrophils all contain β-adrenoceptors and, to a lesser extent, α-adrenoceptors (see review: Madden and Felten, 1995). As was the case with the other hormones, results vary depending on experimental design. Depelchin and Letesson (1981) reported that when EPI was injected (i.p.) into mice six hours before SRBC injection, the antibody response was hastened; however, EPI injection two days before the immune challenge reduced the speed and magnitude of the antibody response. Denervation studies (using 6-hydroxydopamine) reportedly reduced the delayed-type hypersensitivity reaction, IL-2 secretion, cytotoxic T-cell activity, and T-dependent antibody responses, but increased T-independent antibody production (Besedovsky et al., 1979; Sanders and Powell-Oliver, 1992; see review: Madden and Felten, 1995). Madden and Felten (1995) stated that immune regulation by catecholamines is not simply a matter of hormonal effects on individual cells, but that the timing, type of immune cells targeted, and complexity of the immune response contribute to the apparent duality of the effects. Other reviewers agree with this assessment (Madden and Livnat, 1991; Roszman and Carlson, 1991; Black, 1994).

6.3.4   Glucocorticoids

As has been indicated, more is known about the effects of GC than any other stress-induced immune regulator; however, all of the mechanisms through which it acts are far from elucidated. Virtually all of the immune processes illustrated in Figure 6.2 can be interrupted by GC. Glucocorticoids can inhibit the differentiation of circulating monocytes into tissue-dwelling macrophages (Rinehart et al., 1982), as well as inhibit macrophage production of IL-1 and self-antigens necessary for antigen presentation to T-cells (Hirschberg et al., 1982). Glucocorticoids can also reduce the production of IL-2, INF-γ, macrophage activating factor (MAF), and colony stimulating factor (CSF) by T-cells (Gillis et al., 1979; Kelso and Munck, 1984). In addition, GC can depress T-cell proliferation by inhibiting the synthesis of mRNA for IL-2 and INF-γ in T-cells (Arya et al., 1984), and suppress antibody production by interfering with the early stages of B-cell activation (Cupps et al., 1985). Furthermore, GC treatment or stress can alter the number and composition of circulating leukocytes by cytolysis (Homo et al., 1980) or redistribution of cells to other lymphoid organs (Cohen, 1972; Steplewski and Vogel, 1986).

Stress and GC can also enhance disease resistance (Gisler et al., 1971; Okimura and Nigo, 1986; also see review: Sheridan et al., 1994) and enhance some measures of immune function, such as the expression of IL-1 receptors in lymphocytes (Akahoshi et al., 1988) and antibody production in response to the T-dependent pokeweed mitogen (Cooper et al., 1979; Cupps et al., 1984). As was discussed for the peptide hormones, the effects of GC treatment on immune response will vary depending on the species and physical state of the experimental animal (Claman, 1972; Cupps et al., 1984), timing of the hormone treatment relative to immune challenge (Cupps and Fauci, 1982; Monjan and Collector, 1977), or the immune function assayed (Goodwin and Atluru, 1986). Of significance during an immune response when T-cells and B-cells are proliferating is the finding that GC effects vary depending on phase of the cell cycle (Crabtree et al., 1980; Hsu and DeFranco, 1995).

As indicated above, glucocorticoids have diverse actions on various tissues, including the cells of the immune system. Bamberger *et al.* (1996) listed eight factors that determine tissue sensitivity to GC. First, the availability of GC within the cell can be reduced through enzymatic biotransformation via 11β-hydroxysteroid dehydrogenase (Funder *et al.*, 1988) or by a ligand effect modulator that transports GC out of the cell (Kralli *et al.*, 1995); second and third, the number and affinity of glucocorticoid receptors (GR) in the cell can be altered (Miller *et al.*, 1990; Karl *et al.*, 1993); fourth, alterations in ligand-induced conformational changes in GR that affect its ability to bind DNA (Robertson *et al.*, 1995); fifth, state of phosphorylation of the GR (Mendel *et al.*, 1986; Hu *et al.*, 1994); sixth, alteration in nuclear translocation of the activated receptor; seventh, factors that regulate GR binding to DNA (Cavanaugh and Simons, 1994); and eighth, interaction with other nuclear activators or repressors. Another factor that may regulate sex-specific or species-specific GC sensitivity is the hormone buffering of plasma GC-binding globulin proteins, which can alter the amount of available GC by a factor of 25 (Bradley *et al.*, 1976; McDonald *et al.*, 1986).

The effects of steroid hormones are generally mediated through saturable, high affinity, specific receptors in the cytosol or nucleus; the presence of specific GR in mammalian leukocytes is well established (Roth *et al.*, 1985; Plaut, 1987). Glucocorticoid receptors that have not bound hormone occur as heteromeric proteins composed of a single binding molecule and five stress proteins (sp; also known as heat-shock proteins) (Pratt, 1993; Smith and Toft, 1993). Two 90 kDa stress proteins (sp90) appear to be responsible for maintaining the conformation of the receptor so that it will readily bind hormone, but will not bind DNA (Hutchison *et al.*, 1994; Czar *et al.*, 1994). Interestingly, an sp56 associated with the GC receptor is an immunophilin (Tai *et al.*, 1992), which is involved in intracellular protein folding. Immunophilins also bind immunosuppressive compounds such as cyclosporin A, which suppresses T-cell activation by blocking signal transduction that normally results in transcription of IL-2 and the IL-2 receptor genes (Schreiber, 1991; Schreiber and Crabtree, 1992). The significance of the GR–immunophilin–cyclosporin A association is not known; however, upon binding the hormone, the stress proteins are released from the GR. The hormone–receptor complex is activated and binds to another, activated GR to form a homodimer that translocates to the nucleus and binds to DNA at the glucocorticoid response element (GRE) where it regulates transcription (Cavanaugh and Simons, 1994; Katzenellenbogen *et al.*, 1996). Other, non-classical modes of steroid hormone action, such as changing membrane fluidity or modulating membrane neurotransmitter receptors, have also been proposed (see reviews: Brann *et al.*, 1995; Wehling, 1994).

Many of GC's actions appear to inhibit protein synthesis, specifically cytokine production (Guyre *et al.*, 1988). This action seems contradictory to the classical mode of GC action which is for the activated GR to bind DNA and enhance transcription (Katzenellenbogen *et al.*, 1996). One obvious explanation for these negative effects is for GC to enhance the transcription of a protein that is itself inhibitory. Auphan *et al.* (1995) and Scheinman *et al.* (1995) have shown that GC enhances the transcription of a protein identified as IκBβ, which in turn suppresses an important promoter of cytokine synthesis called NF-κB. There also exist negative glucocorticoid response elements (nGRE) that inhibit transcription; however, this mode of action must be less efficient than the classical mode, as the nGRE requires binding by three GRs rather than the classical homodimer (Drouin *et al.*, 1993). Another inhibitory mechanism of GC action is for the activated receptor to bind to a transcription factor rather than the DNA. One such factor to which GR binds is activating protein-1 (AP-1), which can either enhance or suppress transcription (Pearce and Yamamoto, 1993). A second type of GR (termed GRβ) exists and can inhibit GC action (Bamberger *et al.*, 1995). The amino acid sequence of the C-terminus of GRβ differs from that of GRα, such that Grβ cannot bind hormone and is transcriptionally inactive (Bamberger *et al.*, 1996). However, Grβ does inhibit the effects of GC in a dose-dependent manner, perhaps by competing with the GRα for the glucocorticoid response element (Bamberger *et al.*, 1995).

One example of the mechanisms by which GC inhibits immune responses is its suppression of IL-2 transcription in T-cells, which is thought to be mediated by both enhancing the transcription of IκBβ and/ or impairing AP-1 function (Northrop *et al.*, 1992; Vacca *et al.*, 1992; Scheinman *et al.*, 1995) but not by transcriptional interference from GRβ (Bamberger *et al.*, 1997). On the contrary, IL-2 and IL-4 reduced the affinity with which GR binds hormone, and induced GRβ—thus, reducing T-cell sensitivity to GC (Kam *et al.*, 1993; Leung *et al.*, 1997).

6.4   Immune system effects on endocrine functioning

That immune factors can influence the endocrine system has been known since the beginning of the 20th century when disorders of the reproductive and adrenal systems were treated with thymic extracts (Anderson, 1932 as cited in Hall *et al.*, 1985). Nonetheless, it has only been in the past 25 years that researchers have begun to elucidate the pathways through which the immune system can influence the activity of the endocrine system. In the 1970s, Besedovsky *et al.* (1975) reported that *in vivo* antigen stimulation resulted in elevated plasma GC titers concomitant with the peak antibody response. Subsequently, Munck *et al.* (1984) proposed that the adaptive role of GC is to down-regulate physiological systems activated by stress, so that those systems do not overreact and cause tissue damage. Continuing work by Blalock and colleagues (see: Blalock, 1994) and Besedovsky (see: Besedovsky and Del Ray, 1996) has elucidated the interaction between the immune, endocrine, and central nervous systems. In this scenario, immune cells not only receive information from the HPA axis, but also act as sensory organs that communicate with the endocrine and nervous systems (Blalock *et al.*, 1985; Blalock, 1994; Besedovsky and Del Ray, 1996). Figure 6.4

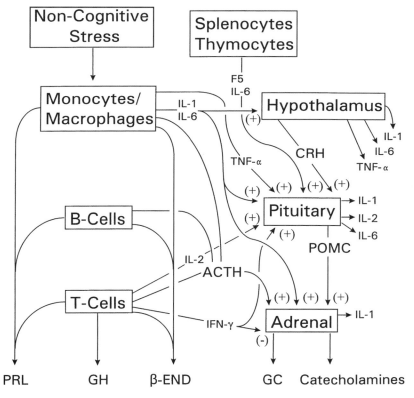

Figure 6.4   Activation of the immune system by non-cognitive stress (i.e. antigen challenge) and the resulting expression of immune cytokines and endocrine hormones by the immune system and the endocrine system, including the release of thymic factor V (F5). Many of the compounds secreted by the immune system act in an autocrine or paracrine manner which is not illustrated in the figure. Although not all studies agree, indications of suppression (−) or activation (+) are based on the predominant conclusions of research reviewed in the text. Please refer to Figures 6.1 and 6.2 for definitions of abbreviations.

illustrates influences of the immune system on the HPA axis including the effects of immune cytokines and the production of endocrine products by immune cells and immune products by the endocrine system. Combining Figure 6.4 with Figure 6.3 demonstrates the complexity of immune–endocrine interactions.

6.4.1 Immune cytokines and CRH

There is little doubt that immune factors can activate the HPA axis. In fact CRH mRNA has been located in the spleen and thymus (Aird *et al.*, 1993). Interleukin-1 can activate the HPA axis; however, there is disagreement as to whether this activation takes place at the hypothalamus or the pituitary (Blalock, 1994; Besedovsky and Del Ray, 1996). Work with ACTH-deficient children suggested that central nervous system involvement may be required to get *in vivo* activation of the HPA axis via the immune system. Normal children were compared to ACTH-deficient children after injections of insulin or typhoid vaccine and the percent of peripheral mononuclear lymphocytes positive for ACTH-like substance was measured. Insulin-induced hypoglycemia resulted in a transient increase in ACTH-positive cells in normal children but not ACTH-deficient children while typhoid vaccination resulted in a higher percentage of ACTH-positive cells in the deficient children but not normal children (Meyer *et al.*, 1987). The authors stated that ACTH-deficient individuals also suffer hypothalamic damage, and that the differences in responses may indicate that the CNS is a necessary component for lymphoid stimulation of the HPA axis.

Besedovsky *et al.* (1985) proposed a glucocorticoid increasing factor (GIF) of lymphoid origins that acts upon the brain. Supernatants from antigen-stimulated, human peripheral blood lymphocyte cultures were injected into rats and caused dose-dependent increases in plasma levels of corticosterone and ACTH. It was also reported that when the rats were treated with dexamethasone or were hypophysectomized prior to injection of culture supernatants, ACTH and corticosterone did not increase (Besedovsky *et al.*, 1985). However, Vahouny *et al.* (1983) were unable to stimulate corticosteroid production *in vitro* using the same system to generate culture supernatants. Besedovsky *et al.* (1983) previously reported that these supernatants decreased the NE content of the hypothalamus and suggested that this may be the mode of action of GIF since NE has an inhibitory effect on corticotropin releasing hormone (Besedovsky *et al.*, 1985).

Woloski *et al.* (1985) reported that supernatants containing IL-1 and IL-6 produced by peripheral blood monocytes in culture had no effect on adrenal cells, but resulted in a dose-dependent increase in ACTH production from pituitary tumor cells. In this study, IL-1 was equally effective, and IL-6 was 3-fold more effective than CRH in stimulating ACTH release. When recombinant IL-1 was injected into mice, it resulted in dose- and time-dependent increases in plasma levels of ACTH and corticosterone (Besedovsky *et al.*, 1986). Furthermore, when culture supernatants from human lymphocytes infected with Newcastle disease virus were treated with anti-IL-1 antibody, they lost the ability to stimulate *in vivo* production of ACTH and corticosterone (Besedovsky *et al.*, 1986). Interleukin-1 acts on the immune system by stimulating T-cells to produce IL-2. When athymic mice, which have no T-cells, were injected with IL-1, the ACTH and corticosterone levels increased, eliminating the possibility that IL-1 was acting through T-cells (Besedovsky *et al.*, 1986). This is significant considering that IL-2, like IL-6, is a very powerful ACTH secretogogue (Karanth and McCann, 1991) and receptors for all three cytokines have been identified in the pituitary (Besedovsky and Del Ray, 1996).

Another line of research has shown that an extract of the thymus gland has CRH activity. Thymosin fraction 5 (F5) is a family of peptides that have a role in the proliferation and maturation of T-cells in the thymus and can partially replace or potentiate T-cells during an immune response (Talmadge, 1984; Zatz and Goldstein, 1985). The administration of what might be pharmacological doses of F5 resulted in dose- and time-dependent increases in blood levels of ACTH, β-endorphin, and cortisol in primates (Healy *et al.*, 1983). The fact that F5 could not stimulate GC production from isolated adrenal glands (Vahouny *et al.*, 1983) supports the likelihood that F5 acts on the HPA above the level of the pituitary.

6.4.2   *Immune cytokines and POMC derivatives*

There is considerable evidence that ACTH plays a role in the interaction between immune and endocrine systems. In fact, analysis by Stefano and Smith (1996) suggests that ACTH might be the key endocrine substance regulating the immune system. In their system, low level production of ACTH from the pituitary and immune cells has endocrine, paracrine and autocrine action to tonally inhibit the immune system. Upon stimulation by non-cognitive stress (i.e. microorganism), enzymes degrade ACTH, freeing the immune cells to release cytokines, which activate and enhance the immune response. These same cytokines (e.g. IL-1, IL-2, IL-6) will ultimately stimulate the HPA axis leading to the release of GC, which will down-regulate the immune response and, through negative feedback, cause the stress-induced, elevated ACTH to return to background levels. Early work in this area (Besedovsky *et al.*, 1975) demonstrated that the ability of rats to generate antibody-producing cells in response to an immunization peaked concomitantly with a significant elevation in serum corticosterone levels and depression in serum thyroxine levels. In order to verify that this regulation was the result of an immune factor, the medium in which rat splenic lymphocytes were cultured with mitogen was injected into allogenic rats and caused a significant dose-dependent increase in plasma corticosterone levels (Besedovsky *et al.*, 1981). These experiments suggested that activated immune cells secrete cytokine(s) that activate the HPA axis or that immune cells secrete molecules of the HPA axis. We have already discussed the effects of immune cytokines on the HPA axis, and there is evidence that immune cells also secrete substances similar, if not identical to, secretogogues of the HPA axis.

Smith *et al.* (1986) demonstrated that POMC-derived endorphins and ACTH could be induced from non-stimulated, human peripheral leukocytes by the addition of CRH and arginine-vasopressin (AVP). Singly these hormones had dose-dependent effects and together, acted synergistically to increase output of ACTH- and β-endorphin-like factors, responses similar to those seen when CRH and AVP stimulated pituitary cells (Smith *et al.*, 1986). The *de novo* synthesis of ACTH from lymphocytes was supported by the findings that its secretion could be blocked by actinomycin D and cycloheximide (Blalock and Smith, 1982), and that stimulated splenocytes express the POMC gene (Westly *et al.*, 1986). Further research revealed similarities between ACTH and interferon. Antiserum for INF-γ neutralized ACTH activity and vice versa (Blalock and Smith, 1980). The similarity between ACTH and INF-γ was also seen when ACTH was added *in vitro* to lymphocyte cultures stimulated by T-independent or T-dependent antigens. INF-γ and ACTH had similar kinetics of suppression, had greater impact on T-dependent than T-independent responses, and suppressed early events in the antibody response (Johnson *et al.*, 1982). Despite the cross-reactivity of ACTH and INF-γ, and similarities in bioactivity, these are not products of a single gene as the amino acid sequence of human INF does not include the ACTH or endorphin sequences (Smith and Blalock, 1981).

6.4.3   Prolactin and growth hormone

As we have indicated, immune disruption in hypophysectomized animals can be reversed by treatment with prolactin and growth hormone (Bernton *et al.*, 1991; Kelley, 1991). Weigent *et al.* (1991) pointed out that determining the role of GH (and PRL) is difficult because the lymphocytes produce the hormones themselves and we have no information on the regulation of the hormone production in lymphocytes. Nonetheless, it is known that lymphocytes produce both hormones (Hiestand *et al.*, 1986; Weigent *et al.*, 1991) and that in all likelihood the immune-derived hormones act in an autocrine and/or paracrine manner to drive cellular proliferation (Bernton *et al.*, 1991; Weigent *et al.*, 1991).

6.4.4 Glucocorticoids

There is no published evidence that GC is produced by immune cells, although Ottaviani and Franceschi (1997) report in unpublished data that there is a GC-like molecule in hemocytes from freshwater snails. It has also been found that the GC precursor, pregnenolone is synthesized in thymic epithelial cells, but not T-cells, of neonatal mice (Vacchio *et al.*, 1994). Because pregnenolone synthesis declined with age, it was suggested that the GC derived from these cells acts through apoptosis to remove GC-sensitive cells during the development of self-tolerance (Vacchio *et al.*, 1994). Similarly, Lechner *et al.* (1997) reported that steroidogenic enzymes necessary for GC production were present in the murine thymus and the chicken thymus and bursa. However, whether the ability to produce GC resided in lymphocytes or epithelial cells was not determined.

6.5 Phylogeny of stress-induced immune–endocrine interaction

The driving force behind research into stress-induced immune modulation in mammals is the need to understand human health. Foremost among the reasons for developing non-mammalian models of stress-induced immune modulation and the attendant immune–endocrine relations is to determine the evolutionary beginnings of these systems and thereby gain more understanding of how the human systems function. Based on the presence of messenger molecules in unicellular organisms and even plants, Roth *et al.* (1985) suggested that the chemical molecules of intercellular communication pre-date vertebrate evolution and, therefore, evolution of the nervous, endocrine or immune systems. Others suggest that the immune and endocrine systems evolved from a single cell similar to the invertebrate hemocyte (Ottaviani and Franceschi, 1997). Another reason for studying non-mammalian models of stress and immune function is the economic importance of some species examined. By far the most research using non-mammalian models has come from the poultry (Dietert and Golemboski, 1994; Marsh and Scanes, 1994) and aquaculture (Iwama *et al.*, 1997) industries, as they try to maximize production efficiency.

In this section we examine non-mammalian models of stress and immune–endocrine interactions — summarizing work with invertebrates, fish, amphibians and birds. Much of this work does not deal with stress, per se, but looks at how the immune and endocrine systems function during development, growth or hormone treatment. Presenting these non-stress studies is reasonable because hormonal and immune altera- tions that occur during these times of change are the same as those elicited by stress. We offer the caveat that care must be taken when making comparisons across phylogenic groups, especially comparisons between ectotherms and endotherms or vertebrates and invertebrates. As an example, there are over 20,000 species of fish, including some that live in water at temperatures below freezing and others that live in water close to boiling (Bond, 1996). Fish are also native to waters with a wide range of salinity and photoperiod (Bond, 1996). There is more variability in the anatomy of the pituitary glands in fish (from cyclostomes to teleosts) than in the remaining vertebrate species (Norris, 1996). Moreover, the activity of the immune and endocrine systems in ectotherms shows seasonal changes independent of the environment or stress (see: Zapata *et al.*, 1992). It would be naive to expect all of the vertebrate and invertebrate physiological systems to behave identically considering these variable environments and endogenous rhythms.

6.5.1   Invertebrates

Virtually all of the research conducted using invertebrate models has addressed the evolutionary origins of immune–endocrine interactions and many have included comparisons with vertebrates. It appears that invertebrates possess all of the components of an HPA axis, perhaps within a single cell. Considerable research attention has been directed at POMC-like compounds and their regulation of immune cells. For example, Cooper *et al.* (1993) demonstrated that endogenous opioids activated both earthworm hemocytes and human granulocytes.

Although numerous studies have looked at various chemical indicators of stress in invertebrates, work with the marine bivalve *Mytilus edulis* has provided one of the few invertebrate models in which the animals receive an identifiable stress (Stefano *et al.*, 1990). In this model, a wooden wedge was placed between the valves to prohibit their closing. If the animal was allowed to maneuver the wedge out and close its valves, there was no apparent stress. However, electrical shocks applied to neural structures prohibited the animal from removing the wedge and resulted in a higher proportion of activated hemocytes than in animals that received either (1) wedge, (2) electrical shock to neural structures, (3) shocks to a non-neural area or (4) wedge and shocks to non-neural areas (Stefano *et al.*, 1990). Treating animals with an opioid analogue or blocker in this and other experiments (Stefano *et al.*, 1989) led the authors to conclude that the stress response was a receptor-mediated action of an endogenous opioid secreted by the hemocytes and acting in an autocrine or paracrine manner.

This group of researchers also demonstrated receptor-mediated CRH immunosuppression (Smith *et al.*, 1992) and identified a biphasic effect from endogenous morphine in the insect *Leucophaea maderae* and humans, as well as *Mytilus* (Stefano *et al.*, 1995). In these experiments, simultaneously exposing invertebrate immunocytes or mammalian monocytes to morphine and an immune stimulant (bacterial cell-wall antigens, LPS) was immunosuppressive. However, cells exposed to morphine for 24 hours prior to treatment with immune stimulant or immune cytokine actually had an enhanced response; *in vivo* experiments using the stress model described above substantiated these *in vitro* results (Stefano *et al.*, 1995). The authors concluded that the long-term exposure to endogenous morphine was important in re-establishing, or priming, the immune cells for further antigen stimulation (Stefano *et al.*, 1995). Interestingly, the time required for this priming to enhance the response (24–48 hours) is the same as that reported for enhanced immune response and disease resistance following stress of chinook salmon *Oncorhynchus tshawytscha* (Maule *et al.*, 1989). Stefano and Smith (1996) have proposed a similar regulatory role for another POMC-derived peptide — ACTH. We previously described this theoretical model of tonal inhibition of the immune system in invertebrates and vertebrates (see section 6.4.2).

Using an *in vitro* model, Ottaviani *et al.* (1992a) demonstrated an HPA-like axis in the freshwater snail *Planorbarius corneus*, except that all of the messenger and effector molecules (CRH, ACTH and catecholamines) are derived from, and have their effects on the snail hemocytes. Invertebrate hemocytes also contain immune messengers, including IL-1, IL-2, and TNF, and these molecules can stimulate the *in vitro* release of catecholamines, perhaps in competition with CRH (Ottaviani *et al.*, 1994, 1995b). As a result of their research with invertebrates, Ottaviani and colleagues proposed that invertebrate hemocytes be considered an 'immune-mobile brain' that receives non-cognitive stimuli and supplies a combined immune–endocrine response (Ottaviani *et al.*, 1992a; Ottaviani and Franceschi, 1996). This hypothesis is compatible with Blalock's (1984) characterization of mammalian immune cells as sensory organs that relay information about non-cognitive stress to the nervous and endocrine systems. Ottaviani *et al.* (1992b) have also shown that ACTH is present in phagocytic cells from the invertebrates through humans; however, while this POMC derivative is found in lymphocytes of anuran amphibians, it is absent from lymphocytes of urodelan amphibians and fish. The authors point out that isotype-switching during the development of an antibody response — the ability to shift immunoglobulin production from IgM to IgG (see: Janeway and Travers, 1994) — also first appears in the anuran amphibians, and speculate that ACTH may have a role in that process. Moreover, Ottaviani and Franceschi (1997) propose that the immune and endocrine systems of mammals evolved from a single cell, similar to the invertebrate hemocyte, which contains functions of both mammalian systems. Ottaviani *et al.* (1997) recently published an extensive comparative review of invertebrate immune–endocrine responses during stress.

6.5.2   Fish

There is a long history of research into the effects of stress on the immune system of fish, and several recent reviews have addressed stress, the endocrine system, and the immune system in fish (Barton and Iwama, 1991; Schreck, 1996; Balm, 1997; Iwama *et al.*, 1997; Wendelaar Bonga, 1997). We believe it is important to again emphasize that there are over 20,000 species of fish and that, although many marine and freshwater species have been used in research on stress and immune function, they are all from the most numerous and most evolutionarily advanced group —the teleosts. As with studies in other vertebrate groups, the results often differ by species, timing and magnitude of stress or treatment, and immune variable examined.

It has been stated frequently that stress in fish is immunosuppressive and reduces disease resistance (Sneiszko, 1974; Wedemeyer, 1974). While there are numerous observations linking stress and disease in fish, experimental confirmation of this relation is quite recent (Maule *et al.*, 1989; Pickering and Pottinger, 1989; Wise *et al.*, 1993; Yin *et al.*, 1995). Early studies with fish mimicked those with mammals, and researchers reported that stress and a variety of treatments and combinations of treatments (e.g. hypophysectomy, injections of NE and NE antagonists, injections of ACTH and GC) caused changes in the numbers and types of circulating leukocytes (Ball and Slicher, 1962; Slicher *et al.*, 1966; Pickford *et al.*, 1971a,b,c). The general pattern of decreased numbers of circulating lymphocytes (primarily B-cells) and increased circulating neutrophils has been reported for acutely stressed catfish *Ictalurus punctatus* (Ellsaesser and Clem, 1986; Bly *et al.*, 1990; Ainsworth *et al.*, 1991), rainbow trout *Oncorhynchus mykiss* (Narnaware and Baker, 1996) and dab *Limanda limanda* (Pulsford *et al.*, 1994). However, the opposite response of increased lymphocytes and decreased neutrophils was reported for Atlantic salmon *Salmo salar* (Thompson *et al.*, 1993).

Stress also affects the functioning of immune cells in fish. Proliferative responses of catfish peripheral blood leukocytes (PBLs) to a T-cell mitogen (ConA) and a B-cell mitogen (LPS) were reduced after stress (Ellsaesser and Clem, 1986; Bly *et al.*, 1990). Ellsaesser and Clem (1986) also reported that the ability of PBLs to generate antibody to T-dependent or T-independent antigens was suppressed. Moreover, they concluded that stress-induced immunosuppression was directed at lymphocytes because the accessory functions of adherent cells (e.g. macrophages) were not affected (Ellsaesser and Clem, 1986). The ability of splenic and pronephric leukocytes to generate antibody-producing cells was also depressed under a variety of stressful conditions in Pacific salmon (Maule et al., 1989; Mazur and Iwama, 1993; Salonius and Iwama, 1993); however, adherent cells appeared to be affected in this genus (Kaattari and Tripp, 1987; Tripp et al., 1987).

Non-specific immune responses in fish are also affected by stress. Although stress had no effect on the phagocytic ability of circulating catfish neutrophils (Ainsworth et al., 1991), the plasma from stressed rainbow trout enhanced the ability of pronephric phagocytes to kill yeast cells (Ruis and Bayne, 1997). This is somewhat in agreement with Pulsford et al. (1994) who reported that the percent of glass-adherent pronephric cells that phagocytosed yeast was significantly greater in dab that were acutely stressed for one hour as compared to controls. However, there was no effect of stress on splenic phagocytes, or in phagocytic indices (number of yeast phagocytosed per cell) from either organ. On the contrary, Narnaware et al. (1994) reported that a 3-hour stress of rainbow trout resulted in a significant decrease in percent phagocytosis and phagocytic index for splenic and pronephric phagocytic cells. Reports on the effects of stress on lysozyme activity in fish are a bit more consistent than those on phagocytosis. Several studies with salmonids have reported that short-term stress (e.g. stress lasting ≤ 2 hours) increased blood lysozyme activity (Mock and Peters, 1990; Thompson et al., 1993; Demers and Bayne, 1997), but longer term stress (≥ 2 hours) decreased lysozyme activity (Mock and Peters, 1990; Yin et al., 1995).

As with mammals, stress-induced elevation in GC (i.e. cortisol) has been implicated in the suppression of immunity and disease resistance in fish. Neither fish nor amphibians have a distinct adrenal gland, but the steroidogenic functions of that organ reside in interrenal cells of the pronephros (also known as head kidney or anterior kidney). Thus, fish and amphibians have a hypothalamic–pituitary–interrenal (HPI) axis. Perhaps the most complete model of stress-induced immune regulation in fish described to date is that for Pacific salmon. Maule et al. (1987, 1989) demonstrated that even moderate increases in plasma cortisol, whether as a result of developmental changes, stress or exogenous GC treatment, reduced the ability of Pacific salmon to generate splenic and pronephric specific antibody-producing cells, either in vivo or in vitro. Elevated plasma cortisol was also responsible for a reduction in disease resistance. Tripp et al. (1987) demonstrated that in vitro, physiologic levels of cortisol caused a dose-dependent immunosuppression of splenic and pronephric cells, and that the cortisol immunosuppression could be abrogated by the addition of medium from non-cortisol-treated, antigen-stimulated cell cultures. Limiting dilution analyses suggested that cortisol inhibits the activation of B-cells, by influencing the release of a cytokine (e.g. IL-1) (Kaattari and Tripp, 1987). Salmonid leukocytes possess specific GR (Maule and Schreck, 1990) and the affinity and number of those GR change as a result of stress or *in vivo* cortisol treatment (Maule and Schreck, 1991). So it appears that in Pacific salmon stress-induced increases in cortisol affect immune functioning via receptor-mediated suppression of a cytokine. Maule *et al.* (1989) also reported immune enhancement and increased disease resistance in Pacific salmon at 24 hours after stress; however, mechanisms of this enhancement have not been elucidated.

A different picture of cortisol's effects on piscine immune systems comes from studies with catfish. As we have indicated, stress had specific effects on several immune responses in catfish, including T-cell and B-cell activities (Ellsaesser and Clem, 1986). *In vivo* cortisol treatment resulted in virtually the same suite of immunosuppressive effects; however, *in vitro* treatment of catfish PBLs with physiologic doses of cortisol had no effect (Ellsaesser and Clem, 1987). Interestingly, neither stress nor *in vitro* cortisol treatment had an effect on catfish neutrophils, but *in vivo* cortisol treatment suppressed phagocytosis (Ainsworth *et al.*, 1991). We are not aware of any studies to detect cortisol receptors in catfish leukocytes. Similar to the studies with catfish, Narnaware *et al.* (1994) found a difference between *in vivo* and *in vitro* GC treatment of phagocytic cells from rainbow trout. Six daily injections of dexamethasone (0.2 mg) reduced the phagocytic index of splenic and pronephric adherent cells as compared to saline-injected controls, but *in vitro* treatment with cortisol for 3 hours had no effect. The use of dexamethasone for several days may explain these differences; when the same researchers treated fish with a single, lower dose (0.05 mg) of cortisol, phagocytic indices were significantly greater than those of saline-injected controls, but did not differ from non-injected fish (Narnaware and Baker, 1996). These researchers also reported that NE injections depressed phagocytosis, but that cortisol or the adrenergic antagonist phentolamine blocked the action of NE. Nevid and Meier (1995) reported that cortisol feeding had no effect on allograft rejection (a T-cell mediated response) in gulf killifish *Fundulus grandis*. In contrast, Pulsford *et al.* (1995) reported that *in vitro* GC treatment suppressed proliferation of dab splenic and nephric lymphocytes but phagocytosis by adherent cells was enhanced by *in vitro* treatment with a moderate dose of GC (150 ng/ml), but was suppressed by a higher dose (320 ng/ml) (Pulsford *et al.*, 1995).

The apparently conflicting effects of GC on immune functioning are further illustrated in experiments examining programmed cell death (apoptosis) in fish leukocytes. Weyts (1998) demonstrated that cortisol selectively induced apoptosis in carp B-cells, but actually inhibited apoptosis in neutrophils. The induction and inhibition of apoptosis could be blocked by the GR blocker RU486, suggesting that both actions were receptor mediated. Alford *et al.* (1994) reported that stress reduced apoptosis of PBLs, but *in vitro* cortisol treatment had no effect. Possible cellular and tissue bases for these disparate results are described in section 6.3.4.

The possibility that immune and endocrine responses are closely related in the genome is suggested by studies in which fish were selectively bred for high or low cortisol response to stress. Rainbow trout selected for a low plasma cortisol response to stress, also had a reduced duration of lymphocytopenia as compared to fish selected for high cortisol response (Pottinger *et al.*, 1994). Similarly, Atlantic salmon selected for low cortisol response also had higher spontaneous serum hemolytic activity and, more important relative to a genetic link, had greater resistance to two fish pathogenic bacteria (Fevolden *et al.*, 1993).

Some of the earliest experiments with fish examined the effects of pituitary hormones on the immune system. However, in most of those studies, injections of ACTH probably acted via the release of GC, and the immune variable considered was change in circulating leukocytes (Ball and Slicher, 1962; Pickford *et al.*, 1971c). In more recent work, *in vitro* ACTH enhanced phagocytic activity in rainbow trout (Bayne and Levy, 1991) similar to its effects on invertebrate hemocytes (Stefano *et al.*, 1995), although the timing of effects differed. It is possible that ACTH in fish acts in an autocrine or paracrine manner, as ACTH mRNA has been detected in fish phagocytes (Ottaviani *et al.*, 1995a). Possible effects of non-cognitive stress (i.e. LPS) on immune-derived POMC peptides were reviewed by Balm (1997). Bayne and colleagues have completed a series of experiments describing autonomic innervation of the spleen (Flory, 1989) and the *in vitro* effects of adrenergic- and cholinergic-receptor agonists on *in vitro* primary antibody response (Flory, 1990), mitogen-stimulated proliferation and phagocytic activity (Flory and Bayne, 1991; Bayne and Levy, 1991) in coho salmon *O. kisutch* and rainbow trout. In summary, β-adrenergic agonists suppressed responses, while α-2 adrenergic and cholinergic agonists enhanced responses except for mitogen proliferation which α-2 adrenergic and cholinergic agonists did not alter.

Plasma levels of the pituitary hormones GH and PRL are altered by stress in fish, as in mammals. Coho salmon plasma PRL increased as a result of acute or chronic stress (Avella *et al.*, 1991); however, PRL had no effect on the ability of coho salmon splenic or pronephric leukocytes to generate antibody-producing cells *in vitro* (M. Avella and C. Schreck, unpublished data). The effects of stress on GH levels varies depending on species and stress (see review: Wendelaar Bonga, 1997), but several studies have shown that GH can have positive effects on the immune responses of fish. In an extensive study of the effects of several hormone treatments, Nevid and Meier (1995) reported that both PRL and GH enhanced allograft rejection in gulf killifish. Furthermore, atropine (muscarinic receptor blocker) had no effect, while naloxone (opioid antagonist) and propranolol (β-adrenergic antagonist) both suppressed rejection. Marc *et al.* (1995) reported that plasma GH correlated positively with plasma lysozyme and respiratory burst activity of pronephric phagocytes during seawater acclimation of brown trout *S. trutta*. Similarly, Kitlen *et al.* (1997) demonstrated increased respiratory burst activity in rainbow trout given GH injections once a week for seven weeks. Narnaware *et al.* (1997) reported increased phagocytosis by splenic and pronephric phagocytes from silver sea bream *Sparus sarba* that received seven, daily GH injections. Interestingly, cytochemical staining for GH receptors in pronephric cells of gilthead sea bream *Sparus aurata* suggested that immature cells (granulocytes and erythroblasts) had a greater number of receptors than did mature monocytes or lymphocytes (Calduch-Giner *et al.*, 1995).

6.5.3   Amphibians

There is a large body of information on the immune systems, endocrine systems, and the effects of stress on the development and metamorphosis of amphibians; however, very few studies specifically examine the effects of stress on immune–endocrine interactions. Those studies that considered stress, generally dealt with the effects of inadequate artificial rearing conditions on immune organs (Dulak and Płytycz, 1989; also see Kinney *et al.*, 1996). Because elevated levels of GC are a feature of amphibian metamorphosis, several studies have examined the effects of *in vivo* GC treatment on immune organs. The morphological results of GC treatment of amphibians are similar to those reported for mammals and fish — thymic involution and peripheral lymphopenia (Tournefier, 1982; Garrido *et al.*, 1987). However, sensitivity to GC in amphibians varies with season (Garrido *et al.*, 1989) as it does with most ectothermic vertebrates (Zapata *et al.*, 1992). Tournefier (1982) demonstrated an enhanced antibody response in the urodelan amphibian *Ambystoma mexicanum* when GC were injected eight days prior to, or on the same day as, antigen injection. Thymectomy also led to an enhanced response, while GC treatment in addition to thymectomy had no additional enhancement. Tournefier (1982) concluded that GC either depleted suppressor T-cells or stimulated helper T-cells. It should be noted that in many of these studies with amphibians, researchers injected what are surely pharmacological doses of GC (e.g. 5–60 mg/animal).

The hypothalamic–pituitary–interrenal (HPI) axis regulates amphibian metamorphosis, and environmental stress accelerates the timing and rate of metamorphosis (see: Denver, 1997; Hayes, 1997). Activation of the HPI axis by environmental stress early in development will accelerate growth and inhibit metamorphosis; however, late in development the same stress will inhibit growth and accelerate metamorphosis (Denver, 1993). The primary glucocorticoid in amphibians is corticosterone (CS), which acts synergistically with thyroid hormone and its receptors to accelerate metamorphosis (Hayes, 1997) and is likely responsible for the dramatic loss of cells in immune organs during metamorphosis (Marx *et al.*, 1987). Research by Ruben and colleagues has addressed the hypothesis that during metamorphosis of the anuran amphibian *Xenopus laevis,* increased endogenous CS down-regulates the immune system to protect cells of the developing adult. Marx *et al.* (1987) demonstrated that, compared to larval and adult stages, there is a 5- to 10-fold increase in CS receptors in thymocytes and splenocytes at the peak of metamorphosis. Subsequently, Ruben *et al.* (1994a,b) reported that *in vitro* and *in vivo* treatment with dexamethasone increased apoptosis of thymic lymphocytes in adult *Xenopus*, but not in metamorphosing animals. They concluded that during metamorphosis the high concentrations of endogenous CS had already removed hormone-sensitive cells. Dexamethasone or CS treatment also suppressed mitogen proliferation, cell viability (Rollins-Smith and Blair, 1993), putative T-helper cell and T-suppressor cell functions, and B-cell functions (Marx *et al.*, 1987). The loss of T-cell functions during metamorphosis may be caused by endogenous CS suppressing the secretion of an IL-2-like substance and inhibiting the expression IL-2 receptors in *Xenopus* lymphocytes (Ruben *et al.*, 1992).

As indicated above, the overriding hypothesis in these studies is that immunosuppression by endogenous CS during metamorphosis acts to protect cells. In fact, changes in the major histocompatibility complex (MHC) of cell-surface antigens suggests that the 'self' identity of the adult differs from that of the larvae (Flajnik *et al.*, 1986); so, the metamorphosing animal must establish a new state of self-tolerance. Recently, Rollins-Smith *et al.* (1997) reported that hypophysectomy of *Xenopus* tadpoles not only interfered with overall animal growth and T-cell expansion, but also that hypophysectomized animals failed to develop the adult MHC pattern. Although the physiological consequences of hypophysectomy are far reaching, these results suggest a possible endocrine influence on the induction of self-antigens in some ways similar to the proposal by Ottaviani *et al.* (1992b) that ACTH secreted by anuran, but not urodelan, lymphocytes has a role in the induction of the evolutionarily advanced process of isotype switching.

6.5.4 Birds

The significant body of research conducted on avians is the result of the economic interests of the poultry industry and also because birds are the penultimate phylogenetic group next to mammals. The immune and endocrine anatomy of birds is very similar to that of mammals, with the exception of the Bursa of Fabricius which is the origin of B-cells in birds. Much of the research with poultry stems from a need to develop high-density rearing enclosures (Dietert and Golemboski, 1994) and as a result, crowding- and heat-stress are seen frequently in the literature. In fact, similar to studies with fish, hens selectively bred for stress-tolerance based on survival, did not exhibit endocrine or immune stress responses when crowded or heat stressed (Hester et al., 1996a,b).

Many of the classic experiments conducted on mammals to examine endocrine effects on the immune system have been duplicated with birds (see review: Marsh and Scanes, 1994), including in vivo and in vitro effects of GC (in this case corticosterone) on leukocyte distribution and immune response. Implants of CS in domestic chickens elevated circulating CS for seven days, but caused peripheral blood lymphocytopenia for 14 days; background and mitogen-stimulated proliferation were reduced by CS treatment in vivo (Davison et al., 1988) and in vitro (Franklin et al., 1987; Davison et al., 1988). Similarly, Siegel et al. (1983) reported that in vivo ACTH treatment several hours prior to antigen challenge suppressed antibody titers when the antigen dose was low, but had no effect on high antigen doses. Fowles et al. (1993) injected mallard ducks Anas platyrhyncos with dexamethasone daily for 28 days and reported reduced primary and secondary antibody responses, decreased phagocytosis, but increased NK-cell activity. Lesions to the baso-medial-hypothalamus of 6-week-old chickens resulted in several temporary T-cell impairments including reduced mitogen proliferation, reduced delayed-type hypersensitivity, and reduced total immunoglobulin. Specific primary, but not memory, antibody responses were also temporarily impaired (Karin et al., 1988). Johnson et al. (1993) surgically hypophysectomized 3-week-old chickens and reported no effect on bursa weight, but the weight of the thymus was reduced, although there was no change in the proportions of putative T-helper cells (CD4+) and T-suppressor cells (CD8+). However, in the peripheral blood there was significant increase in CD8+ cells relative to CD4+ cells; these effects were partially abrogated by treatment with a recombinant chicken GH. Chickens that received twice-daily injections of chicken GH for seven days reportedly had increased NK-cell-like activity (Haddad and Mashaly, 1991). Trout and Mashaly (1994) demonstrated that the effects of heat stress and ACTH injections differed from those reported following hypophysectomy — while there was no effect on B-cells in blood or spleen, both CD4+ and CD8+ cells declined in the blood and increased in the spleen.

Circulating prolactin increases in birds during egg incubation, and recently several studies have explored possible effects of PRL on immunity. Background, but not mitogen-stimulated, lymphocyte proliferation increased concomitantly with increased PRL during incubation of ring doves *Streptopelia risoria* (Ibars *et al.*, 1997). *In vivo* and *in vitro* treatment with exogenous PRL increased phagocytosis and respiratory burst activity of ring dove heterophils (Rodriguez *et al.*, 1996). Barriga *et al.* (1994) also reported that serum from antigen-challenged ring doves had enhanced bactericidal and hemolytic activity. If exogenous PRL was added to the serum, the bactericidal and hemolytic activity was synergistically enhanced over that of the antigen-enhanced serum or normal serum treated with PRL. Interestingly, *in vivo* PRL treatment of chickens had the most immune enhancement when it was administered 4 to 8 hours after dawn (Skwarło-Sonta, 1992). This phenomenon appeared to be the result of interaction with diel changes in endogenous CS (Skwarło-Sonta, 1992).

A number of studies with chickens have examined the effects of non-cognitive stress acting through the immune system to affect endocrine activity. Injection of *Salmonella pullorum* antigen caused a 7- to 10-fold increase in serum CS as compared to PBS-injected controls (Siegel *et al.*, 1985). Adrenal cells from control birds produced significant amounts of CS when incubated with serum or splenic leukocytes from antigen-treated birds, leading the authors to conclude that antigen-stimulated leukocytes produce an ACTH-like substance (Siegel *et al.*, 1985). Trout *et al.* (1988) reported a significant increase in CS about three hours after initiation of either a primary or memory antibody response. The possible influence of the immune system on the endocrine system in chickens was also demonstrated by Mashaly (1984) who reported that bursectomy caused a significant increase in circulating CS for at least 4 weeks.

6.6   Conclusion

At the beginning of this chapter we expressed agreement with Ottaviani and Franceschi (1996) that the stress response must be viewed as a positive, adaptive reaction. We have presented a large number of studies that offer conflicting data — in some, stress or treatment with stress-related hormones enhanced immune responses and in others, stress suppressed responses. We do not believe that these disparate results bring into question the adaptive nature of the stress response, but they do illustrate the difficulty of interpreting outcomes from experimental designs that involve unnatural stresses (e.g. physically restraining a rat, crowding chickens in a cage, or holding fish in a net out of water) that are in no way related to stresses under which the responses evolved. Allowing an animal to respond to a predator would seem to be the most natural of stresses. Similarly, lesioning or ablating tissue (e.g. hypophysectomy) or hormone treatments may help us to understand mechanisms, but the results should not necessarily be considered the final word on how systems respond under natural conditions.

Although it is generally accepted that stress is immunosuppressive, studies with mammals (Gisler *et al.*, 1971; Okimura and Nigo, 1986), fish (Maule *et al.*, 1989), and invertebrates (Stefano *et al.*, 1990) reported an enhancement of the immune response at some time after stress. The same was true of *in vivo* hormone treatment—enhancement or suppression of immune function depended on the timing or dose of treatment. Furthermore, suppression of the immune response may be adaptive. It has been proposed that GC immunosuppression in mammals (Munck *et al.*, 1984), amphibians (Marx *et al.*, 1987; Ruben *et al.*, 1994a,b), and fish (Maule *et al.*, 1987) acts to protect tissue from over-active immune cells. Besedovski and Del Ray (1996) point out that endocrine suppression of immune function during bacterial endotoxic sepsis (i.e. non-cognitive stress) actually protects the individual from its own, overactive immune response. They also suggest that the death of individuals in whom endotoxin levels exceed the capacity of the endocrine and immune systems is evolutionarily significant. The authors speculated that this 'negative self-selection' protects other healthy individuals from those who have become vectors for the pathogen (Besedovski and Del Ray, 1996). This clearly non-Darwinian view of evolution is suggestive of natural selection at a level above the individual—an alternative mode of selection proposed by some (Eldredge and Gould, 1972; also see: Gould, 1982). Breeding studies with non-mammalian species (Fevolden *et al.*, 1993; Hester *et al.*, 1996a,b) suggest a Darwinian evolutionary view in which animals with a low stress response have an adaptive advantage by virtue of increased disease resistance. Independent of evolutionary perspective, there can be no doubt that animals evolved adaptive responses to stress—including stress-induced immune–endocrine interactions.

Acknowledgments

We thank Chris Bayne and Mathilakath Vijayan for reviewing the manuscript. We also thank our colleagues Karen Hans and Lisa Weiland at the Columbia River Research Laboratory for their assistance.

References

Ader, R., Felton, D.L. and Cohen, C. (eds.) (1991) *Psychoneuroimmunology*, 2nd edn, Academic Press, Inc., San Diego.

Ainsworth, A.J., Dexiang, C. and Waterstrat, P.R. (1991) Changes in peripheral blood leukocytes percentages and function of neutrophils in stressed channel catfish. *Journal of Aquatic Animal Health*, **3 (1)** 41-47.

Aird, F., Clevenger, C.V., Prytowsky, M.B. and Redei, E. (1993) Corticotropin-releasing factor mRNA in rat thymus and spleen. *Proceedings of the National Academy of Sciences*, **90** 7104-7106.

Akahoshi, T., Oppenheim, J.J. and Matsushima, K. (1988) Induction of high-affinity interleukin 1 receptor on human peripheral blood lymphocytes by glucocorticoid hormones. *Journal of Experimental Medicine*, **167** 924-936.

Alford III, P.B., Tomasso, J.R., Bodine, A.B. and Kendall, C. (1994) Apoptotic death of peripheral leukocytes in channel catfish: Effect of confinement-induced stress. *Journal of Aquatic Animal Health*, **6 (1)** 64-69.

Arya, S.K., Wong-Staal, F. and Gallo, R.C. (1984) Dexamethasone-mediated inhibition of human T cell growth factor and γ-interferon messenger RNA. *Journal of Immunology*, **133 (1)** 273-276.

Auphan, N., Didonato, J.A., Rosette, C., Helmberg, A. and Karin, M. (1995) Immunosuppression by glucocorticoids: inhibition of NF-κB activity through induction of IκB synthesis. *Science*, **270** 286-290.

Avella, M., Schreck, C.B. and Prunet, P. (1991) Plasma prolactin and cortisol concentrations of stressed coho salmon, *Oncorhynchus kisutch*, in fresh water or salt water. *General and Comparative Endocrinology*, **81** 21-27.

Ball, J.N. and Slicher, A.M. (1962) Influence of hypophysectomy and of an adrenocortical inhibitor (*SU*-4885) on the stress-response of the white blood cells in the teleost fish, *Mollienesia latipinna* Le Sueur. *Nature*, **196** 1331-1332.

Balm, P.H.M. (1997) Immune-endocrine interactions in *Fish Stress and Health in Aquaculture* (eds. G.K. Iwama, A.D. Pickering, J.P. Sumpter and C.B. Schreck), Cambridge University Press, Cambridge, pp 195-221.

Bamberger, C.M., Bamberger, A., de Castro, M. and Chrousos, G.P. (1995) Glucocorticoid receptor β, a potential endogenous inhibitor of glucocorticoid action in humans. *Journal of Clinical Investigation*, **95** 2435-2441.

Bamberger, C.M., Schulte, H.M. and Chrousos, G.P. (1996) Molecular determinants of glucocorticoid receptor function and tissue sensitivity to glucocorticoids. *Endocrine Review*, **17 (3)** 245-261.

Bamberger, C.M., Else, T., Bamberger, A., Beil, F.U. and Schulte, H.M. (1997) Regulation of the human interleukin-2 gene by the α and β isoforms of the glucocorticoid receptor. *Molecular and Cellular Endocrinology*, **136** 23-28.

Barriga, C., Lopez, R. and Rodriguez, A.B. (1994) Haemolytic and bactericidal activity of serum from the ring dove (*Streptopelia risoria*) after treatment with exogenous prolactin. *Journal of Comparative Physiology B*, **164** 499-502.

Barton, B.A. and Iwama, G.K. (1991) Physiological changes in fish from stress in aquaculture with emphasis on the response and effects of corticosteroids. *Annual Review of Fish Diseases*, pp 3-26.

Bayne, C.J. and Levy, S. (1991) The respiratory burst of rainbow trout, *Oncorhynchus mykiss* (Walbaum), phagocytes is modulated by sympathetic neurotransmitters and the 'neuro' peptide ACTH. *Journal of Fish Biology*, **38** 609-619.

Bernton, E.W., Bryant, H.U. and Holaday, J.W. (1991) Prolactin and immune function, in *Psychoneuroimmunology*, 2nd edn, (eds. R. Ader, D.L. Felton and C. Cohen), Academic Press, Inc, San Diego, pp 403-424.

Besedovsky, H.O. and Del Ray, A. (1996) Immune-neuro-endocrine interactions: facts and hypotheses. *Endocrine Reviews*, **17 (1)** 64-102.

Besedovsky, H., Sorkin, E., Keller, M. and Muller, J. (1975) Changes in blood hormone levels during the immune response. *Proceedings of the Society for Experimental Biology and Medicine*, **150** 466-470.

Besedovsky, H.O., Del Rey, A., Sorkin, E., Da Prada, M. and Keller, H.H. (1979) Immuno-regulation mediated by the sympathetic nervous system. *Cellular Immunology*, **48** 346-355.

Besedovsky, H.O., Del Rey, A. and Sorkin, E. (1981) Lymphokine-containing supernatants from Con A-stimulated cells increase corticosterone blood levels. *Journal of Immunology*, **126** 385-387.

Besedovsky, H., Del Rey, A., Sorkin, E., Da Prada, M., Burri, R. and Honegger, C. (1983) The immune response evokes changes in brain noradrenergic neurons. *Science*, **221** 564-566.

Besedovsky, H.O., Del Rey, A.E. and Sorkin, E., Lotz, W. and Schwulera, U. (1985b) Lymphoid cells produce an immunoregulatory glucocorticoid increasing factor (GIF) acting through the pituitary gland. *Clinical and Experimental Immunology*, **59** 622-628.

Besedovsky, H., Del Rey, A., Sorkin, E. and Dinarello, C.A. (1986) Immunoregulatory feedback between interleukin-1 and glucocorticoid hormones. *Science*, **233** 652-654.

Black, P. (1994) Central nervous system-immune system interactions: psychoneurendocrinology of stress and its immune consequences. *Antimicrobial Agents and Chemotherapy*, **38 (1)** 1-6.

Blalock, J.E. (1984) The immune system as a sensory organ. *Journal of Immunology*, **132 (3)** 1067-1070.

Blalock, J.E. (1994) The syntax of immune-neuroendocrine communication. *Immunology Today*, **15 (11)** 504-511.

Blalock, J.E. and Smith, E.M. (1980) Human leukocyte interferon: Structural and biological relatedness to adrenocorticotropic hormone and endorphins. *Proceedings of the National Academy of Sciences*, **77** 5972-5974.

Blalock, J.E. and Smith, E.M. (1982) Human lymphocyte production of neuroendocrine hormone-related substance, in *Human Lymphokine* (eds. A. Kahn, N.O. Hill and D.C. Dumont), Academic Press, Inc., New York, pp 323-332.

Blalock, J.E. and Smith, E.M. (1985) A complete regulatory loop between the immune and neuroendocrine systems. *Federation Proceedings*, **44** 108-111.

Blalock, J.E., Harbour-McMenamin, D. and Smith, E.M. (1985) Peptide hormones shared by the neuroendocrine and immunologic systems. *Journal of Immunology* (suppl), **135** 858-861.

Bly, J.E., Miller, N.W. and Clem, L.W. (1990) A monoclonal antibody specific for neutrophils in normal and stressed channel catfish. *Developmental and Comparative Immunology*, **14 (2)** 211-221.

Bond, C.E. (1996) *Biology of Fishes*, Saunders College Publishing, New York.

Bost, K.L., Clarke, B.L., Xu, J., Kiyono, H., McGhee, J.R. and Pascual, D. (1990) Modulation of IgM secretion and H chain mRNA expression in CH12.LX.C4.5F5 B cells by adrenocorticotropic hormone. *Journal of Immunology*, **145 (12)** 4326-4331.

Bradley, A.J., McDonald, I.R. and Lee, A.K. (1976) Corticosteroid-binding globulin and mortality in a dasyurid marsupial. *Journal of Endocrinology*, **70** 323-324.

Brann, D.W., Hendry, L.B. and Mahesh, V.B. (1995) Emerging diversities in the mechanism of action of steroid hormones. *Journal of Steroid Biochemistry and Molecular Biology*, **52 (2)** 113-133.

Calduch-Giner, J.A., Sitjá-Bobadilla, A., Álvarez-Pellitero, P. and Pérez-Sánchez, J. (1995) Evidence for a direct action of GH on haemopoietic cells of a marine fish, the gilthead sea bream (*Sparus aurata*). *Journal of Endocrinology*, **146** 459-467.

Cannon, W.B., Britton, S.W., Lewis, J.T. and Groeneveld, A. (1927) Studies on the conditions of activity in endocrine glands: the influence of motion and emotion on medulliadrenal secretion. *American Journal of Physiology*, **79** 433-465.

Cavanaugh, A.H. and Simons, Jr., S.S. (1994) Factor-assisted DNA binding as a possible general mechanism for steroid receptors. Functional heterogeneity among activated receptor-steroid complexes. *Journal of Steroid Biochemistry and Molecular Biology*, **48 (5/6)** 433-446.

Chrousos, G.P. and Gold, P.W. (1992) The concepts of stress and stress system disorders. *Journal of the American Medical Association*, **267 (9)** 1244-1252.

Claman, N.H. (1972) Corticosteroids and lymphoid cells. *New England Journal of Medicine*, **287** 388-397.

Clarke, B.L. and Bost, K.L. (1989) Differential expression of functional adrenocorticotropic hormone receptors by subpopulations of lymphocytes. *Journal of Immunology*, **143 (2)** 464-469.

Cohen, J.J. (1972) Thymus-derived lymphocytes sequestered in the bone marrow of hydrocortisone-treated mice. *Journal of Immunology*, **108 (3)** 841-844.

Cooper, D.A., Duckett, M., Petts, V. and Penny, R. (1979) Corticosteroid enhancement of immunoglobulin synthesis by pokeweed mitogen-stimulated human lymphocytes. *Clinical Experimental Immunology*, **37** 145-151.

Cooper, E.L., Leung, M.K., Suzudi, M.M., Vick, K., Cadet, P. and Stefano, G.B. (1993) An enkephalin-like molecule in earthworm coelomic fluid modifies leukocyte behavior. *Developmental and Comparative Immunology*, **17 (3)** 201-210.

Crabtree, G.R., Munck, A. and Smith, K.A. (1980) Glucocorticoids and lymphocytes II. Cell cycle-dependent changes in glucocorticoid receptor content. *Journal of Immunology*, **125** 13-17.

Cupps, T.R., Edgar, L.C., Thomas, C.A. and Fauci, A.S. (1984) Multiple mechanisms of B cell immunoregulation in man after administration of *in vivo* corticosteroids. *Journal of Immunology*, **132 (1)** 170-175.

Cupps, T.R. and Fauci, A.S. (1982) Corticosteroid-mediated immunoregulation in man. *Immunological Reviews*, **65** 133-155.

Cupps, T.R., Gerrard, T.L., Falkoff, R.J.M., Whalen, G. and Fauci, A.S. (1985) Effects of *in vitro* corticosteroids on B cell activation, proliferation and differentiation. *Journal of Clinical Investigation*, **75** 754-761.

Czar, M.J., Owens-Grillo, J.K., Dittmar, K.D., Hutchison, K.A., Zacharek, A.M., Leach, K.L., Deibel, M.R. Jr. and Pratt, W.B. (1994) Characterization of protein-protein interactions determining the heat shock protein (hsp90-hsp70-hsp56) heterocomplex. *Journal of Biological Chemistry*, **269 (15)** 11155-11161.

Dardenne, M., De Moraes, M.C.L., Kelly, A. and Gagnerault, M.C. (1994) Prolactin receptor expression in human hematopoietic tissues analyzed by flow cytoflourometry. *Endocrinology*, **134 (8)** 2108-2114.

Davison, T.F., Misson, B.G., Williamson, R.A. and Rea, J. (1988) Effect of increased circulating corticosterone in the immature fowl on the blasogeic responses of peripheral blood lymphocytes. *Developmental and Comparative Immunology*, **12 (1)** 131-144.

Demers, N.E. and Bayne, C.J. (1997) The immediate effects of stress on hormones and plasma lysozyme in rainbow trout. *Developmental and Comparative Immunology*, **21 (4)** 363-373.

Denver, R.J. (1993) Acceleration of anuran amphibian metamorphosis by corticotropin-releasing hormone-like peptides. *General Comparative Endocrinology*, **91** 38-51.

Denver, R.J. (1997) Proximate mechanisms of phenotypic plasticity in amphibian metamorphosis. *American Zoology*, **37** 172-184.

Depelchin, A. and Letesson, J.J. (1981) Adrenaline influence on the immune response. I. Accelerating or suppressor effects according to the time of application. *Immunological Letters*, **3** 199-205.

Dietert, R.R. and Golemboski, K.A. (1994) Environment-immune interactions. *Poultry Science*, **73** 1062-1076.

Drouin, J., Sun, Y.L., Chamberland, M., Gauthier, Y., De Lean, A., Nemer, M. and Schmidt, T.J. (1993) Novel glucocorticoid receptor complex with DNA element of the hormone-repressed POMC gene. *EMBO*, **12 (1)** 145-156.

Dulak, J. and Płytycz, B. (1989) The effect of laboratory environment on the morphology of the spleen and the thymus in the yellow-bellied toad, *Bombina variegata* (L.). *Developmental and Comparative Immunology*, **13 (1)** 49-56.

Duvaux-Miret, O., Stefano, G.B., Smith, E.M., Dissous, C. and Capron, A. (1992) Immunosuppression in the definitive and intermediate hosts of the human parasite *Schistosoma mansoni* by release of immunoactive neuropeptides. *Proceedings of the National Academy of Sciences*, **89** 778-781.

Edwards III, C.K., Ghiasuddin, S.M., Schepper, J.M., Yunger, L.M. and Kelley, K.W. (1988) A newly defined property of somatotropin: Priming of macrophages for production of superoxide anion. *Science*, **239** 769-771.

Eldredge, N. and Gould, S.J. (1972) Punctuated equilibria: an alternative to phyletic gradualism, in *Models in Paleobiology* (ed. T.J.M. Schopf), Freeman Cooper, San Francisco, pp 82-115.

Ellsaesser, C.F. and Clem, L.W. (1986) Haematological and immunological changes in channel catfish stressed by handling and transport. *Journal of Fish Biology*, **28** 511-521.

Ellsaesser, C.F. and Clem, L.W. (1987) Cortisol-induced hematologic and immunologic changes in channel catfish (*Ictalurus punctatus*). *Comparative Biochemistry and Physiology*, **88A** 589-594.

Felten, S.Y. and Felten, D.L. (1991) Innervation of lymphoid tissue, in *Psychoneuroimmunology*, 2nd edn (eds. R. Ader, D.L. Felton and C. Cohen), Academic Press, Inc., San Diego, pp 27-69.

Fevolden, S.E., Nordmo, R., Refstie, T. and Røed, K.H. (1993) Disease resistance in Atlantic salmon (*Salmo salar*) selected for high or low responses to stress. *Aquaculture*, **109** 215-224.

Flajnik, M.F., Kaufman, J.F., Hsu, E., Manes, M., Parisot, R. and Du Pasquier, L. (1986) Major histocompatibility complex-encoded class I molecules are absent in immunologically competent *Xenopus* before metamorphosis. *Journal of Immunology*, **137** 3891-3899.

Flory, C.M. (1989) Autonomic innervation of the spleen of the coho salmon, *Oncorhynchus kisutch*: a histochemical demonstration and preliminary assessment of its immunoregulatory role. *Brain, Behavior, and Immunity*, **3** 331-334.

Flory, C.M. (1990) Phylogeny of neuroimmunoregulation: effects of adrenergic and cholinergic agents on the *in vitro* antibody response of the rainbow trout, *Oncorhynchus mykiss*. *Developmental and Comparative Immunology*, **14** 283-294.

Flory, C.M. and Bayne, C.J. (1991) The influence of adrenergic and cholinergic agents on the chemiluminescent and mitogenic responses of leukocytes from the rainbow trout, *Oncorhynchus mykiss*. *Developmental and Comparative Immunology*, **15** 135-142.

Fowles, J.R., Fairbrother, A., Fix, M., Schiller, S. and Kerkvliet, N.I. (1993) Glucocorticoid effects on natural and humoral immunity in mallards. *Developmental and Comparative Immunology*, **17 (2)** 165-178.

Franklin, R.A., Davila, D.R. and Delley, K.W. (1987) Chicken serum inhibits lectin-induced proliferation of autologous splenic mononuclear cells (42472). *Proceedings of the Society for Experimental Biology and Medicine*, **184** 225-233.

Funder, J.W., Pearce, P.T., Smith, R. and Smith, A.I. (1988) Mineralocorticoid action: target tissue specificity is enzyme, not receptor, mediated. *Science*, **242** 583-585.

Garrido, E., Gomariz, R.P., Leceta, J. and Zapata, A. (1987) Effects of dexamethasone on the lymphoid organs of *Rana Perezi*. *Developmental and Comparative Immunology*, **11 (2)** 375-384.

Garrido, E., Gomariz, R.P., Leceta, J. and Zapata, A. (1989) Different sensitivity to the dexamethasone treatment of the lymphoid organs of *Rana perezi* in two different seasons. *Developmental and Comparative Immunology*, **13 (1)** 57-64.

Gillis, S., Crabtree, G.R. and Smith, K.A. (1979) Glucocorticoid-induced inhibition of T cell growth factor produciton. II. The effect on the *in vitro* generation of cytolytic T cells. *Journal of Immunology*, **123 (4)** 1632-1638.

Gisler, R.H., Bussard, A.E., Mazie, J.C. and Hess, R. (1971) Hormonal regulation of an immune response. I. Induction of an immune response *in vitro* with lymphoid cells from mice exposed to acute systemic stress. *Cellular Immunology*, **2** 634-645.

Goodwin, J.S. and Atluru, D. (1986) Mechanism of action of glucocorticoid-induced immunoglobulin production: role of lipoxygenase metabolites of arachidonic acid. *Journal of Immunology*, **136** 3455-3460.

Gould, S.J. (1982) Darwinism and the expansion of evolutionary theory. *Science*, **216** 380-387.

Guyre, P.M., Girard, M.T., Morganelli, P.M. and Manganiello, P.D. (1988) Glucocorticoid effects on the production and actions of immune cytokines. *Journal of Steroid Biochemistry*, **30 (1-6)** 89-93.

Haddad, E.E. and Mashaly, M.M. (1991) Chicken growth hormone, triiodothyronine and thyrotropin releasing hormone modulation of the levels of chicken natural cell-mediated cytotoxicity. *Developmental and Comparative Immunology*, **15 (1/2)** 65-72.

Hadden, J.W., Hadden, E.M. and Coffey, R.G. (1991) First and second messengers in the development and function of thymus-dependent lymphocytes, in *Psychoneuroimmunology*, 2nd edn (eds. R. Ader, D.L. Felton and C. Cohen), Academic Press, Inc., San Diego, pp 529-560.

Hall, N.R., McGillis, J.P., Spangelo, B.L. and Goldstein, A.L. (1985) Evidence that thymosins and other biologic response modifiers can function as neuroactive immunotransmitters. *Journal of Immunology* (suppl), **135** 806s-811s.

Hayes, T.B. (1997) Steroids as potential modulators of thyroid hormone activity in anuran metamorphosis. *American Zoology*, **37** 185-194.

Healy, D.L., Hodgen, G.D., Schulte, H.M., Chrousos, G.P., Loriaux, D.L., Hall, N.R. and Goldstein, A.L. (1983) The thymus-adrenal connection: thymosin has corticotropin-releasing activity in primates. *Science*, **222** 1353-1355.

Hester, P.Y., Muir, W.M., Craig, J.V. and Albright, J.L. (1996a) Group selection for adaptation to multiple-hen cages: hematology and adrenal function. *Poultry Science*, **75** 1295-1307.

Hester, P.Y., Muir, W.M. and Craig, J.V. (1996b) Group selection for adaptation to multiple-hen cages: humoral immune response. *Poultry Science*, **75** 1315-1320.

Hiestand, P.C., Mekler, P., Nordmann, R. and Permmongkol, C. (1986) Prolactin as a modulator of lymphocyte responsiveness provides a possible mechanism of action for cyclosporin. *Proceedings of the National Academy of Sciences*, **83** 2599-2603.

Hirschberg, H., Hirschberg, T., Nausieainen, H., Braathen, L.R. and Joffe, E. (1982) The effects of corticosteroid on the antigen presenting properties of human monocytes and endothelial cells. *Clinical Immunology and Immunopathology*, **23** 577-585.

Homo, F., Picard, F., Durant, S., Gagne, D., Simon, J., Dardenne, M. and Duval, D. (1980) Glucocorticoid receptors and their functions in lymphocytes. *Journal of Steroid Biochemistry*, **12** 433-443.

Hsu, S. and DeFranco, D.B. (1995) Selectivity of cell cycle regulation of glucocorticoid receptor function. *Journal of Biological Chemistry*, **270 (7)** 3359-3364.

Hu, L.-M., Bodwell, J., Hu, J.-M., Ortí, E. and Munck, A. (1994) Glucocorticoid receptors in ATP-depleted cells. *Journal of Biological Chemistry*, **269 (9)** 6571-6577.

Hutchison, K.A., Dittmar, K.D. and Pratt, W.B. (1994) All of the factors required for assembly of the glucocorticoid receptor into a functional heterocomplex with heat shock protein 90 are preassociated in a self-sufficient protein folding structure, a "foldosome". *Journal of Biological Chemistry*, **269 (45)** 27894-27899.

Ibars, C.B., Rodriguez, A.B., Skwarlo-Sonta, K. and Lea, R.W. (1997) Mitogenic effect of naturally occurring elevated plasma prolactin on ring dove lymphocytes. *Developmental and Comparative Immunology*, **21 (1)** 47-58.

Irwin, M. and Jones, L. (1991) Life stress, depression and reduced natural cytotoxicity: clinical findings and putative mechanisms, in *Stress and Immunity* (eds. N. Plotnikoff, A. Murgo, R. Faith and J. Wybran), CRC Press, Boca Raton, Florida, pp 109-128.

Iwama, G.K., Pickering, A.D., Sumpter, J.P. and Schreck, C.B. (eds) (1997) *Fish Stress and Health in Aquaculture*, Cambridge University Press, Cambridge.

Janeway, C.A., Jr. and Travers, P. (1994) *Immunobiology: The Immune System in Health and Disease*, Current Biology Ltd., New York.

Johnson, B.E., Scanes, C.G., King, D.B. and Marsh, J.A. (1993) Effect of hypophysectomy and growth hormone on immune development in the domestic fowl. *Developmental and Comparative Immunology*, **17 (4)** 331-340.

Johnson, E.W., Blalock, J.E. and Smith, E.M. (1988) ACTH receptor induction of leukocyte cyclic AMP. *Biochemical and Biophysical Research Communications*, **157 (3)** 1205-1211.

Johnson, H.M., Smith, E.M., Torres, B.A. and Blalock, J.E. (1982) Regulation of the *in vitro* antibody response by neuroendocrine hormones. *Proceedings of the National Academy of Sciences*, **79** 4171-4174.

Johnson, H.M., Torres, B.A., Smith, E.M., Dion, L.D. and Blalock, J.E. (1984) Regulation of lymphokine (γ-interferon) production by corticotropin. *Journal of Immunology*, **123 (1)** 246-250.

Kaattari, S.L. and Tripp, R.A. (1987) Cellular mechanisms of glucocorticoid immunosuppression in salmon. *Journal of Fish Biology*, **31 (suppl A)** 129-132.

Kam, J.C., Szefler, S.J., Surs, W., Sher, E.R. and Leung, D.Y.M. (1993) Combination IL-2 and IL-4 reduces glucocorticoid receptor-binding affinity and T cell response to glucocorticoids. *Journal of Immunology*, **151 (7)** 3460-3466.

Karanth, S. and McCann, S.M. (1991) Anterior pituitary hormone control by interleukin 2. *Proceedings of the National Academy of Sciences*, **88** 2961-2965.

Karin, N., Heller, E.D., Snapir, N., Robinzon, B. and Friedman, A. (1988) The effect of electrolytic lesions in the baso-medial-hypothalamus on the immune response of the chicken. *Developmental and Comparative Immunology*, **12 (4)** 833-842.

Karl, M., Lamberts, S.W., Detera-Wadleigh, S.D., Encio, I.J., Stratakis, C.A., Hurley, D.M., Accili, D. and Chrousos, G.P. (1993) Familial glucocorticoid resistance caused by a splice site deletion in the human glucocorticoid receptor gene. *Journal of Clinical Endocrinology and Metabolism*, **76** 683-689.

Katzenellenbogen, J.A., O'Malley, B.W. and Katzenellenbogen, B.S. (1996) Tripartite steroid hormone receptor pharmacology: interaction with multiple effector sites as a basis for the cell- and promoter-specific action of theses hormones. *Molecular Endocrinology*, **10 (2)** 119-131.

Kelley, K.W. (1991) Growth hormone in immunobiology, in *Psychoneuroimmunology*, 2nd edn (eds. R. Ader, D.L. Felton and C. Cohen), Academic Press, Inc., San Diego, pp 377-402.

Kelley, K.W. and Dantzer, R. (1991) Growth hormone and prolactin as natural antagonists of glucocorticoids in immunoregulation, in *Stress and Immunity* (eds. N. Plotnikoff, A. Murgo, R. Faith and J. Wybran), CRC Press, Boca Raton, Florida, pp 433-452.

Kelso, A. and Munck, A. (1984) Glucocorticoid inhibition of lymphokine secretion by alloreactive T lymphocyte clones. *Journal of Immunology*, **133 (2)** 784-791.

Kiess, W. and Butenandt, O. (1985) Specific growth hormone receptors on human peripheral mononuclear cells: Reexpression, identification, and characterization. *Journal of Clinical Endocrinology and Metabolism*, **60** 740-746.

Kinney, K.S., Felten, S.Y. and Cohen, N. (1996) Sympathetic innervation of the amphibian spleen: developmental studies in *Xenopus laevis*. *Developmental and Comparative Immunology*, **20 (1)** 51-60.

Kitlen, J.W., Hejbøl, E.K., Zinck, T., Varming, K., Byatt, J.C. and McLean, E. (1997) Growth performance and respiratory burst activity in rainbow trout treated with growth hormone and vaccine. *Fish and Shellfish Immunology*, **7** 297-304.

Kralli, A., Bohen, S.P. and Yamamoto, K.R. (1995) LEM1, an ATP-binding-cassette transporter, selectively modulates the biological potency of steroid hormones. *Proceedings of the National Academy of Sciences*, **92** 4701-4705.

Lechner, O., Oliveira dos Santos, A.J., Dietrich, H. and Wick, G. (1997) Lymphoid tissues in mice and chickens produce glucocorticoid hormones. *Developmental and Comparative Immunology*, **21 (2)** 156.

Leonard, B.E. and Song, C. (1996) Stress and the immune system in the etiology of anxiety and depression. *Pharmacology Biochemistry and Behavior*, **54 (1)** 299-303.

Leung, D.Y.M., Hamid, Q., Vottero, A., Szefler, S.J., Surs, W., Minshall, E., Chrousos, G.P. and Klemm, D.J. (1997) Association of glucocorticoid insensitivity with increased expression of glucocorticoid receptor β. *Journal of Experimental Medicine*, **186 (9)** 1567-1574.

Madden, K.S. and Felten, D.L. (1995) Experimental basis for neural-immune interactions. *Physiological Reviews*, **75** 77-106.

Madden, K.S. and Livnat, S. (1991) Catecholamine action and immunologic reactivity, in *Psychoneuroimmunology*, 2nd edn (eds. R. Ader, D.L. Felton and C. Cohen), Academic Press, Inc., San Diego, pp 283-310.

Mandler, R.N., Biddison, W.E., Mandler, R. and Serrate, S.A. (1986) β-Endorphin augments the cytolytic activity and interferon production of natural killer cells. *Journal of Immunology*, **136** 934-939.

Marc, A.M., Quentel, C., Severe, A., Le Bail, P.Y. and Boeuf, G. (1995) Changes in some endocrinological and non-specific immunological parameters during seawater exposure in the brown trout. *Journal of Fish Biology*, **46** 1065-1081.

Marsh, J.A. and Scanes, C.G. (1994) Neuroendocrine-immune interactions. *Poultry Science*, **73** 1049-1061.

Marx, M., Ruben, L.N., Nobis, C. and Duffy, D. (1987) Compromised T-cell regulatory functions during anuran metamorphosis: the role of corticosteroids, in *Developmental and Comparative Immunology* (eds. E.L. Cooper, C. Langlet and J. Bierne.), Alan R. Liss, Inc. New York, USA, pp 129-140.

Mashaly, M.M. (1984) Bursectomy and its influence on circulating corticosterone, triiodothyronine, and thyroxine in immature male chickens. *Poultry Science*, **63** 798-800.

Maule, A.G. and Schreck, C.B. (1990) Glucocorticoid receptors in leukocytes and gill of coho salmon. *General and Comparative Endocrinology*, **77** 448-455.

Maule, A.G. and Schreck, C.B. (1991) Stress and cortisol treatment changed affinity and number of glucocorticoid receptors in leukocytes and gill of coho salmon. *General and Comparative Endocrinology*, **84** 83-93.

Maule, A.G., Schreck, C.B. and Kaattari, S.L. (1987) Changes in the immune system of coho salmon (*Oncorhynchus kisutch*) during the parr-to-smolt transformation and after implantation with cortisol. *Canadian Journal of Fisheries and Aquatic Science*, **44** 161-166.

Maule, A.G., Tripp, R.A., Kaattari, S.L. and Schreck, C.B. (1989) Stress alters immune function and disease resistance in chinook salmon (*Oncorhynchus tshawytscha*). *Journal of Endocrinology*, **120** 135-142.

Mazur, C.F. and Iwama, G.K. (1993) Handling and crowding stress reduces number of plaque-forming cells in atlantic salmon. *Journal of Aquatic Animal Health*, **5 (2)** 98-101.

McDonald, I.R., Lee, A.K., Than, K.A. and Martin, R.W. (1986) Failure of glucocorticoid feedback in males of a population of small marsupials (*Antechinus swainsonii*) during the period of mating. *Journal of Endocrinology*, **108** 63-68.

Mendel, D.B., Bodwell, J.E. and Munck, A. (1986) Glucocorticoid receptors lacking hormone-binding activity are bound in nuclei of ATP-depleted cells. *Nature*, **324** 478-480.

Meyer III, W.J., Smith, E.M., Richards, G.E., Cavallo, A., Morrill, A.C. and Blalock, E.J. (1987) *In vivo* immunoreactive adrenocorticotropin (ACTH) production by human mononuclear leukocytes from normal and ACTH-deficient individuals. *Journal of Clinical Endocrinology and Metabolism*, **64** 98-105.

Miller, A.H., Spencer, R.L., Stein, M. and McEwen, B.S. (1990) Adrenal steroid receptor binding in spleen and thymus after stress or dexamethasone. *American Journal of Physiology*, **259** 405-412.

Mock, A. and Peters, G. (1990) Lysozyme activity in rainbow trout, *Oncorhynchus mykiss* (Walbaum), stressed by handling transport, and water pollution. *Journal of Fish Biology*, **37** 873-885.

Monjan, A.A. and Collector, M.I. (1977) Stress induced modulation of the immune response. *Science*, **196** 307-308.

Mukherjee, P., Mastro, A.M. and Hymer, W.C. (1990) Prolactin induction of interleukin-2 receptors on rat splenic lymphocytes. *Endocrinology*, **126 (1)** 88-94.

Munck, A. and Guyre, P.M. (1991) Glucocorticoids and immune function, in *Psychoneuroimmunology*, 2nd edn (eds. R. Ader, D.L. Felton and C. Cohen), Academic Press, Inc., San Diego, pp 447-474.

Munck, A., Guyre, P.M. and Holbrook, N.J. (1984) Physiological functions of glucocorticoids in stress and their relations to pharmacological actions. *Endocrine Reviews*, **5** 25-44.

Narnaware, Y.K. and Baker, B.I. (1996) Evidence that cortisol may protect against the immediate effects of stress on circulating leukocytes in the trout. *General and Comparative Endocrinology*, **103** 359-366.

Narnaware, Y.K., Baker, B.I. and Tomlinson, M.G. (1994) The effect of various stresses, corticosteroids and adrenergic agents on phagocytosis in the rainbow trout *Oncorhynchus mykiss*. *Fish Physiology and Biochemistry*, **13 (1)** 31-40.

Narnaware, Y.K., Kelly, S.P. and Woo, N.Y.S. (1997) Effect of injected growth hormone on phagocytosis in silver sea bream (*Sparus sarba*) adapted to hyper- and hypo-osmotic salinities. *Fish and Shellfish Immunology*, **7** 515-517.

Nevid, N.J. and Meier, A.H. (1995) Timed daily administrations of hormones and antagonists of neuroendocrine receptors alter day-night rhythms of allograft rejection in the gulf kilifish, *Fundulus Grandis*. *General and Comparative Endocrinology*, **97** 327-339.

Norris, D.O. (1996) *Vertebrate Endocrinology*, 3rd edn, Academic Press, Inc., San Diego.

Northrop, J.P., Crabtree, G.R. and Mattila, P.S. (1992) Negative regulation of interleukin 2 transcription by the glucocorticoid receptor. *Journal of Experimental Medicine*, **175** 1235-1245.

Okimura, T. and Nigo, Y. (1986) Stress and immune responses. I. Suppression of T cell function in restraint-stressed mice. *Japanese Journal of Pharmacology*, **40** 505-511.

Ottaviani, E. and Franceschi, C. (1996) The neuroimmunology of stress from invertebrates to man. *Progress in Neurobiology*, **48** 421-440.

Ottaviani, E. and Franceschi, C. (1997) The invertebrate phagocytic immunocyte: clues to a common evolution of immune and neuroendocrine systems. *Immunology Today*, **18 (4)** 169-174.

Ottaviani, E., Caselgrandi, E., Petraglia, F. and Franceschi, C. (1992a) Stress response in the freshwater snail *Planorbarius corneus* (L.) (Gastropoda, Pulmonata): interaction between CRF, ACTH, and biogenic amines. *General and Comparative Endocrinology*, **87** 354-360.

Ottaviani, E., Franceschi, A., Cossarizza, A. and Frenceschi, C. (1992b) ACTH-like molecules in lymphocytes. A study in different vertebrate classes. *Neuropeptides*, **23** 215-219.

Ottaviani, E., Franchini, A., Caselgrandi, E., Cossarizza, A. and Franceschi, C. (1994) Relationship between corticotropin-releasing factor and interleukin-2: evolutionary evidence. *Federation of European Biochemical Societies*, **351** 19-21.

Ottaviani, E., Capriglione, T. and Franceschi, C. (1995a) Invertebrate and vertebrate immune cells express pro-opiomelanocortin (POMC) mRNA. *Brain, Behaviour, and Immunity*, **9** 1-8.

Ottaviani, E., Caselgrandi, E. and Franceschi, C. (1995b) Cytokines and evolution: *in vitro* effects if IL-1α, IL-1β, TNF-α and TNF-β on an ancestral type of stress response. *Biochemical and Biophysical Research Communications*, **207 (1)** 288-292.

Ottaviani, E., Franchini, A. and Franceschi, C. (1997) Pro-opiomelanocortin-derived peptides, cytokines, and nitric oxide in immune responses and stress: an evolutionary approach. *International Review of Cytology*, **170** 79-141.

Pearce, D. and Yamamoto, K.R. (1993) Mineralocorticoid and glucocorticoid receptor activities distinguished by nonreceptor factors at a composite response element. *Science*, **259** 1161-1165.

Pickering, A.D. and Pottinger, T.G. (1989) Stress responses and disease resistance in salmonid fish: Effects of chronic elevation of plasma cortisol. *Fish physiology and Biochemistry*, **7 (1-4)** 253-258.

Pickford, G.E., Srivastava, A.K., Slicher, A.M. and Pang, P.K.T. (1971a) The stress response in the abundance of circulating leucocytes in the killifish, *Fundulus heteroclitus*. I. The cold-shock sequence and the effects of hypophysectomy. *Journal of Experimental Zoology*, **177** 89-96.

Pickford, G.E., Srivastava, A.K., Slicher, A.M. and Pang, P.K.T. (1971b) The stress response in the abundance of circulating leucocytes in the killifish, *Fundulus heteroclitus*. II. The role of catecholamines. *Journal of Experimental Zoology*, **177** 97-108.

Pickford, G.E., Srivastava, A.K., Slicher, A.M. and Pang, P.K.T. (1971c) The stress response in the abundance of circulating leucocytes in the killifish, *Fundulus heteroclitus*. III. The role of the adrenal cortex and a concluding discussion of the leucocyte-stress syndrome. *Journal of Experimental Zoology*, **177** 109-118.

Plaut, M. (1987) Lymphocyte hormone receptors. *Annual Review of Immunology*, **5** 621-669.

Plotnikoff, N., Murgo, A., Faith, R. and Wybran, J. (eds.) (1991) *Stress and Immunity*, CRC Press, Boca Raton, Florida.

Pottinger, T.G., Moran, T.A. and Morgan, J.A.W. (1994) Primary and secondary indices of stress in the progeny of rainbow trout (*Oncorhynchus mykiss*) selected for high and low responsiveness to stress. *Journal of Fish Biology*, **44** 149-163.

Pratt, W.B. (1993) The role of heat shock proteins in regulating the function, folding, and trafficking of the glucocorticoid receptor. *Journal of Biological Chemistry*, **268 (29)** 21455-21458.

Pulsford, A.L., Lemaire-Gony, S., Tomlinson, M., Collingwood, N. and Glynn, P.J. (1994) Effects of acute stress on the immune system of the dab, *Limanda limanda*. *Comparative Biochemistry and Physiology*, **109C** 129-139.

Pulsford, A.L., Crampe, M., Langston, A. and Glynn, P.J. (1995) Modulatory effects of disease, stress, copper, TBT, and vitamin E on the immune system of flatfish. *Fish and Shellfish Immunology*, **5 (8)** 631-643.

Rinehart, J.J., Wuest, D. and Acherman, G.A. (1982) Corticosteroid alteration of human monocyte to macrophage differentiation. *Journal of Immunology*, **129** 1436-1440.

Robertson, M.M., Bodine, P.V., Hsu, T.C., Alnemri, E.S. and Litwack, G. (1995) Modulator inhibits nuclear translocation of the glucocorticoid receptor in the human leukemic cell line CEM C-7, *Cancer Research*, **55** 548-556.

Rodriguez, A.B., Barriga, C. and Lea, R.W. (1996) Effect of prolactin, *in vivo* and *in vitro*, upon heterophil phagocytic function in the ring dove (*Streptopelia risoria*). *Developmental and Comparative Immunology*, **20 (6)** 451-457.

Rollins-Smith, L.A. and Blair, P.J. (1993) The effects of corticosteroid hormones and thyroid hormones on lymphocyte viability and proliferation during development and metamorphosis of *Xenopus laevis*. *Differentiation*, **54** 155-160.

Rollins-Smith, L.A., Davis, A.T. and Reinert, L.K. (1997) Effects of early hypophysectomy on development of the immune system of *Xenopus laevis*. *Developmental & Comparative Immunology*, **21 (2)** 152.

Roszman, T.L. and Carlson, S.L. (1991) Neurotransmitters and molecular signaling, in *Psychoneuroimmunology*, 2nd edn (eds. R. Ader, D.L. Felton and C. Cohen), Academic Press, Inc., San Diego, pp 311-336.

Roth, J., LeRoith, D., Collier, E.S., Weaver, N.R., Watkinson, A., Cleland, C.F. and Glick, S.M. (1985) Evolutionary origins of neuropeptides, hormones, and receptors: possible applications to immunology. *Journal of Immunology*, **135 (2)** 816-819.

Ruben, L.N., Scheinman, M.A., Johnson, R.O., Shiigi, S., Clothier, R.H. and Balls, M. (1992) Impaired T cell functions during amphibian metamorphosis: IL-2 receptor expression and endogenous ligand production. *Mechanisms of Development*, **37** 167-172.

Ruben, L.N., Buchholz, D.R., Ahmadi, P., Johnson, R.O., Clothier, R.H. and Shiigi, S. (1994a) Apoptosis in thymus of adult *Xenopus laevis*. *Developmental and Comparative Immunology*, **18 (3)** 231-238.

Ruben, L.N., Ahmadi, P., Johnson, R.O., Buchholz, D.R., Clothier, R.H. and Shiigi, S. (1994b) Apoptosis in the thymus of developing *Xenopus laevis*. *Developmental and Comparative Immunology*, **18 (4)** 343-353.

Ruis, M.A.W. and Bayne, C.J. (1997) Effects of acute stress on blood clotting and yeast killing by phagocytes of rainbow trout. *Journal of Aquatic Animal Health*, **9 (3)** 190-195.

Russell, H.D., Kibler, R., Matrisian, L., Larson, D.F., Poulos, B. and Magun, B. (1985) Prolactin receptors on human T and B lymphocytes: Antagonism of prolactin binding by cyclosporine. *Journal of Immunology*, **134** 3027-3031.

Salonius, K. and Iwama, G.K. (1993) Effects of early rearing environment on stress response, immune function, and disease resistance in juvenile coho (*Oncorhynchus kisutch*) and chinook salmon (*O. tshawytscha*). *Canadian Journal of Fisheries and Aquatic Science*, **50** 759-766.

Sanders, V.M. and Powell-Oliver, F.E. (1992) β_2-Adrenoceptor stimulation increases the number of antigen-specific precursor B lymphocytes that differentiate into IgM-secreting cells without affecting burst size. *Journal of Immunology*, **148 (6)** 1822-1828.

Scheinman, R.I., Cogswell, P.C., Lofquist, A.K. and Baldwin, A.S., Jr. (1995) Role of transcriptional activation of IκBα in mediation of immunosuppression by glucocorticoids. *Science*, **270** 283-286.

Schreck, C.B. (1996) Immunomodulation: Endogenous factors in *The Fish Immune System: Organism, Pathogen, and Environment* (eds. G. Iwama and T. Nakanishi), Academic Press, Inc., San Diego, pp 311-337.

Schreiber, S.L. (1991) Chemistry and biology of the immunophilins and their immunosuppressive ligands. *Science*, **251** 283-287.

Schreiber, S.L. and Crabtree, G.R. (1992) The mechanism of action for cyclosporin A and FK506. *Immunology Today*, **13** 136-142.

Selye, H. (1936) A syndrome produced by diverse nocuous agents. *Nature*, **138** 32.

Selye, H. (1976) *The Stress of Life,* 2nd edn, McGraw-Hill Book Co., New York.

Shavit, Y., Lewis, J.W., Treman, G.W., Gale, R.P. and Liebeskind, J.C. (1984) Opioid peptides mediate the suppressive effect of stress on natural killer cell cytotoxicity. **223** 188-190.

Sheridan, J.F., Dobbs, C., Brown, D. and Zwilling, B. (1994) Psychoneuroimmunology: stress effects on pathogenesis and immunity during infection. *Microbiology Reviews*, **7 (2)** 200-212.

Siegel, H.S., Latmer, J.W. and Gould, N.R. (1983) Concentration of *Salmonella pullorum* antigen and the immunosuppressive effect of adrenocorticotropin in growing chickens. *Poultry Science*, **62** 897-903.

Siegel, H.S., Gould, N.R. and Latimer, J.W. (1985) Splenic leukocytes from chickens injected with *Salmonella pullorum* antigen stimulate production of corticosteroids by isolated adrenal cells (42037). *Proceedings of the Society for Experimental Biology and Medicine*, **178** 523-530.

Skwarło-Sonta, K. (1992) Prolactin as an immunoregulatory hormone in mammals and birds. *Immunology Letters*, **33** 105-122.

Slicher, A.M., Pickford, G.E. and Pang, P.K.T. (1966) Effects of "training" and of volume and composition of the injection fluid on stress-induced leukopenia in the mummichog. *The Progressive Fish-Culturist*, **28** 216-219.

Smith, D.F. and Toft, D.O. (1993) Steroid receptors and their associated proteins. *Molecular Endocrinology*, **7 (1)** 4-11.

Smith, E.M. and Blalock, J.E. (1981) Human lymphocyte production of corticotropin and endorphin-like substances: association with leukocyte interferon. *Proceedings of the National Academy of Sciences*, **78** 7530-7534.

Smith, E.M., Morrill, A.C., Meyer III, W.J. and Blalock, J.E. (1986) Corticotropin releasing factor induction of leukocyte-derived immunoreactive ACTH and endorphins. *Nature*, **321** 881-882.

Smith, E.M., Hughes, T.K., Cadet, P. and Stefano, G.B. (1992) Corticotropin-releasing factor-induced immunosuppression in human and invertebrate immunocytes. *Cellular and Molecular Neurobiology*, **12** 473-481.

Sneiszko, S.F. (1974) The effects of environmental stress on outbreaks of infectious diseases of fish. *Journal of Fish Biology*, **6** 197-208.

Stefano, G.B. and Smith, E.M. (1996) Adrenocorticotropin - a central trigger in immune responsiveness: tonal inhibition of immune activation. *Medical Hypotheses*, **46** 471-478.

Stefano, G.B., Cadet, P. and Scharrer, B. (1989) Stimulatory effects of opiod neuropeptides on locomotory activity and conformational changes in invertebrate and human immunocytes: evidence for a subtype of δ receptor. *Proceedings of the National Academy of Sciences*, **86** 6307-6311.

Stefano, G.B., Cadet, P., Dokun, A. and Scharrer, B. (1990) A neuroimmunoregulatory-like mechanism responding to stress in the marine bivalve *Mytilus edulis. Brain, Behavior, and Immunity*, **4** 323-329.

Stefano, G.B., Leung, M.K., Bilfinger, T.V. and Scharrer, B. (1995) Effect of prolonged exposure to morphine on responsiveness of human and invertebrate immunocytes to stimulatory molecules. *Journal of Neuroimmunology*, **63** 175-181.

Steplewski, Z. and Vogel, W.H. (1986) Total leukocyte, T cell subpopulation and natural killer cell activity in rats exposed to restraint stress. *Life Sciences*, **38** 2419-2427.

Tai, P.-K.K., Albers, M.W., Chang, H., Faber, L.E. and Schreiber, S.L. (1992) Association of a 59-kilodalton immunophilin with the glucocorticoid receptor complex. *Science*, **256** 1315-1318.

Talmadge, J.E. (1984) Thymosin: immunomodulatory and therapeutic characteristics, in *Chemical Regulation of Immunity in Veterinary Medicine*, A.R. Liss. Inc., New York, pp 457-465.

Thompson, I., White, A., Fletcher, T.C., Houlihan, D.F. and Secombes, C.J. (1993) The effect of stress on the immune response of atlantic salmon (*Salmo salar* L.) fed diets containing different amounts of vitamin C. *Aquaculture*, **114** 1-18.

Tournefier, A. (1982) Corticosteroid action on lymphocyte subpopulations and humoral immune response of axolotl (urodele amphibian). *Immunology*, **46** 155-162.

Tripp, R.A., Maule, A.G., Schreck, C.B. and Kaattari, S.L. (1987) Reversal of cortisol-mediated suppression of salmonid lymphocyte responses by culture supernatants. *Developmental and Comparative Immunology*, **11** 565-576.

Trout, J.M. and Mashaly, M.M. (1994) The effects of adrenocorticotropic hormone and heat stress on the distribution of lymphocyte populations in immature male chickens. *Poultry Science*, **73** 1694-1698.

Trout, J.M., Mashaly, M.M. and Siegel, H.S. (1988) Changes in the profiles of circulating white blood cells, corticosterone, T_3 and T_4 during the initiation of humoral immunity in immature male chickens. *Developmental and Comparative Immunology*, **12 (2)** 331-346.

Vacca, A., Felli, M.P., Farina, A.R., Martinotti, S., Maroder, M., Screpanti, I., Meco, D., Petrangeli, E., Frati, L. and Gulino, A. (1992) Glucocorticoid receptor-mediated suppression of the interleukin 2 gene expression through impairment of the cooperativity between nuclear factor of activated T cells and AP-1 enhancer elements. *Journal of Experimental Medicine*, **175** 637-646.

Vacchio, M.S., Papadopoulos, V. and Ashwell, J.D. (1994) Steroid production in the thymus: implications for thymocyte selection. *Journal of Experimental Medicine*, **179** 1835-1846.

Vahouny, G.V., Kyeyune-Nyombi, E., McGillis, J.P., Tare, N.S., Huang, K.Y., Tombes, A.L., Goldstein, A.L. and Hall, N.R. (1983) Thymosin peptides and lymphokines do not directly stimulate adrenal corticosteroid production *in vitro*. *Journal of Immunology*, **130** 791-794.

Webster, E.L. and de Souza, E.B. (1988) Corticotropin-releasing factor receptors in mouse spleen: identification, autoradiographic localization and regulation by divalent cations and guanine nucleotides. *Endocrinology*, **122** 609-617.

Wedemeyer, G. (1974) Stress as a predisposing factor in fish diseases. Fish Disease Leaflet 38. Fish and Wildlife Service, Washington, DC.

Wehling, M. (1994) Nongenomic actions of steroid hormones. *Trends in Endocrinology and Metabolism*, **5 (8)** 347-353.

Weigent, D.A., Blalock, J.E. and LeBoeuf, R.D. (1991) An antisense oligodeoxynucleotide to growth hormone messenger ribonucleic acid inhibits lymphocyte proliferation. *Endocrinology*, **128 (4)** 2053-2057.

Wendelaar Bonga, S.E. (1997) The stress response in fish. *Physiological Reviews*, **77** 591-625.

Westly, H.J., Kleiss, A.J., Kelley, K.W., Wong, P.K.Y. and Yuen, P.H. (1986) Newcastle disease virus-infected splenocytes express the proopiomelanocortin gene. *Journal of Experimental Medicine*, **163** 1589-1594.

Weyts, F.A.A. (1998) Corticosteroids and interleukin-1, messengers for communication between the endocrine and immune system in carp. Ph.D. Dissertation, Wageningen Institute of Animal Sciences, Agricultural University, Wageningen, The Netherlands.

Williamson, S.A., Knight, R.A., Lightman, S.L. and Hobbs, J.R. (1987) Differential effects of β-endorphin fragments on human natural killing. *Brain, Behavior, and Immunity*, **1** 329-225.

Wise, D.J., Schwedler, T.E. and Otis, D.L. (1993) Effects of stress on susceptibility of naive channel catfish in immersion challenge with *Edwardsiella ictaluri*. *Journal of Aquatic Animal Health*, **5 (2)** 92-97.

Woloski, B.M.R.N.J., Smith, E.M., Meyer III, W.J., Fuller, G.M. and Blalock, J.E. (1985) Corticotropin-releasing activity of monokines. *Science*, **230** 1035-1037.

Wybran, J., Appelboom, T., Famaey, J.-P. and Gov, A. (1979) Suggestive evidence for receptors for morhine and metenkephalin on normal human blood T lymphocytes. *Journal of Immnunology*, **123** 1068-1070.

Yin, Z., Lam, T.J. and Sin, Y.M. (1995) The effects of crowding stress on the non-specific immune response in fancy carp (*Cyprinus carpio* L.). *Fish and Shellfish Immunology*, **5** 519-529.

Zapata, A.G., Varas, A. and Torroba, M. (1992) Seasonal variations in the immune system of lower vertebrates. *Immunology Today*, **13** 142-147.

Zatz, M.M. and Goldstein, A.L. (1985) Mechanism of action of thymosin. I. Thymosin fraction 5 increases lymphokine production by mature murine T cells responding in a mixed lymphocyte reaction. *Journal of Immunology*, **134** 1032-1038.

7   Impact of stress on animal toxicology

Malin Celander

7.1   Introduction

Living organisms are continuously confronted with foreign substances
(xenobiotics), which include natural chemicals and anthropogenic (man-
made) chemicals. These comprise natural products produced by moulds,
plants and animals, and synthetic products, including many drugs,
pesticides and pollutants. Lipophilic xenobiotics may accumulate to toxic
levels if they are not efficiently excreted. The elimination of xenobiotics
often depends on their conversion to water-soluble compounds by a
process known as biotransformation, which is catalysed by various
enzymes.

Toxicology is a wide topic, and there are many textbooks and reviews
that describe various aspects of toxicology and pharmocogenetics. This
chapter focuses on xenobiotic metabolizing enzymes, and the cytochrome
P450 superfamily in vertebrates in particular. The possible impact of
physiological stress (glucocorticoid hormones and synthetic derivatives)
on responses to chemical stress (aromatic organic hydrocarbons) in two
distinct phylogenetic groups, mammals and fish, will be discussed.

7.2   Drug metabolizing enzymes

Drug metabolizing enzymes (DMEs) are defined as enzymes that
metabolize drugs, endobiotics, xenobiotics, carcinogens, drugs, pesticides
and other environmental pollutants (Nebert, 1994). DMEs are present
both in prokaryotes and in eukaryotes, and it has been suggested that the
eukaryotic genes have evolved from prokaryotic ancestral genes. It is
believed that the genes coding for these enzymes evolved for metabolism
of endogenous molecules, and that these genes have diversified more
recently in response to the adverse effects of foreign chemicals (Nebert
and Gonzalez, 1987; Gonzalez and Nebert, 1990). It has been proposed
that DMEs play important roles in maintaining steady-state levels of
endogenous ligands involved in ligand-modulated transcription of genes
effecting homeostasis, growth, differentiation and neuroendocrine functions (Nebert, 1991). To date, relatively little is known about the

---

A list of abbreviations used in this chapter may be found on p. 270.

endogenous functions of these enzymes. However, the roles of numerous DMEs in the biotransformation of foreign substances, and the involvement of these enzymes in toxicity and chemical carcinogenesis have received enormous attention in terrestrial as well as in aquatic animals. This has been summarized in a number of excellent reviews during the last decade (e.g. Nebert and Gonzalez, 1987; Gonzalez, 1989; Okey, 1990; Guengerich and Shimada, 1991; Stegeman, 1993; Stegeman and Hahn, 1994; Di Giulio et al., 1995; Maurel, 1996; Miller et al., 1996; Parkinson, 1996).

Biotransformation of lipophilic substances is mediated by the concerted action of several DMEs. These enzymes are usually classified as either 'Phase I' or 'Phase II' enzymes. Phase I reactions are sometimes called functionalization or activation reactions, because a functional group, usually a hydroxyl group, is being inserted in the substrate which then becomes activated. This activated metabolite can in some situations be more toxic than the original substrate. However, this metabolite is normally conjugated with an endogenous molecule, such as glucuronic acid, glutathione or sulfate, through Phase II reactions, which also are called conjugation reactions (Nebert et al., 1996).

Whether Phase I and Phase II metabolism result in a less toxic end-product or not, these reactions usually result in the formation of a more water-soluble product, that can be more readily excreted from the cell (Nebert et al., 1996). Thus, biotransformation usually results in increased excretion rates of foreign substances, which reduces the risk for accumulation of these substances to toxic levels in the organism.

7.2.1   Phase I reactions

Phase I can be catalysed by cytochrome P450 (CYP) monooxygenases, flavin-containing monooxygenases, hydrolases, lipoxygenases, cyclooxygenases, peroxidases, oxidases, monoamine oxidases, dioxygenases and reductases (Nebert, 1994). Phase I reactions are dominated by the CYP superfamily, which usually generate oxygenated metabolites (Nebert et al., 1996). The CYP enzymes appear to be the most numerous of all DMEs, and they also exhibit the broadest range of substrate specificities (Nebert, 1991). In addition to hydroxylation, CYP enzymes also catalyse other oxidative reactions such as epoxidation, N-, S- and O-dealkylation, deamination, sulfoxidation and desulfuration (Nebert and Gonzalez, 1987).

The CYP enzymes do not act alone. Several other enzymes are involved in the CYP redox cycle, including reductase enzymes such as NADPH-cytochrome P450 reductase and NADH-cytochrome b_5 reductase. The catalytic cycle is initiated when a substrate (RH) binds to the CYP, which usually results in conversion of the prosthetic heme Fe^{3+} in the catalytic site of the CYP enzyme from a low-spin to a high-spin Fe^{3+}. This Fe^{3+} is next reduced by an electron from the electron donor NADPH, via the NADPH-cytochrome P450 reductase enzyme, and subsequently molecular oxygen (O_2) is bound to the CYP–substrate complex. This is a critical step as the CYP catalytic cycle may be interrupted here, which results in the formation of a reactive oxygen species ($O_2^{-\bullet}$, superoxide). If not interrupted, the CYP catalytic redox cycle will proceed and a second electron is added, sometimes from the electron donor NADH via cytochrome b_5 reductase. The subsequent steps involve formation of hydrogen peroxide (H_2O_2), followed by cleavage of the O–O bound, formation of a substrate-radical ($R^{\bullet}$) and finally the hydroxylation of this substrate-radical and the release of the product (ROH) from the oxidized CYP enzyme, which then becomes ready for another redox cycle (Poulos and Ragg, 1992). These reactions are summarized in Figure 7.1.

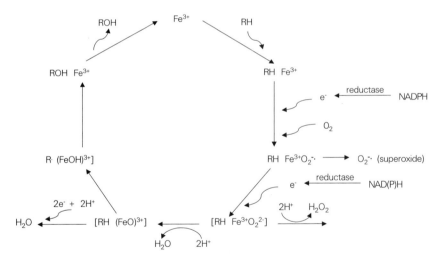

Figure 7.1 The cytochrome P450 catalytic cycle as described in section 7.2.1. Adapted from Poulos and Raag (1992).

7.2.2 The CYP superfamily

The CYP superfamily consists of several CYP genes that all are related to one another and are thought to have evolved from the same bacterial ancestral gene, having existed more than 3.5 billion years ago (Nelson *et al.*, 1993). Diversification of the CYP superfamily in terrestrial animals is believed to be driven (in part) by animal–plant 'warfare' (Gonzalez and Nebert, 1990). The numerous genes of the CYP superfamily are organized into gene families and gene subfamilies, as has been recommended by the P450 nomenclature committee. As a rule, a CYP amino acid sequence from one gene family is defined as usually having less than 40% amino acid sequence identity to that of any other gene family. Whereas genes within a gene subfamily usually share greater than 60% identity in amino acid sequence (Nebert et al., 1987, 1991; Nelson et al., 1993, 1996). The 'Nelson Lab Homepage' provides a continuous updating of the CYP superfamily (drnelson.utmem.edu/nelsonhomepage.html).

Of 74 distinct CYP gene families reported so far, 14 have been identified in mammals (Nelson et al., 1996). These consist of inducible and constitutively expressed CYP genes. Generally, the constitutively expressed CYP enzymes catalyse reactions involving endogenous substrates and play important roles in the synthesis, activation and degradation of steroids and steroid-derived compounds as well as fatty acids and fatty acid-derived compounds. These CYP enzymes often have restricted substrate specificity. The inducible CYP enzymes, on the other hand, possess considerably wider and overlapping substrate specificities. The inducible CYP forms are predominantly found within gene family CYP1, CYP2, CYP3 or CYP4. These inducible CYP forms are essential in the metabolism of foreign lipophilic compounds and play important roles in pharmacology, toxicology and in chemical carcinogenesis (Gonzalez, 1989; Guengerich and Shimada, 1991; Gonzalez and Gelboin, 1994; Maurel, 1996; Miller et al., 1996; Parkinson, 1996; Kelly et al., 1997).

CYP enzymes are membrane-bound hemoproteins of about 48 to 60 kDa, each containing approximately 500 amino acids. In animals, most CYP proteins are found in the smooth endoplasmic reticulum. However, a few CYP enzymes, predominantly some of those involved in steroid biosynthesis and metabolic pathways, are located in the inner membrane of the mitochondria (Nebert and Gonzalez, 1987). CYP expression has been identified both in hepatic and extrahepatic tissues such as kidney, intestine, lung, gonads, adrenal, pituitary, prostate, brain, skin, leukocytes, spleen and the cardiovasculature (e.g. Dees et al., 1982; Gonzalez, 1989; Okey, 1990; Lund et al., 1991). Although the contribution of extrahepatic CYP compared to hepatic metabolism of xenobiotics seems low, the in situ formation of metabolites in certain tissues may influence target organ sensitivity, responsiveness and toxicity (Lund et al., 1991).

There are substantial differences in the degree of expression between various CYP genes depending on several biotic factors, including hormones, as well as several abiotic factors such as xenobiotics (Gonzalez, 1989; Okey, 1990; Lund et al., 1991). In this chapter, questions regarding the impact of adrenal stress hormones (glucocorti-coids) on the expression of xenobiotic metabolizing members of the CYP superfamily in vertebrates will be discussed.

7.2.3 *Xenobiotic metabolizing CYP enzymes*

As previously mentioned, the inducible CYP genes are predominantly found in gene families CYP1, CYP2, CYP3 or CYP4. The enzymes belonging to these CYP families play important roles in the oxidative metabolism of numerous xenobiotics, naturally occurring as well as those of anthropogenic origin. These compounds include hydrocarbons formed through, for example, volcanic activities and/or combustion processes, pro-carcinogens, plant products (phytoalexins), drugs, pesticides and other organic environmental pollutants. In addition to foreign substances, these CYP enzymes also metabolize a wide variety of endobiotics, such as steroid hormones, fatty acids, alcohol and ketones (Gonzalez, 1989; Okey, 1990; Capdevila *et al.*, 1992; Maurel, 1996; Parkinson, 1996).

The mammalian CYP1 gene family comprises two subfamilies, CYP1A and CYP1B, both highly inducible by polycyclic aromatic hydrocarbons (PAHs) and planar halogenated aromatic hydrocarbons (PHAHs), including planar PCBs and dioxins. The mammalian CYP2 gene family is diverse and comprises at least eight subfamilies. Various types of substances including phenobarbital (PB), DDT, non-planar PCBs, ethanol, ketones and several therapeutic drugs have been shown to activate transcription of certain mammalian CYP2 genes or stabilize certain proteins within this gene family. In contrast to the diverse CYP2 gene family, only one subfamily so far has been identified in the CYP3 gene family. However, the diversity in terms of structurally different substances that act as inducers and/or substrates to members of this subfamily is extraordinary. Thus, mammalian members of the CYP3A subfamily are inducible by a wide variety of substances, including steroids, natural products, carcinogens, pesticides, environmental pollu-tants and numerous therapeutic drugs. The CYP4 gene family members in mammals metabolize fatty acids and are predominantly inducible by peroxisome proliferators such as clofibrate but also by phthalates and certain PCBs. In mammals, three subfamilies belonging to the CYP4 gene family have so far been identified (Nelson *et al.*, 1996).

The inducible mammalian CYP gene families and some of their substrates are listed in Table 7.1. Many of these substrates also activate the expression of the genes coding for the CYP enzymes that metabolize them (Nebert and Gonzalez, 1987; Okey, 1990; Maurel, 1996; Parkinson, 1996). It should be emphasized that only a few substrates for each gene family are provided in Table 7.1. There are probably thousands of

Table 7.1 Examples of substrates to the inducible CYP gene families in mammals

Gene family	Subfamilies	Substrates
CYP1	1A, 1B	PAH, PHAH, pesticides, estrogen, bilirubin, arachidonic acid, caffeine, indoles, flavonoids
CYP2	2A, 2B, 2C, 2D, 2E, 2F, 2G, 2J	alcohol, ketones, drugs, steroids, arachidonic acid, caffeine, pesticides
CYP3	3A	steroids, drugs, PAH, pesticides, caffeine
CYP4	4A, 4B, 4F	lauric acid, arachidonic acid, phthalates, PCBs

substrates for these enzymes. In addition to specific inducers, gene expression of several xenobiotic metabolizing CYP forms also is regulated by hormones, including insulin, ACTH, growth hormones and steroid hormones (Lund *et al.*, 1991).

The aquatic environment is continuously subjected to environmental pollutants including PAHs and PHAHs. This is probably the main reason why the piscine CYP system is the foremost investigated non-mammalian CYP system today. The induction of CYP1A in fish is a well established biomarker, 'an early warning signal', routinely used to estimate exposure to anthropogenic aromatic organic pollutants in the aquatic environment (Stegeman and Hahn, 1994). CYP1A cDNAs have been isolated from several fish species (Heilmann *et al.*, 1988; Leaver *et al.*, 1993; Berndtson and Chen, 1994; Morrison *et al.*, 1995, 1998; Roy *et al.*, 1996). These genes all show slightly greater similarities to the mammalian CYP1A1 genes than the CYP1A2 genes (Morrison *et al.*, 1995, 1998). Fish CYP1A genes are believed to have emerged from ancestral CYP1A1 at the time of fish/terrestrial animal divergence, 380 million years ago (MYA). Between that time and when birds split from mammals, 320 MYA, CYP1A2 arose by gene duplication (Nebert and Gonzalez, 1987; Jaiswal *et al.*, 1987).

In addition to the CYP1 gene family, fish representatives of the CYP2, CYP3 and CYP4 gene families also have been isolated. A CYP2B like *N*-terminal fragment has been sequenced from the marine fish *Stenotomus chrysops* (Klotz *et al.*, 1986). Furthermore, cDNAs isolated from two different fish species, rainbow trout (*Onchorhynchus mykiss*) and killifish (*Fundulus heteroclitus*), have been designated to novel CYP2 subfamilies: CYP2K (Buhler *et al.*, 1994; Oleksiak, M.F. and Stegeman, J.J., personal communication), CYP2M (Yang *et al.*, 1995), CYP2N and CYP2P (Oleksiak, M.F. and Stegeman, J.J., personal communication). Members of the CYP3A subfamily also have been isolated from these two fish species (Celander and Stegeman, 1997; Gen Bank accession number U96077). Finally, a member of the CYP4 gene family, isolated from rainbow trout liver has been designated to a novel subfamily; CYP4T (Falckh *et al.*, 1997). Many CYP genes, in particular CYP genes within the CYP2 gene family, are thought to have emerged with terrestrial animals. Certain CYP genes conceivably could have evolved in separate directions in fish compared to that in mammals. Whether the novel subfamilies of the CYP2 and CYP4 gene families identified in fish are unique to this taxa remains to be verified. Nevertheless, great similarities seem to exist between mammals and fish, in particular within the CYP1 and the CYP3 gene families. In this chapter, the regulatory effects of glucocorticoid steroid hormones on inducible CYP forms, and in particular that on members of the CYP1A and CYP3A subfamilies in mammals and in fish will be discussed.

7.2.4   Phase II reactions

Phase II reactions are mediated by different enzymes, belonging to distinct gene superfamilies. Phase II enzymes often include UDP-glucuronosyl transferases (UGT), glutathione transferases (GST), sulfotransferases, transaminases, acetyltransferases, methyltransferases, acyltransferases, quinone reductases, aldoketoreductases, carboxylesterases, NAD(P)-dependent alcohol and steroid dehydrogenases, glycosylases, glucuronidases and various hydrolases and esterases (Nebert, 1994).

These enzymes participate in the alteration of certain lipophilic substances, and in particular those generated by the Phase I reactions. Phase I metabolism, however, can sometimes elicit increased toxicity in the cell as a result of generation of reactive oxidized intermediates, such as hydroxy or epoxide derivatives as well as formation of reactive oxygen species (Nebert et al., 1996). The hydroxylated intermediates generated by Phase I reactions also can be conjugated with polar endogenous molecules, such as glutathione, glucuronic acid, sulfates, amino acids or acetates by Phase II reactions, yielding a hydrophilic product that can more easily be excreted from the cells (Nebert and Gonzalez, 1987). Epoxides are highly unstable compounds that may cause severe damage to the organism, by binding to cellular macromolecules such as proteins, RNA and DNA. Fortunately, these epoxide metabolites can be deactivated by the enzyme epoxide hydrolase (EH) to less reactive diols. Alternatively, epoxides also can be directly be conjugated with endogenous glutathione by the GST enzyme in Phase II (Raney et al., 1992). Biotransformation of the ultimate pro-carcinogen benzo[a]pyrene (B[a]P) is illustrated in Figure 7.2.

7.3   The aryl hydrocarbon receptor

Most of the toxic effects caused by exposure to PAH/PHAH are mediated by an endogenous cytosolic receptor, the aryl hydrocarbon receptor

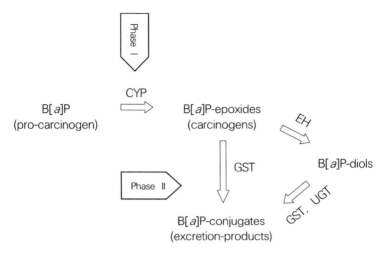

Figure 7.2 Biotransformation of benzo[*a*]pyrene (B[*a*]P). In Phase I, cytochromes P450 (CYP) activate the pro-carcinogen B[*a*]P to carcinogenic metabolites, B[*a*]P-epoxides. These epoxides can be further hydroxylated to B[*a*]P-diols by the enzyme epoxide hydrolase (EH). In Phase II, the B[*a*]P-diols are conjugated with endogenous molecules such as glutathione by glutathione transferase (GST) or glucuronic acid by UDP-glucuronosyl transferase (UGT). Alternatively, B[*a*]P-epoxides can also be directly conjugated with glutathione by the GST enzyme in Phase II.

(AHR). The AHR has been shown to be involved in the regulation of several gene products including Phase I genes, such as CYP1A1, CYP1A2 and CYP1B1. This receptor also activates transcription of several Phase II genes, such as NAD(P)H:menadione oxidoreductase (NMO-1), a cytosolic 'class 3' aldehyde dehydrogenase (ALDH-3), a 4-methylumbelliferone specific UDP glucuronosyltransferase (UGT *06) and a 2,4-dinitro-1-chlorobenzene specific glutathione transferase (GST-Ya). In addition to specific DME genes, the AHR also is involved in regulation of genes coding for proteins that participate in the control of cell growth such as plasminogen activator inhibitor, transforming growth factors-α and β_2, c-fos, Jun-B, c-jun and Jun-D, δ-aminolevulinic acid synthase (Hankinson, 1995).

7.3.1 The AHR signal transduction pathway

The signal transduction pathway for PAH/PHAH inducible proteins includes the action of the AHR (Poland and Knutson, 1982; Whitlock, 1993; Hankinson, 1995). The AHR is normally present in an inactive form in the cytosol, associated with 90-kDa heatshock proteins (hsp90).

Upon ligand binding by, for example, PAHs or PHAHs, the hsp90 dissociate from the AHR. The ligand–AHR complex is next translocated into the nucleus where it associates with its dimerization partner; the aryl hydrocarbon receptor nuclear translocator (ARNT) protein to become activated. The ligand–AHR–ARNT complex activates specific response elements called dioxin (or xenobiotic) response elements (DREs or XREs) near the promotor region of specific genes, resulting in enhanced transcription of these genes (Denison *et al.*, 1988; Landers and Bunce, 1991; Whitlock *et al.*, 1996; Hahn, 1998) (Figure 7.3).

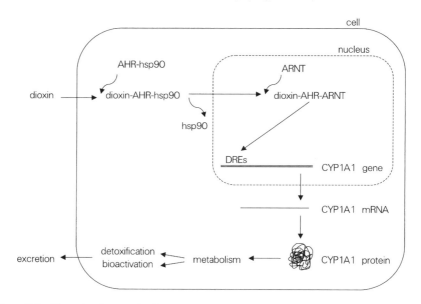

Figure 7.3 The signal transduction pathway for CYP1A1 induction. A polyaromatic hydrocarbon or a polyhalogenated aromatic hydrocarbon, such as dioxin, passively diffuses through the plasma membrane and binds to the cytosolic aryl hydrocarbon receptor (AHR), which is subsequently transformed to its active form. Activation of the AHR involves the dissociation of the two 90-kDa heatshock proteins (hsp90) in the cytosol and formation of a heterodimer between the AHR and the aryl hydrocarbon receptor nuclear translocator (ARNT) protein in the nucleus. Binding of the dioxin–AHR–ARNT complex to dioxin response elements (DREs) in the promotor region of the CYP1A1 gene initiates transcription of this gene. Enhanced CYP1A1 gene expression results in increases in CYP1A1 metabolism, which promotes detoxification or activation of CYP1A1 substrates. CYP1A1 metabolism generally facilitates the formation of more water-soluble compounds that can be excreted more easily from the cell.

The AHR contains a basic helix–loop–helix motif and a region designated as Per-ARNT-Sim. The Per-ARNT-Sim region exhibits sequence homology with Per (a *Drosophila* circadian rhythm protein), ARNT (see above) and Sim (a *Drosophila* developmental regulatory protein) (Ema *et al.*, 1992; Whitlock *et al.*, 1996). The AHR is an ancient protein that appeared in evolution at least 450–510 MYA (Hahn *et al.*, 1997). Phylogenetic analyses, including representatives of early diverging vertebrates (jawless, cartilaginous and bony fish), showed that the AHR has been well conserved during vertebrate evolution, suggesting important endogenous functions of this protein (Hahn *et al.*, 1997). AHR and ARNT orthologues have recently been discovered in the nematode *Caenorhabditis elegans*, indicating that the AHR signalling complex evolved before nematodes and mammals diverged more than 500 MYA. However, the AHR orthologue from *C. elegans* was not activated by classical vertebrate AHR ligands (Powell-Coffman *et al.*, 1998).

AHR-deficient mice exhibited liver- and immune system dysfunctions, further indicating important physiological roles for this ubiquitous receptor. It has been proposed that the AHR plays a role in hepatic development (Fernandez-Salguero *et al.*, 1995; Schmidt *et al.*, 1996). However, the endogenous ligand for the AHR has not yet been identified. To date, the most specific ligand to the AHR described is 2,3,7,8-tetrachlorodibenzo-*p*-dioxin (TCDD) (Poland and Knutson, 1982). Other classes of AHR ligands include, PAHs such as B[*a*]P, phytoalexins such as carotenoids, flavonoids and indole derivatives and more recently metabolites of benzimidazoles, clinically used as gastric proton-pump inhibitors have been suggested as putative ligands for the AHR (e.g. Rannug *et al.*, 1995; Dzeletovic *et al.*, 1997; Gradelet *et al.*, 1997). Thus, in addition to environmental pollutants, dietary compounds and therapeutic drugs also activate the AHR function.

7.3.2   The AHR gene battery

The murine AHR has been demonstrated to regulate two Phase I genes, Cyp1a1 and Cyp1a2, and four Phase II genes, Nmo-1, Aldh-3, UGT *06 and Gst-Ya (Nebert *et al.*, 1990). These six DME genes together constitute the 'AHR gene battery' (Nebert and Gonzalez, 1987).

The genes belonging to the AHR gene battery are coordinately positively controlled by the AHR. There also are complex interrelationships between the genes within this gene battery. For example, Cyp1a1 or Cyp1a2 activity mediates a down-regulation of the expression of Phase II genes (RayChaudhuri *et al.*, 1990). Moreover, the Nmo-1 gene is involved in the negative regulation of all four Phase II enzymes, but not of the Phase I genes (Nebert *et al.*, 1993). This complex pattern of 'cross-talk' among the various genes of the AHR gene battery has been speculated to exist in order to ensure optimal biotransformation capacity following oxidative stress, to restore normal physiological steady-state levels of the endogenous ligand (Nebert, 1994). Thus, these genes are believed to play important roles in reproduction, development, toxicity, cancer and oxidative stress (Nebert, 1989, 1991, 1994). However, as previously mentioned, the endogenous ligand for the AHR has yet not been identified.

In addition to AHR ligands, regulation of the AHR gene battery also seems to be under the influence of hormones. Effects of stress hormones, i.e. glucocorticoid hormones on gene regulation of various DMEs, including members of the AHR gene battery will be discussed next.

7.4 Stress hormones and DMEs

Adrenal glucocorticoid hormones and/or synthetic derivatives have been shown to affect various DMEs in vertebrates *in vitro* as well as *in vivo*. For simplicity, glucocorticoids and synthetic derivatives will hereafter be abbreviated as GCs, if specific names not are provided. GCs have been described as positive- or negative modulators of the induction of certain DMEs by specific inducers. This section focuses on the effects of GCs on the regulation of the AHR gene battery, the GC-inducible and metabolizing CYP3A subfamily. Finally, the effects of GC on the modulation of CYP2B inducibility will be discussed briefly.

7.4.1 *Regulation of the AHR gene battery by glucocorticoids*

GCs have been shown to act on the expression of certain DMEs, including members of the AHR gene battery. The effects of GCs have been most thoroughly investigated for the CYP1A subfamily, which will be discussed in detail in section 7.5. Treatment of cultured rat hepatocytes with dexamethasone (DEX), resulted in a 2- to 3-fold potentiation of the PAH-induced CYP1A1, GST-Ya and UGT *06 gene expression and a 60 to 80% suppression of the PAH-induced NMO-1 and ALDH-3 gene expression (Xiao *et al.*, 1995). Thus, the AHR gene battery, in addition to being regulated by AHR agonists, also appears to be under the influence of GCs. However, both positive and negative GC-mediated regulatory effects appeared to exist for different genes within the AHR gene battery (Prough *et al.*, 1996a,b). Studies using transient transfection of gene constructs, containing the 5'-flanking promotor region or intronic regions of CYP1A1, GST-Ya and ALDH-3 genes from rat revealed interactions between GR and canonical GRE consensus sequences in these genes (Hines *et al.*, 1988; Mathis *et al.*, 1989; Prough *et al.*, 1996a,b; Falkner *et al.*, 1998). These findings suggest that specific GREs are involved in the GC-dependent regulation of certain genes within the AHR gene battery.

The effects of GCs on regulation of the AHR gene battery seem to vary depending on developmental stages. In fetal rat hepatocytes, treatment with DEX resulted in potentiation of the NMO-1 protein content (Sherratt *et al.*, 1990), whereas in adult rat hepatocytes, DEX treatment resulted in a repression of NMO-1 gene expression (Xiao *et al.*, 1995). Steroid hormones are involved in neonatal programming of the constitutive expression of some CYP forms involved in steroid synthesis in the adult rat (Einarsson *et al.*, 1973). Levels of circulating GCs in the fetal rat are higher than that in the adult rat. Immediately following parturition, GC levels rapidly decline and reach a minimum between 4 and 10 days postpartum. Thereafter, GC levels start to increase steadily until rats are about 30 days of age and are maintained around this level throughout life (Greengard, 1975). *In vivo* studies in fetal (21-day gestational age), neonatal (5-day-old) and adolescent (30-day-old) rats demonstrated that the regulation of AHR gene battery by exogenous GCs (DEX) clearly was dependent on developmental stages. In neonatal rats, where the endogenous levels of circulating GCs was lowest (30% that of adult rat), addition of DEX resulted in potentiation of induction of CYP1A1, GST-Ya and NMO-1 (Linder and Prough, 1993). In adolescent rats, where the levels of endogenous GCs are higher, treatment with DEX resulted in no significant potentiation of CYP1A1 or CYP1A2 induction, whereas addition of DEX resulted in a pronounced decrease of the PAH-mediated induction of GST-Ya and NMO-1 (Linder and Prough, 1993). This discrepancy in responses conceivably could be an effect of endogenous GCs on the regulation of these genes (Xiao *et al.*, 1995). It is possible that fluctuations of circulating GC levels, as a result of physiological stress, also could have effects on regulation of DME gene expression. Future studies should address questions concerning whether fluctuations of levels of endogenous circulating GCs are mirrored in expression of genes within the AHR gene battery.

7.4.2 *The glucocorticoid inducible CYP3A subfamily*

Expression of hepatic CYP3A in mammals can be induced several-fold by GCs (Schuetz and Guzelian, 1984). Slight increases in hepatic CYP3A also have been demonstrated in a fish species, rainbow trout, treated with cortisol *in vivo* (Celander *et al.*, 1989a). Phylogenetic analyses suggest that the CYP3A gene has been well conserved during vertebrate evolution (Celander and Stegeman, 1997). However, the induction response to GCs in trout appears to be considerably weaker than that reported in mammals, which implies regulatory differences in CYP3A expression between these two vertebrate groups.

It has been suggested that the GC inducible CYP3A genes are part of the glucocorticoid-responsive battery of genes in mammals (Schuetz *et al.*, 1984). Although, time-course and dose-response relationships differ between induction of CYP3A and that of a typical GC-responsive gene, tyrosine aminotransferase (TAT) (Schuetz *et al.*, 1984; Schuetz and Guzelian, 1984; Burger *et al.*, 1992). Paradoxically, GCs such as the synthetic GC DEX, as well as anti-GCs, such as the synthetic pregnenolone 16α-carbonitrile (PCN), have been demonstrated to induce expression of CYP3A, whereas TAT activity only is induced by GCs (Schuetz *et al.*, 1984; Schuetz and Guzelian, 1984; Burger *et al.*, 1992). It has been suggested that induction of CYP3A proceeds by a non-classical GR-mediated pathway (Schuetz *et al.*, 1984; Schuetz and Guzelian, 1984; Burger *et al.*, 1992; Quattrochi *et al.*, 1995; Huss *et al.*, 1996). A possible GR-independent induction of hepatic CYP3A1 gene expression was demonstrated with metyrapone in rats, and this response was shown to be further potentiated in the presence of DEX (Wright *et al.*, 1996). DEX and PCN earlier was shown to activate the rat CYP3A1 gene expression *in vitro* through the same response element. Moreover, this response element was demonstrated to confer the synergistic effect of PCN on CYP3A1 induction by DEX (Quattrochi *et al.*, 1995). A GR responsive enhancer has been identified in the promotor region of the human CYP3A5 gene, suggesting the participation of the GR in the activation of CYP3A5 expression by DEX (Schuetz *et al.*, 1996). Non-steroidal substances, such as the macrolide antibiotics rifampicin (RIF), troleandomycin (TAO) and erythromycin, commonly used as therapeutic drugs, also have been demonstrated to be potent inducers of CYP3A expression in mammals (Daujat *et al.*, 1991a). Interestingly, RIF was demonstrated to be capable of activating the human GR, either by direct activation of the GR itself, or indirectly through GR-associated 56-kDa heatshock proteins (Calleja *et al.*, 1998). Obviously, the induction of CYP3A gene expression is complex and might differ between different CYP3A genes. At present, the direct or indirect involvement of the GR in CYP3A induction cannot yet be excluded.

A novel orphan steroid receptor named the pregnane X receptor (PXR) recently was described in the mouse. This receptor was shown to be activated by endogenous steroids, such as pregnenolone and progesterone, as well as by synthetic GCs and anti-GCs. It has been proposed that this PXR may mediate non-classical GC signalling pathways (Kliewer *et al.*, 1998). Thus, it is possible that the non-classical GR-mediated pathway for induction of CYP3A expression is mediated by the PXR, and that this response further can be potentiated by GCs, through a classical GR-mediated pathway. Future studies should address questions regarding regulatory relationships between various classes of substances that influence the CYP3A expression, as well as a possible role of the PXR receptor in CYP3A gene regulation.

The CYP3A is the major CYP form in livers of mammals and fish (Maurel, 1996; Celander *et al.*, 1996a). CYP3As expression also is prominent in extrahepatic cells, such as epithelial cells within the gastrointestinal tract, kidneys and lungs or gills (De Waziers *et al.*, 1990; Kolars *et al.*, 1992; Husøy *et al.*, 1994; Ghosh *et al.*, 1995; Anttila *et al.*, 1997; Celander, M., Moore, M.J. and Stegeman, J.J., unpublished data). In addition to the digestive and respiratory tract, CYP3A expression also has been demonstrated in the cardiovasculature. Thus, CYP3A mRNA was detected in endothelial cells from the human umbilical vein using a reverse transcriptase polymerase chain reaction technique (Farin *et al.*, 1994). A possible involvement of CYP3A in blood pressure regulation was suggested in spontaneously hypertensive rats where renal CYP3A activities, measured as corticosterone 6β-hydroxylation, positively correlated with systolic blood pressure (Ghosh *et al.*, 1995). Furthermore, CYP3A-mediated bioactivation of nitroglycerine was demonstrated in rat aorta microsomes (Yuan *et al.*, 1997). In a marine mammalian species, the pilot whale (*Globicephala melas*), immunohistochemical analyses revealed the presence of CYP3A immunoreactive proteins in smooth muscle cells of large arteries and arterioles (Celander, M., Moore, M.J. and Stegeman, J.J., unpublished data).

CYP3A enzymes are responsible for hydroxylation of steroids, including GCs and sex steroids (Waxman *et al.*, 1988, 1991; Ged *et al.*, 1989; Gentile *et al.*, 1996; Hammond *et al.*, 1997). CYP3A predominantly metabolize steroids at the 6β-position (Waxman *et al.*, 1988). CYP3A enzymes also metabolize/activate an immense number of non-steroidal xenobiotics including natural products, environmental pollutants and therapeutic drugs (Maurel, 1996; Parkinson, 1996). Certain drug–drug interactions have been suggested to be a result of CYP3A metabolism (Pichard *et al.*, 1992; Halpert *et al.*, 1994; Kostrubsky *et al.*, 1995, 1997). Furthermore, CYP3A enzymes have been shown to activate several known pro-carcinogens (Guengerich and Shimada, 1991; Maurel, 1996), and expression of CYP3A genes has been observed in malignant tumours (Murray *et al.*, 1995). However, the role of CYP3A metabolism in chemical carcinogenesis still remains to be verified.

The strategic cellular localization of these proteins implies a central role of CYP3As for fine-tuning of steroid hormone levels *in situ*, as well as in the biochemical defence against foreign compounds. Furthermore, CYP3A activities also are involved in activation of pro-toxicants/ carcinogens and in activation of vasoactive compounds, which also could have important implications for the toxicity of CYP3A substrates.

Induction of CYP3A activities by GCs conceivably could affect the animals catalytic capacity for other steroids and the clearance of xenobiotics and/or activation of pro-carcinogens and therapeutic agents. Future studies should address questions concerning whether fluctuations of GC levels as a result of physiological stress also could induce or enhance the expression of CYP3A genes.

7.4.3   Modulation of CYP2B induction by glucocorticoids

Studies in cultures of fetal rat hepatocytes revealed that addition of DEX to the medium resulted in adult-like expression of CYP2B and CYP3A genes in these cells (Kremers et al., 1981; Roelandt et al., 1995). In adult rat hepatocytes, DEX treatment resulted in a biphasic effect on the β-naphthoflavone- (BNF) mediated induction of members of the CYP1A subfamily, as well as on the PB-mediated induction of members of the CYP2B subfamily (Sidhu and Omiecinski, 1995). Addition of DEX at low concentrations (1 to 10 nM) resulted in potentiation of the BNF-mediated induction of CYP1A1 and CYP1A2 and a potentiation of the PB-mediated induction of CYP2B1 and CYP2B2 expression. In contrast, addition of DEX at higher concentrations (1 µM) resulted in a slight repression of the BNF-mediated CYP1A1 induction (but not CYP1A2 induction) and a profound down-regulation of PB-mediated CYP2B1 and CYP2B2 induction. Expression of CYP3A1 in these cells was not regulated in a similar biphasic fashion, as this gene was fully responsive even at high levels of DEX (Sidhu and Omiecinski, 1995). This suggests that the GC-dependent modulation of CYP2B induction by PB differs from the non-classical GR-mediated CYP3A1 induction. Instead, the modulation of CYP2B1/2 induction in rat hepatocytes appears to proceed by similar mechanisms to that for the modulation of CYP1A1 induction. However, differences exist between CYP1A and CYP2B genes in their response to high levels of GCs. To date, effects of GCs on DMEs have been most thoroughly investigated for the synergistic effect of GCs on CYP1A induction, which will be discussed next.

7.5   Glucocorticoids and CYP1A induction

The most pronounced effects of GCs on modulation of induction responses by specific inducers have been those observed on CYP1A induction by AHR agonists. The first report on the synergistic effects of GCs and PAHs on monooxygenase activities, i.e. aryl hydrocarbon hydroxylase (AHH) activities in a rat hepatoma cell line (H-4-II-E) was presented by Wiebel and Singh (1980). The most comprehensive descriptions of the GC-dependent potentiation of CYP1A1 induction in mammalian systems have been provided by Prough and colleagues in several papers (Mathis *et al.*, 1986a,b, 1989; Hines *et al.*, 1988; Prough *et al.*, 1989, 1996b; Sherratt *et al.*, 1989, 1990; Linder and Prough, 1993; Xiao *et al.*, 1995). Potentiation of CYP1A induction also has been described hepatic cells from non-mammalian vertebrates, such as fish (Devaux *et al.*, 1992; Celander *et al.*, 1996b, 1997a). The following paragraphs summarize the highlights from these various studies as well as those by others.

7.5.1   *Dose-response relationships*

Dose-response relationships between doses of GCs and monooxygenase activities measured as AHH, ethoxycoumarin *O*-deethylase (ECOD) or ethoxyresorufin *O*-deethylase (EROD) activities have been established in mammalian hepatocytes (Kremers *et al.*, 1981; Edwards *et al.*, 1984; Mathis *et al.*, 1986a,b). Dose-response relationships between doses of GCs and EROD activities also have been shown in fish cells, including rainbow trout hepatocytes (Devaux *et al.*, 1992) and a fish hepatoma cell line, the *Poeciliopsis lucida* hepatocellular carcinoma (PLHC-1) cell line (Celander *et al.*, 1996b, 1997a).

Ethoxyresorufin is a specific substrate for CYP1A enzymes (Burke *et al.*, 1977, 1985). AHH and ECOD activities are mainly mediated by CYP1A enzymes, but also may be catalysed by other CYP enzymes. For example, B[*a*]P, which is used as the substrate for measuring AHH activities, is known to be metabolized by both CYP1A and CYP3A enzymes (Guengerich and Shimada, 1991). Ethoxycoumarin is a substrate for a number of CYP enzymes including members of the CYP1, CYP2 and CYP3 gene families (e.g. Boobis *et al.*, 1986; Celander *et al.*, 1989b; Klotz *et al.*, 1986; Fry *et al.*, 1992; Celander *et al.*, 1996a). Thus, the dose relationships between doses of GCs and monooxygenase activities, in particular AHH and ECOD activities, also could involve CYP forms other than CYP1As. However, the primary involvement of CYP1A enzymes in the GC-dependent increase of monooxygenase activities was confirmed by positive correlation of these activities to CYP1A gene expression, measured as CYP1A mRNA and/or protein levels (Mathis *et al.*, 1989; Sidhu and Omiecinski, 1995; Celander *et al.*, 1996b, 1997a). In the absence of AHR agonists, the GCs alone had little or no effect on CYP1A expression (Mathis *et al.*, 1986a; Celander *et al.*, 1996b). This indicates that the enhancement of CYP1A induction by AHR agonists in the presence of GCs was not an additive effect of GCs, but rather a potentiation of the CYP1A induction. Moreover, the apparent efficacy (i.e. maximal induction response) for CYP1A induction was increased when DEX was added to the culture media (Mathis *et al.*, 1986a,b, 1989; Celander *et al.*, 1996b). The potentiation seems to be a result of increased expression of the CYP1A gene, which was confirmed by increases in *de novo* synthesis of CYP1A1 in rat hepatocytes (Mathis *et al.*, 1986a). The capacity of GCs to potentiate CYP1A induction seems to vary between different GR agonists. The rank order in which various GCs, all at 1 μM, potentiated CYP1A expression in cultured fetal rat hepatocytes was DEX > cortisol > corticosterone (Mathis *et al.*, 1986a). In the fish PLHC-1 cell line, the rank order in which various GCs, all at 10 μM, potentiated CYP1A expression was DEX > cortisol > prednisone ≥ RU 38486 (Celander *et al.*, 1996b). Thus, DEX was more efficient in enhancing CYP1A expression than the same amount of cortisol, both in mammalian and in fish cells, which is consistent with the hierarchy of affinity of these steroids for the adult rat GR (Mathis *et al.*, 1986a). Interestingly, RU 38486 (RU 486) which is described as a progesterone and GR antagonist in mammals, appears to act as a partial GR agonist in the fish cell line (Celander *et al.*, 1996b). The GR agonist concentration-dependence for potentiation of EROD induction in PLHC-1 differed also and was dependent on exposure times. At 24 h exposure, potentiation was obtained with 0.01 μM DEX, whereas at 48 h, a dose of DEX three orders of magnitude higher (10 μM) was required to obtain a degree of potentiation comparable to that seen at 24 h, for reasons unknown (Celander *et al.*, 1996b). However, the metabolism of DEX cannot yet be excluded as a cause of this time dependency. It should be noted that in stressed fish the concentration of circulating GCs is around 0.1 μM (Biron and Benfey, 1994; Narnaware *et al.*, 1994). Thus, in fish cells as well as in mammalian cells, the potentiation of CYP1A induction *in vitro* occurs with concentrations of GCs that are in the same range as that reported in the plasma from stressed animals.

In mammalian cells of hepatic origin and in rainbow trout hepatocytes, the degree of potentiation of CYP1A induction varied between 2- and 5-fold (Mathis *et al.*, 1986a,b, 1989; Hines *et al.*, 1988; Devaux *et al.*, 1992; Sidhu and Omiecinski, 1995). In the PLHC-1 cells, the magnitude of the GC-dependent potentiation of CYP1A induction could be up to 20-fold. In addition to doses of GCs, the degree of this potentiation in PLHC-1 cells was shown also to be strongly dependent on the doses of the AHR agonist, with greatest potentiation occurring at sub-maximal doses of the AHR agonists. Thus, addition of DEX resulted in up to a 20-fold potentiation of EROD induction at sub-maximal doses of TCDD (0.1 nM). This is in contrast to PLHC-1 cell cultures treated with maximally inducing doses of TCDD (1 nM), where the same amount of DEX elicited only a 2-fold enhancement of EROD induction. At supra-maximal doses of TCDD (100 nM) the potentiation was negligible (Celander *et al.*,

1996b). Similar results were obtained when TCDD was replaced with a considerably less potent PAH-type inducer such as BNF. Thus, the effect of DEX treatment in PLHC-1 cells was most pronounced, up to 19-fold, at sub-maximal doses of BNF and the presence of DEX generally increased the potency of the AHR agonist by one order of magnitude (Celander *et al.*, 1997a). The greater influence of GCs in the CYP1A induction response observed in PLHC-1 cells could have important consequences for animals in the environment, where exposure to CYP1A inducers is common and generally at sub-maximal levels.

In vitro studies in mammalian and fish hepatic cells have demonstrated great impact of GCs on the CYP1A induction response, and complex dose-response relationships between doses of both GCs and AHR agonists. It is possible that increased levels of circulating GCs as a result of physiological stress could result in enhanced induction of CYP1A expression. This has toxicological implications as elevated CYP1A activities may result in increased risk for formation of carcinogenic intermediates or reactive oxygen species, which could have negative consequences for the organisms. Future investigations should address the question of whether fluctuations of circulating GCs levels as a result of stress are paralleled by changes in CYP1A induction responses *in vivo*.

7.5.2 Time-course relationships

There was a rapid decline in CYP1A expression over time in cultures of PLHC-1 cells treated with BNF. This probably reflects efficient metabolism of BNF by the CYP1A enzyme. However, as CYP1A expression decreases, the effect of DEX increases in these cultures. The magnitude of potentiation of EROD induction differed substantially between doses of BNF and times of exposure. Similar to TCDD-treated cells, the effects of DEX were more pronounced in cells treated with sub-maximal doses of BNF, but also at longer exposure times. For example, in cells dosed with $1\,\mu M$ BNF the potentiation of EROD induction was none at 6 h, 2-fold at 24 h and 19-fold at 48 h post dosing (Celander *et al.*, 1997a). The reason for this time dependency in reaching maximal degree of potentiation is not known and at this stage we only can speculate. One explanation for the greater potentiation with time observed in PLHC-1 treated with BNF could be a result of BNF reaching sub-maximal concentration for EROD induction as a result of CYP1A metabolism. Another possibility could be that GC-mediated potentiation involves a time-requiring process. A delay in potentiation of induction of CYP1A activities has also been reported in a rat hepatoma cell line (H4IIEC3/T) treated with DEX and TCDD and it was suggested that this potentiation involved a time-consuming process, possibly an induction of AHR content by DEX (Wiebel and Cikryt, 1990). However, GC-dependent potentiation also occurs in rat hepatocytes treated with rapidly metabolized PAHs, which suggests that the AHR is not the limiting factor and that induction of AHR by DEX is probably of less importance for obtaining potentiation of CYP1A induction (Xiao *et al.*, 1995). Another possibility could be slower CYP1A protein turnover in the presence of DEX, suggesting regulation of CYP1A expression at a post-transcriptional level. It earlier has been suggested that a post-transcriptional mechanism could be of some importance in regulating hepatic CYP1A2 mRNA levels in the rat (Pasco *et al.*, 1988; Silver and Krauter, 1988; Silver *et al.*, 1990). However, more recently it was shown, using four CYP1A2-specific intronic run-on probes, that all increases in hepatic CYP1A2 mRNA levels in rats can be totally accounted for by transcriptional activation of this gene (Pasco *et al.*, 1993), and not by post-transcriptional mechanisms as was suggested earlier. However, the questions regarding differences in time dependency between GC-dependent potentiation of the mammalian CYP1A1 and CYP1A2 genes and the piscine CYP1A gene requires further investigations before it can be fully understood. Thus, there seem to exist complex dose-response and time-course relationships for the GC-dependent potentiation of CYP1A by AHR agonists. Future studies should investigate how and whether typical plasma profiles of circulating GCs, similar to those following acute stress, could influence the CYP1A induction response.

7.5.3 A classical GR-mediated pathway

The GC-dependent potentiation of CYP1A1 induction by AHR agonists is believed to proceed by a classical glucocorticoid receptor (GR) pathway. There are several lines of evidence in support of this theory: (I) The response is specific for GR agonists. (II) The response is paralleled to that of a classical GR-mediated response. (III) The response is reduced in the presence of GR antagonists. (IV) Functioning GR response elements (GREs) have been identified in the mammalian CYP1A1 genes. These various findings are discussed in the following paragraphs.

(i) Potentiation of CYP1A induction has been demonstrated with steroids that are known to bind to the GR such as cortisol, corticosterone, DEX, prednisone, RU 28362 and RU 38486 (Mathis *et al.*, 1986a; Celander *et al.*, 1996b). Other GCs, including a precursor of corticosterone (deoxycorticosterone) as well as other classes of steroids such as estradiol, progesterone and testosterone had no effect on CYP1A induction by benzanthracene in fetal rat or human hepatocytes (Mathis *et al.*, 1986a,b). Furthermore, the steroids PCN or spironolactone and the macrolide antibiotics RIF or TAO all failed to potentiate CYP1A induction in the PLHC-1 cells (Celander *et al.*, 1996b). Although, the antibiotic RIF has been shown to potentiate the induction of CYP1A in cultures of rabbit hepatocytes, in the presence of cyclohexamide (Daujat *et al.*, 1991b). Recent studies have shown that RIF is capable of activating the human GR (Calleja *et al.*, 1998). If similar mechanisms also operate in rabbit hepatocytes, it is possible that the RIF-dependent potentiation of CYP1A observed in rabbit hepatocytes proceeds by a GR-mediated pathway. Thus, potentiation of CYP1A induction in fish and mammalian hepatic cells seems to be restricted to substances that interact with the GR.

(ii) The concentration of DEX required for half-maximal induction of CYP1A1 protein content and activity was similar to that required for half-maximal induction of TAT activity in cultured fetal rat hepatocytes (Mathis *et al.*, 1986a). In human fetal hepatocytes the dose of DEX required for half-maximal induction of potentiation of CYP1A1 potentiation, 5 nM, is similar to the apparent K_D of binding of DEX to the GR (Mathis *et al.*, 1986b). Increases in TAT activities were also observed in hepatic fish cells with concentrations of DEX that elicited potentiation of CYP1A induction (Devaux *et al.*, 1992; Celander *et al.*, 1996b). Thus, potentiation of CYP1A induction in fish and in mammalian cells appears to be paralleled with a traditional GR-mediated response, the induction of TAT activity, suggesting a classical GR-mediated pathway.

(iii) The GC-mediated potentiation of CYP1A induction was reduced or abolished in the presence of GR antagonists. In rat hepatocytes, addition of the GR antagonist cortisol 21-mesylate abolished the potentiation of CYP1A1 induction (Mathis *et al.*, 1986b). Addition of GR antagonists, such as PCN or RU 38486, to cultures of PLHC-1 cells decreased the GC-mediated potentiation by approximately 50% (Celander *et al.*, 1996b). These GR antagonists all are specific to the type II GR. In contrast, addition of spironolactone, which is specific for the type I GR, had no effect on the DEX-mediated potentiation in PLHC-1 cells (Celander *et al.*, 1996b). These data suggest that the GC-dependent potentiation of CYP1A induction is mediated by the type II GR.

(iv) Sequence analyses revealed the presence of putative GR consensus hexanucleotide sequences [TGT(C/T)CT] in intron I of both the rat and human CYP1A1 genes (Kimura *et al.*, 1984; Hines *et al.*, 1985; Kawajiri *et al.*, 1986). The most convincing piece of evidence for the involvement of the GR in the potentiation of CYP1A induction by AHR agonists was provided in two separate studies performed in human and rat hepatocytes (Hines *et al.*, 1988; Mathis *et al.*, 1989). Deleting most of intron I in the human CYP1A1 gene eliminated the DEX synergism, without affecting the response to an AHR agonist (Hines *et al.*, 1988). Furthermore, SouthWestern blot analysis and exonuclease footprinting demonstrated that intronic GREs in the rat CYP1A1 gene was capable of binding to the GR *in vitro* (Mathis *et al.*, 1989). Thus, potentiation of CYP1A1 induction in mammals involves the increased transcription of the CYP1A1 gene, presumably via the GR and GRE consensus sequences identified in mammalian CYP1A1 genes. The potentiation of CYP1A induction in fish is probably mediated by similar mechanisms, and putative GREs have been identified in teleost CYP1A genes (Berndtson and Chen, 1994; Roy *et al.*, 1996). However, whether these piscine GREs are functional remains to be verified.

In summary, circumstantial evidence, provided from *in vitro* studies in mammalian or fish cells of hepatic origin, indicate that the GC-dependent potentiation of CYP1A induction by AHR agonists proceeds by a classical type II GR pathway. One could speculate whether this particular GR-mediated response, triggered by exposure to PAH/PHAH, could influence other GR-mediated responses in the same cells. This recently has been demonstrated in the rat where treatment with an AHR agonist *in vivo* resulted in changes in the activities of key enzymes of the gluconeogenic and the sterol synthetic pathways, implying a combined involvement of the AHR and GR in response to AHR agonists (Boll *et al.*, 1998). Knowledge of possible interactions between various GR-mediated processes will increase our understanding of various mechanisms of toxicity or the possible interference of environmental pollutants with traditional stress responses.

7.5.4   Potentiation of CYP1A induction in vivo

The vast majority of investigations of GCs on CYP1A inducibility have been performed in isolated cells in culture. Usually there is a close correlation between *in vitro* and *in vivo* studies. However, discrepancies between results obtained *in vitro* and those obtained *in vivo* sometimes occurs. Nevertheless, *in vitro* studies are important for understanding the nature of certain mechanisms in isolated systems. Moreover, results from *in vitro* experiments often provide the basis for further *in vivo* experiments. Although, *in vitro* studies are important to investigate isolated mechanisms, *in vivo* studies are required to fully understand integrative physiological processes.

Treatment of late-fetal rats with GCs *in vivo* resulted in increases of total CYP content (Leakey and Fouts, 1979). The perinatal period is critical to the quantitative and qualitative development of DMEs and is regulated in parts by GCs (Kremers, 1986). As mentioned above (section 7.4.1) studies performed in neonatal rats *in vivo* showed that the effect of exogenous GCs on CYP1A induction by AHR agonists was more pronounced when levels of endogenous circulating GCs were low (Linder and Prough, 1993). A more pronounced effect of DEX treatment in animals with low endogenous GCs, was also supported by data from adrenalectomized rats. Adrenalectomized rats, i.e. rats depleted of endogenous GCs, displayed DEX-dependent potentiation of CYP1A1 induction *in vivo* (Sherratt *et al.*, 1989). Because potentiation of CYP1A1 induction *in vivo* was significant only at low levels of endogenous GCs, such as in neonatal rats and in adrenalectomized adult rats, it has been proposed that the full extent of induction of CYP1A may be directly associated with the endogenous levels of circulating GCs. (Linder and Prough, 1993).

Future *in vivo* studies should address questions of whether changes in GC levels could possibly affect the sensitivity of the animal towards various types of toxicants. Knowledge of the effects of increases in GCs levels in fetal, juvenile and adult animals *in vivo* could provide important information about the sensitivity to certain toxicants during various life stages, which is important for the risk assessment of specific chemicals. Stress hormones have been shown to enhance the induction of CYP1A *in vitro* as well as *in vivo*, and it is plausible that stress could further stimulate drug metabolism. Enhancement of CYP1A activities could result in a more rapid detoxification, preventing accumulation of CYP1A substrate to toxic levels. However, enhancement of CYP1A activities could also result in increased toxicity, as a result of increased generation of activated toxicants/carcinogens. Thus, whether GC potentiation of CYP1A induction would be beneficial for the animal, depends on the nature of the CYP1A substrates the animal is being exposed to.

7.5.5   *Potentiation of CYP1A induction in extrahepatic cells*

The GC-dependent potentiation of CYP1A induction by AHR has been thoroughly investigated in cells of hepatic origin, whereas information of that in extrahepatic cells is scant. Although potentiation occurs in hepatic cells, a different microenvironment of transcription factors in other cell types could alter that GR agonist response. Lack of effect of DEX on the induction of CYP1A by a PAH has been reported in rat lung and kidney (Sherratt *et al.*, 1989).

The vascular endothelium is a major target for CYP1A induction *in vivo* in mammals as well as in fish (Dees *et al.*, 1982; Anderson *et al.*, 1987; Stegeman *et al.*, 1989). The endothelium is the single-cell layer that lines all blood vessels and constitutes capillaries. The vascular endothelium is an important site for CYP1A induction and it also is continuously exposed to circulating GCs. CYP1A1 expression in cultures of porcine aorta endothelial cells (PAEC) was shown to be highly induced *in vitro* by treatment with AHR agonists (Stegeman *et al.*, 1995). Addition of GCs resulted in potentiation of that response in cultures of PAEC and human aorta endothelial cells (HAEC), which suggest that GC-mediated potentiation of CYP1A1 induction by TCDD also occurs in endothelial cells (Celander *et al.*, 1997b). The potentiation of CYP1A1 in these endothelial cells shows great resemblance to that in mammalian hepatic cells, with up to a 3-fold degree of potentiation with GCs. Similar to hepatic cells, the potentiation of EROD induction occurred in a biphasic fashion, with a maximum at 1 μM DEX in cultures of PAEC. The additional increase in EROD activity in HAEC treated with DEX was abolished in the presence of the GR agonist RU 38486, suggesting that this response involves the action of the GR. The degree of the GC-mediated potentiation in PAEC changed over time, being more pronounced after 48 h than after 24 h, for reasons unknown (Celander *et al.*, 1997b). As mentioned above, the magnitude of the potentiation of CYP1A induction in a fish cell line (PLHC-1) was greater at sub-maximal doses of TCDD (Celander *et al.*, 1996b). Thus, it is possible that the increased degree of potentiation observed in PAEC over time is a consequence of declining levels of TCDD to sub-maximal in these cells. Such a decline could result from the metabolism of TCDD and/or redistribution of the TCDD molecules within the cells. Another possible explanation for the observed temporal effect could involve post-transcriptional stabilization of CYP1A1 expression in the presence of GCs. A delay in reaching maximal GC-mediated potentiation of CYP1A induction has been reported in hepatoma cell lines from two different vertebrate groups treated with DEX (Wiebel and Cikryt, 1990; Celander *et al.*, 1997a). However, further studies are required to explain the time dependency of the GR agonist-mediated potentiation of CYP1A induction, and whether potentiation of CYP1A1 is also significant in the vascular endothelium *in vivo*. Enhanced CYP1A1 activities could promote activation of protoxicants or promutagens, which may result in endothelial cell dysfunction and injuries (Thirman *et al.*, 1994). AHR agonists/CYP1A substrates may stimulate the formation of reactive oxygen species in endothelial cells (Toborek *et al.*, 1995). Thus, potentiation of CYP1A1 induction by stress hormones could have consequences for the toxicokinetics of AHR agonists and CYP1A1 substrates in the vascular endothelium *in situ*. Future studies should address questions concerning possible interaction between stress hormones and the effect of stress and AHR-mediated responses in the cardiovasculature.

7.6 Conclusions

In this chapter the regulatory effects of adrenal stress hormones such as GCs and synthetic derivatives on several DME genes have been discussed, and in particular DREs that are involved in the metabolism of aromatic hydrocarbons. Great attention has been directed towards the GC-dependent potentiation of CYP1A induction by AHR agonists and the majority of these studies have been performed in isolated hepatic cell cultures *in vitro*. However, recent studies have begun to disclose effects of GCs on the induction response of CYP1A *in vivo*. The GR-mediated potentiation of CYP1A induction by AHR agonists has been reported in fetal mammalian hepatocytes, in adult mammalian hepatocytes, in mammalian hepatoma cell lines, in fish hepatocytes, in a fish hepatoma cell line and also in cultures of mammalian aorta endothelial cells. Thus, this response seems to be a widespread response that appeared early in vertebrate evolution, prior the emergence of the mammalian line. However, whether it is an adaptive feature to physiological stress requires further *in vivo* investigations before it can be fully established. Nevertheless, so far all results point in one direction, showing that the induction of CYP1A gene expression by AHR agonists is greatly enhanced in the presence of GR agonists. This was demonstrated *in vitro* at concentrations of GCs reported *in vivo* in the bloodstream in stressed animals. Thus, this implies that the GR-mediated potentiation of CYP1A induction could be activated following physiological stress. In addition to CYP1A, GCs also induce and/or modulate inducibilities of several phase I and phase II genes. However, the mechanism by which various DME genes are regulated by GCs might differ between different gene families. Conceivably, there could be cross-regulatory linkages between the various genes that include the activation of the GR, although this so far has been poorly investigated. Biotransformation of lipophilic organic substances comprises the concerted action of several DMEs and it is no surprise that stress hormones could have pleiotropic effects on these different gene families in order to ensure optimal biotransformation of foreign compounds. Stressed animals have greater metabolic rates than unstressed resting animals, and as the need for energy increases the intake of ingested or inhaled foreign compounds increases. This higher exposure to xenobiotics in turn increases the pressure on the xenobiotic-biotransformation machinery. Thus, it is possible that the stimulatory effect of GCs on the expression of certain DME genes is an adaptive response to physiological stress, developed to prevent increased accumulation of foreign compounds to toxic levels in the animal.

Acknowledgements

Financial support was provided by the Göteborg University, the Swedish Council for Forest and Agricultural Research (SJFR), the Swedish

Natural Research Council (NFR) and the Carl Trygger Foundation. I also would like to thank Drs. Mark Hahn and John Stegeman at the Woods Hole Oceanographic Institution, Massachusetts USA, Dr. Daniel W. Nebert, University of Cincinatti Medical Center, Ohio, USA and Dr. Russel A. Prough, University of Louisville, Kentucky, USA for comments on this manuscript.

Abbreviations

AH	aryl hydrocarbon
AHH	aryl hydrocarbon hydroxylase
AHR	aryl hydrocarbon receptor
ALDH-3	aldehyde dehydrogenase 'class 3'
ARNT	aryl hydrocarbon receptor nuclear translocator
B[a]P	benzo[a]pyrene
BNF	β-naphthoflavone
CYP	cytochrome P450
DEX	dexamethasone
DME	drug metabolizing enzyme
DRE	dioxin response element
EH	epoxide hydrolase
ECOD	ethoxycoumarin O-deethylase
EROD	ethoxyresorufin O-deethylase
GC	glucocorticoid
GR	glucocorticoid receptor
GRE	glucocorticoid response element
GST	glutathione transferase
GST-Ya	2,4-dinitro-1-chlorobenzene specific GST
HAEC	human aorta endothelial cells
hsp90	90-kDa heatshock proteins
MYA	million years ago
NAD(P)H	nicotine amide dinucleotide (phosphate) reduced
NMO-1	NAD(P)H:menadione oxidoreductase (EC 1.6.99.2)
PAH	polycyclic aromatic hydrocarbon
PAEC	porcine aorta endothelial cells
PB	phenobarbital
PCB	polychlorinated biphenyl
PCN	pregnenolone 16α-carbonitrile
PHAH	planar halogenated aromatic hydrocarbon
PLHC-1	*Poeciliopsis lucida* hepatocellular carcinoma
PXR	pregnane X receptor
RIF	rifampicin

TAO	troleandomycin
TAT	tyrosine aminotransferase
TCDD	2,3,7,8-tetrachlorodibenzo-*p*-dioxin
UGT	UDP-glucuronosyl transferase
UGT *06	4-methylumbelliferone specific UGT
XRE	xenobiotic response element

References

Anderson, L.M., Ward, J.M., Park, S.S., Jones, A.B., Junker, J.L., Gelboin, H.V. and Rice, J.M. (1987) Immunohistochemical determination of inducibility phenotype with a monoclonal antibody to a methylcholanthrene-inducible isozyme of cytochrome P-450. *Cancer Research*, **47** 6079-6085.

Anttila, S., Hukkanen, J., Hakkola, J., Stjernvall, T., Beaune, P., Edwards, R.J., Boobis, A.R., Pelkonen, O. and Raunio, H. (1997) Expression and localization of CYP3A4 and CYP3A5 in human lung. *American Journal of Respiration and Cell Molecular Biology*, **16** 242-249.

Berndtson, A.K. and Chen, T.T. (1994) Two unique *CYP1* genes are expressed in response to 3-methylcholanthrene treatment in rainbow trout. *Archives of Biochemistry and Biophysics*, **310 (1)** 187-195.

Biron, M. and Benfey, T.J. (1994) Cortisol, glucose and hematocrit changes during acute stress, cohort sampling, and the diel cycle in diploid and triploid brook trout (*Salvelinus fontinalis* Mitchill). *Fish Physiology and Biochemistry*, **13** 153-160.

Boll, M., Webster, L.W.D., Font, M. and Stampfl, A. (1998) The enzyme inducers 3-methylcholanthrene and phenobarbital affect the activities of glucocorticoid hormone-regulated enzymes in rat liver and kidney. *Toxicology*, **126** 127-136.

Boobis, A.R, Whyte, C. and Davies, D.S. (1986) Selective induction and inhibition of the components of 7-ethoxycoumarin *O*-deethylase activity in the rat. *Xenobiotica*, **16 (3)** 233-238.

Buhler, D.R., Yang, Y.-H., Dreher, T.W., Miranda, C.L. and Wang, J.-L. (1994) Cloning and sequencing of the major rainbow trout constitutive cytochrome P450 (CYP2K1): identification of a new cytochrome P450 gene subfamily and its expression in mature rainbow trout liver and trunk kidney. *Archives of Biochemistry and Biophysics*, **312 (1)** 45-51.

Burger, H.-J., Schuetz, J.D., Schuetz, E.G. and Guzelian, P.S. (1992) Paradoxical transcriptional activation of rat liver cytochrome P-450 3A1 by dexamethasone and the antiglucocorticoid pregnenolone 16α-carbonitrile: analysis by transient transfection into primary monolayer cultures of adult rat hepatocytes. *Proceedings of the National Academy of Sciences, USA*, **89** 2145-2149.

Burke, M.D., Prough, R.A. and Mayer, R.T. (1977) Characteristics of a microsomal cytochrome P-488-mediated reaction ethoxyresorufin O-deethylation. *Drug Metabolism and Disposition*, **5 (1)** 1-8.

Burke, M.D., Thompson, S., Elcombe, C.R., Halpert, J., Haaparanta, T. and Mayer, R.T. (1985) Ethoxy-, pentoxy- and benzyloxyphenoxazones and homologues: a series of substrates to distinguish between different induced cytochromes P-450. *Biochemical Pharmacology*, **34 (18)** 3337-3345.

Calleja, C., Pascussi, J.M., Mani, J.C., Maurel, P. and Vilarem, M.J. (1998) The antibiotic rifampicin is a nonsteroidal ligand and activator of the human glucocorticoid receptor. *Nature Medicine*, **4 (1)** 92-96.

Capdevila, J.H., Falck, J.R. and Estabrook, R.W. (1992) Cytochrome P450 and the arachidonate cascade. *FASEB Journal*, **6** 731-736.

Celander, M. and Stegeman, J.J. (1997) Isolation of a cytochrome P450 3A cDNA sequence (CYP3A30) from the marine teleost *Fundulus heteroclitus* and phylogenetic analyses of *CYP3A* genes. *Biochemical and Biophysical Research Communications*, **236** 306-312.

Celander, M., Ronis, M. and Förlin, L. (1989a) Initial characterization of a constitutive cytochrome P-450 isoenzyme in rainbow trout liver. *Marine Environmental Research*, **28** 9-13.

Celander, M., Förlin, L. and Andersson, T. (1989b) Cytochrome P-450 mediated O-dealkylation of 7-alkoxycoumarins in liver microsomes from rainbow trout (*Salmo gairdneri*). *Fish Physiology and Biochemistry*, **6 (4)** 199-205.

Celander, M., Buhler, D.R., Förlin, L., Goksøyr, A., Miranda, C.L., Woodin, B.R. and Stegeman, J.J. (1996a) Immunochemical relationships of cytochrome P4503A-like proteins in teleost fish. *Fish Physiology and Biochemistry*, **15 (4)** 323-332.

Celander, M., Hahn, M.E. and Stegeman, J.J. (1996b) Cytochromes P450 (CYP) in the *Poeciliopsis lucida* hepatocellular carcinoma cell line (PLHC-1): dose-response and time-dependent glucocorticoid potentiation of CYP1A without induction of CYP3A. *Archives of Biochemistry and Biophysics*, **329 (1)** 113-122.

Celander, M., Bremer, J., Hahn, M.E. and Stegeman, J.J. (1997a) Glucocorticoid-xenobiotic interactions: dexamethasone-mediated potentiation of cytochrome P4501A induction by β-naphthoflavone in a fish hepatoma cell line (PLHC-1). *Environmental Toxicology and Chemistry*, **16 (5)** 900-907.

Celander, M., Weisbrod, R. and Stegeman, J.J. (1997b) Glucocorticoid potentiation of cytochrome P4501A1 induction by 2,3,7,8-tetrachlorodibenzo-*p*-dioxin in porcine and human endothelial cells in culture. *Biochemical and Biophysical Research Communications*, **232** 749-753.

Daujat, M., Pichard, L., Fabre, I., Pineau, T., Fabre, G., Bonfils, C. and Maurel, P. (1991a) Induction protocols for cytochromes P450IIIA *in vivo* and in primary cultures of animal and human hepatocytes. *Methods in Enzymology*, **206** 345-353.

Daujat, M., Clair, P., Astier, C., Fabre, I., Pineau, T., Yerle, M., Gellin, J. and Maurel, P. (1991b) Induction, regulation and messenger half-life of cytochromes *P*450 IA1, IA2 and IIIA6 in primary cultures of rabbit hepatocytes CYP1A1, 1A2 and 3A6 chromosome location in the rabbit and evidence that post-transcriptional control of gene 1A2 does not involve mRNA stabilization. *European Journal of Biochemistry*, **200** 501-510.

Dees, J.H., Masters, B.S.S., Muller-Eberhard, U. and Johnson, E.F. (1982) Effect of 2,3,7, 8-tetrachlorodibenzo-*p*-dioxin and phenobarbital on the occurrence and distribution of four cytochrome P-450 isozymes in rabbit, kidney, lung, and liver. *Cancer Research*, **42** 1423-1432.

Denison, M.S., Fisher, J.M. and Whitlock, J.P., Jr. (1988) The DNA recognition site for the dioxin-Ah receptor complex. *Journal of Biological Chemistry*, **263 (33)** 17221-17224.

Devaux, A., Pesonen, M., Monod, G. and Andersson, T. (1992) Glucocorticoid-mediated potentiation of P450 induction in primary culture of rainbow trout hepatocytes. *Biochemical Pharmacology*, **43 (4)** 898-901.

De Waziers, I., Cugnenc, P.H., Yang, C.S., Leroux, J.-P. and Beaune, P.H. (1990) Cytochrome P 450 isoenzymes, epoxide hydrolase and glutathione transferases in rat human hepatic and extrahepatic tissues. *Journal of Pharmacology and Experimental Therapeutics*, **253 (1)** 387-394.

Di Giulio, R.T., Benson, W.H., Sanders, B.M. and Van Veld, P.A. (1995) Biochemical mechanisms: adaptation, and toxicity, in *Fundamentals of Aquatic Toxicology*, Second edition (ed. G.M. Rand), Taylor and Francis, Washington DC, USA.

Dzeletovic, N., McGuire, J., Daujat, M., Tholander, J., Ema, M., Fujii-Kuriyama, Y., Bergman, J., Maurel, P. and Poellinger, L. (1997) Regulation of dioxin receptor function by omeprazole. *Journal of Biological Chemistry*, **272 (19)** 12705-12713.

Edwards, A.M., Glistak, M.L., Lucas, C.M. and Wilson, P.A. (1984) 7-Ethoxycoumarin deethylase activity as a convenient measure of liver drug metabolizing enzymes: regulation in cultured rat hepatocytes. *Biochemical Pharmacology*, **33 (9)** 1537-1546.

Einarsson, K., Gustafsson, J.-Å. and Stenberg, Å. (1973) Neonatal imprinting of liver microsomal hydroxylation and reduction of steroids. *Journal of Biological Chemistry*, **248 (14)** 4987-4997.

Ema, M., Sogawa, K., Watanabe, N., Chujoh, Y., Matsushita, N., Gotoh, O., Funae, Y. and Fujii-Kuriyama, Y. (1992) cDNA cloning and structure of mouse putative Ah receptor. *Biochemical and Biophysical Research Communications*, **184 (1)** 246-253.

Falckh, P.H.J., Wu, Q.K. and Ahokas, J.T. (1997) CYP4T1-a cytochrome P450 expressed in rainbow trout (*Oncorhynchus mykiss*) liver. *Biochemical and Biophysical Research Communications*, **236** 302-305.

Falkner, K.C., Rushmore, T.H., Linder, M.W. and Prough, R.A. (1998) Negative regulation of the rat glutathione *S*-transferase A2 gene by glucocorticoids involves a canonical glucocorticoid consensus sequence. *Molecular Pharmacology*, **53** 1916-1927.

Farin, F.M., Pohlman, T.H. and Omiecinski, C.J. (1994) Expression of cytochrome P450s and microsomal epoxide hydrolase in primary cultures of human umbilical vein endothelial cells. *Toxicology and Applied Pharmacology*, **124** 1-9.

Fernandez-Salguero, P.M., Pineau, T., Hilbert, D.M., McPhail, T., Lee, S.S.T., Kimura, S., Nebert, D.W., Rudikoff, S., Ward, J. and Gonzalez, F.J. (1995) Immune system impairment and hepatic fibrosis in mice lacking the dioxin-binding Ah receptor. *Science*, **268** 722-726.

Fry, J.R., Garle, M.J. and Lal, K. (1992) Differentiation of cytochrome P-450 inducers on the basis of 7-alkoxycoumarin *O*-deethylase activities. *Xenobiotica*, **22 (2)** 211-215.

Ged, C., Rouillon, J.M., Pichard, L., Combalbert, J., Bressot, N., Bories, P., Michel, H. Beaune, P. and Maurel, P. (1989) The increase in urinary excretion of 6β-hydroxycortisol as a marker of human hepatic cytochrome P450IIIA induction. *British Journal of Clinical Pharmacology*, **28 (4)** 373-387.

Gentile, D.M., Tomlinson, E.S., Maggs, J.L., Park, B.K. and Back, D.J. (1996) Dexamethasone metabolism by human liver *in vitro*. Metabolic identification and inhibition of 6-hydroxylation. *Journal of Pharmacology and Experimental Therapeutics*, **277 (1)** 105-112.

Ghosh, S.S., Basu, A.K., Ghosh, S., Hagley, R., Kramer, L., Schuetz, J., Grogan, W.M., Guzelian, P. and Watlington, C.O. (1995) Renal and hepatic family 3A cytochromes P450 (CYP3A) in spontaneously hypersensitive rats. *Biochemical Pharmacology*, **50 (1)** 49-54.

Gonzalez, F.J. (1989) The molecular biology of cytochrome P450s. *Pharmacological Reviews*, **40 (4)** 243-288.

Gonzalez, F.J. and Gelboin, H.V. (1994) Role of human cytochromes P450 in the metabolic activation of chemical carcinogens and toxins. *Drug Metabolism Reviews*, **26 (1-2)** 165-183.

Gonzalez, F.J. and Nebert, D.W. (1990) Evolution of the P450 superfamily: animal-plant "warfare", molecular drive, and human genetic differences in drug oxidation. *Trends in Genetics*, **6** 182-186.

Gradelet, S., Astorg, P., Pineau, T., Canivenc, M.-C., Siess, M.-H., Leclerc, J. and Lesca, P. (1997) Ah receptor-dependent CYP1A induction by two carotenoids, canthaxanthin and β-apo-8'-carotenal, with no affinity for the TCDD binding site. *Biochemical Pharmacology*, **54** 307-315.

Greengard, O. (1975) Steroids and the maturation of rat tissues. *Journal of Steroid Biochemistry*, **6** 639-642.

Guengerich, F.P. and Shimada, T. (1991) Oxidation of toxic and carcinogenic chemicals by human cytochrome P-450 enzymes. *Chemical Research in Toxicology*, **4 (4)** 391-407.

Hahn, M.E. (1998) The aryl hydrocarbon Receptor: a comparative perspective. *Comparative Biochemistry and Physiology*, *C*, **121** 23-53 (Special issue on forms and functions of cytochrome P450.)

Hahn, M.E., Karchner, S.I., Shapiro, M.A. and Perera, S.A. (1997) Molecular evolution of two vertebrate aryl hydrocarbon (dioxin) receptors (AHR1 and AHR2) and the PAS family. *Proceedings of the National Academy of Sciences, USA,* **94** 13743-13748.

Halpert, J.R., Guengerich, F.P., Bend, J.R. and Correia, M.A. (1994) Selective inhibitors of cytochromes P450. *Toxicology and Applied Pharmacology,* **125** 163-175.

Hammond, D.K., Zhu, B.T., Wang, M.Y., Ricci, M.J. and Liehr, J.G. (1997) Cytochrome P450 metabolism of estradiol in hamster liver and kidney. *Toxicology and Applied Pharmacology,* **145 (1)** 54-60.

Hankinson, O. (1995) The aryl hydrocarbon receptor complex. *Annual Review of Pharmacology and Therapeutics,* **35** 307-340.

Heilmann, L.J., Sheen, Y.Y., Bigelow, S.W. and Nebert, D.W. (1988) Trout P450IA1: cDNA and deduced protein sequence, expression in liver, and evolutionary significance. *DNA,* **7 (6)** 370-387.

Hines, R.N., Levy, J.B., Conrad, R.D., Iversen, P.L., Shen, M.-L., Renli, A.M. and Bresnick, E. (1985) Gene structure and nucleotide sequence for rat cytochrome *P*-450c. *Archives of Biochemistry and Biophysics,* **237 (2)** 465-476.

Hines, R.N., Mathis, J.M. and Jacob, C.S. (1988) Identification of multiple regulatory elements on the human cytochrome P450IA1 gene. *Carcinogenesis,* **9 (9)** 1599-1605.

Husøy, A.-M., Myers, M.S., Willis, M.L., Collier, T.K., Celander, M. and Goksøyr, A. (1994) Immunohistochemical localization of CYP1A and CYP3A-like isozymes in hepatic and extrahepatic tissues of Atlantic cod (*Gadus morhua* L.), a marine teleost. *Toxicology and Applied Pharmacology,* **129** 294-308.

Huss, J.M., Wang, S.I., Astrom, A., McQuiddy, P. and Kasper, C.B. (1996) Dexamethasone responsiveness of a major glucocorticoid-inducible CYP3A gene is mediated by elements unrelated to a glucocorticoid receptor binding motif. *Proceedings of the National Academy of Sciences, USA,* **93** 4666-4670.

Jaiswal, A.K., Nebert, D.W., McBride, O.W. and Gonzalez, F.J. (1987) Human P3450: cDNA and complete protein sequence, repetitive Alu sequences in the 3'nontranslated region, and localization of gene chromosome 15. *Journal of Experimental Pathology,* **3 (1)** 1-17.

Kawajiri, K., Watanabe, J., Gotoh, O., Tagashira, Y., Sogawa, K. and Fujii-Kuriyama, Y. (1986) Structure and drug inducibility of the human cytochrome P-450c gene. *European Journal of Biochemistry,* **159** 219-225.

Kelly, J.D., Eaton, D.L., Guengerich, F.P. and Coulombe, R.A., Jr. (1997) Aflatoxin B$_1$ activation in human lung. *Toxicology and Applied Pharmacology,* **144** 88-95.

Kimura, S., Gonzalez, F.J. and Nebert, D.W. (1984) The murine *Ah* locus comparison of the complete cytochrome P$_1$-450 and P$_3$-450 cDNA nucleotide and amino acid sequences. *Journal of Biological Chemistry,* **259 (17)** 10705-10713.

Kliewer, S.A., Moore, J.T., Wade, L., Staudinger, J.L., Watson, M.A., Jones, S.A., McKee, D.D., Oliver, B.B., Willson, T.M., Zetterström, R.H., Perlmann, T. and Lehmann, J. (1998) An orphan nuclear receptor activated by pregnanes defines a novel steroid signaling pathway. *Cell,* **92** 73-82.

Klotz, A.V., Stegeman, J.J., Woodin, B.R., Snowberger, E.A., Thomas, P.E. and Walsh, C. (1986) Cytochrome *P*-450 isozyme from the marine teleost *Stenotomus chrysops:* their roles in steroid hydroxylation and the influence of cytochrome b$_5$. *Archives of Biochemistry and Biophysics,* **249 (2)** 326-338.

Kolars, J.C., Schmiedlin-Ren, P., Dobbins III, W.O., Schuetz, J., Wrighton, S.A. and Watkins, P.B. (1992) Heterogeneity of cytochrome P450IIIA expression in rat gut epithelia. *Gastroenterology,* **102** 1186-1198.

Kostrubsky, V.E., Wood, S.G., Bush, M.D., Szakacs, J., Bement, W.J., Sinclair, P.R., Jeffery, E.H. and Sinclair, J.F. (1995) Acute hepatotoxicity of acetaminophen in rats treated with ethanol plus isopentanol. *Biochemical Pharmacology,* **50 (11)** 1743-1748.

Kostrubsky, V.E., Lewis, L.D., Wood, S.G., Sinclair, P.R., Wrighton, S.A. and Sinclair, J.F. (1997) Effect of taxol on cytochrome P450 3A and acetaminophen toxicity in cultured rat hepatocytes: comparison to dexamethasone. *Toxicology and Applied Pharmacology*, **142** 79-86.

Kremers, P. (1986) Drug metabolism in cultured fetal hepatocytes, in *Research in Isolated and Cultured Hepatocytes* (eds. A. Guillouzo and C. Guguen-Guillouzo), J. Libbey-Inserm, London, Paris, pp 285-312.

Kremers, P., Goujon, F., De Graeve, J., Van Cantfort, J. and Gielen, J.E. (1981) Multiplicity of cytochrome P-450 in primary fetal hepatocytes in culture. *European Journal of Biochemistry*, **116** 67-72.

Landers, J.P. and Bunce, N.J. (1991) The *Ah* receptor and the mechanism of dioxin toxicity. *Biochemical Journal*, **276** 273-87.

Leakey, J.E.A. and Fouts, J.R. (1979) Precocious development of cytochrome *P*-450 in neonatal rat liver after glucocorticoid treatment. *Biochemical Journal*, **182** 233-235.

Leaver, M.J., Pirrit, L. and George, S.G. (1993) Cytochrome P450 1A1 cDNA from plaice (*Pleuronectes platessa*) and induction of P450 1A1 mRNA in various tissues by 3-methylcholanthrene and isosafrole. *Molecular Marine Biology and Technology*, **2 (6)** 338-345.

Linder, M.W. and Prough, R.A. (1993) Developmental aspects of glucocorticoid regulation of polycyclic aromatic hydrocarbon-inducible enzymes in rat liver. *Archives of Biochemistry and Biophysics*, **302 (1)** 92-102.

Lund, J., Zaphiropoulos, P.G., Mode, A., Warner, M. and Gustafsson, J.-Å. (1991) Hormonal regulation of cytochrome P-450 gene expression. *Advances in Pharmacology*, **22** 325-354.

Mathis, J.M., Prough, R.A., Hines, R.N., Bresnick, E. and Simpson, E.R. (1986a) Regulation of cytochrome *P*-450c by glucocorticoids and polycyclic aromatic hydrocarbons in cultured fetal rat hepatocytes. *Archives of Biochemistry and Biophysics*, **246 (1)** 439-448.

Mathis, J.M., Prough, R.A. and Simpson, E.R. (1986b) Synergistic induction of monooxygenase activity by glucocorticoids and polycyclic aromatic hydrocarbons in human fetal hepatocytes in primary monolayer culture. *Archives of Biochemistry and Biophysics*, **244 (2)** 650-661.

Mathis, J.M., Houser, W.H., Bresnick, E., Cidlowski, J.A., Hines, R.N., Prough, R.A. and Simpson, E.R. (1989) Glucocorticoid regulation of the rat cytochrome P450c (P450IA1) gene: receptor binding within intron I. *Archives of Biochemistry and Biophysics*, **269 (1)** 93-105.

Maurel, P. (1996) The CYP3 family, in *Cytochromes P450 Metabolic and Toxicological Aspects* (ed. C. Ioannides), CRC Press, Inc., Boca Raton, FL, USA.

Miller, M.S., Juchau, M.R., Guengerich, F.P., Nebert, D.W. and Raucy, J.L. (1996) Symposium overview drug metabolic enzymes in developmental toxicology. *Fundamentals of Applied Toxicology*, **34** 165-175.

Morrison, H.G., Oleksiak, M.J., Cornell, N.W., Sogin, M.L. and Stegeman, J.J. (1995) Identification of cytochrome *P*-450 1A (CYP1A) genes from two teleost fish, toadfish (*Opsanus tau*) and scup (*Stenotomus chrysops*), and phylogenetic analyses of CYP1A genes. *Biochemical Journal*, **308** 97-104.

Morrison, H.G., Weil, E.J., Karchner, S.I., Sogin, M.L. and Stegeman, J.J. (1998) Molecular cloning of CYP1A from the estuarine fish *Fundulus heteroclitus* and phylogenetic analysis of CYP1 genes: update with new sequences. *Comparative Biochemistry and Physiology*, C, **121** 231-240.

Murray, G.I., Taylor, V.E., McKay, J.A., Weaver, R.J., Ewen, S.W., Melvin, W.T. and Burke, M.D. (1995) The immunohistochemical localization of drug-metabolizing enzymes in prostate cancer. *Journal of Pathology*, **177 (2)** 147-152.

Narnaware, Y.K., Baker, B.I. and Tomlinson, M.G. (1994) The effect of various stresses, corticosteroids and adrenergic agents on phagocytosis in the rainbow trout *Oncorhynchus mykiss*. *Fish Physiology and Biochemistry*, **13** 31-40.

Nebert, D.W. (1989) The *Ah* locus: genetic differences in toxicity, cancer mutation and birth defects. *Critical Reviews in Toxicology*, **20** 153-174.

Nebert, D.W. (1991) Proposed role of drug-metabolizing enzymes: regulation of steady state levels of the ligands that effect growth, homeostasis, differentiation, and neuroendocrine functions. *Molecular Endocrinology*, **5** 1203-1214.

Nebert, D.W. (1994) Drug-metabolizing enzymes in ligand-modulated transcription. *Biochemical Pharmacology*, **47 (1)** 25-37.

Nebert, D.W. and Gonzalez, F.J. (1987) P450 Genes: Structure, evolution, and regulation. *Annual Review of Biochemistry*, **56** 945-993.

Nebert, D.W., Adesnik, M., Coon, M.J., Estabrook, R.W., Gonzalez, F.J., Guengerich, F.P., Gunsalus, I.C., Johnson, E.F., Kemper, B., Levin, W., Phillips, I.R., Sato, R. and Waterman, M.R. (1987) The P450 gene superfamily: recommended nomenclature. *DNA*, **6 (1)** 1-11.

Nebert, D.W., Petersen, D.D. and Fornace, A.J., Jr. (1990) Cellular responses to oxidative stress: the [*Ah*] gene battery as a paradigm. *Environmental Health Perspectives*, **88** 13-25.

Nebert, D.W., Nelson, D.R., Coon, M.J., Estabrook, R.W., Feyereisen, R., Fujii-Kuriyama, Y., Gonzalez, F.J., Guengerich, F.P., Gunsalus, I.C., Johnson, E.F., Loper, J.C., Sato, R., Waterman, M.R. and Waxman, D.J. (1991) The P450 superfamily: update on new sequences, gene mapping, and recommended nomenclature. *DNA Cell Biology*, **10 (1)** 1-14.

Nebert, D.W., Puga, A. and Vasiliou, V. (1993) Role of the Ah receptor and the dioxin-inducible [*Ah*] gene battery in toxicity, cancer, and signal transduction. *Annals of the New York Academy of Sciences*, **685** 624-640.

Nebert, D.W., McKinnon, R.A. and Puga, A. (1996) Human drug-metabolizing enzyme polymorphisms: effects on risk of toxicity and cancer. *DNA Cell Biology*, **15 (4)** 273-280.

Nelson, D.R., Kamataki, T., Waxman, D.J., Guengerich, F.P., Estabrook, R.W., Feyereisen, R., Gonzalez, F.J., Coon, M.J., Gunsalus, I.C., Gotoh, O., Okuda, K. and Nebert, D.W. (1993) The P450 superfamily: update on new sequences, gene mapping, accession numbers, early trivial names of enzymes, and nomenclature. *DNA Cell Biology*, **12 (1)** 1-51.

Nelson, D.R., Koymans, L., Kamataki, T., Stegeman, J.J., Feyereisen, R., Waxman, D.J., Waterman, M.R., Gotoh, O., Coon, M.J., Estabrook, R.W., Gunsalus, I.C. and Nebert, D.W. (1996) P450 superfamily: update on new sequences, gene mapping, accession numbers and nomenclature. *Pharmacogenetics*, **6** 1-42.

Okey, A.B. (1990) Enzyme induction in the cytochrome P-450 system. *Pharmacology and Therapeutics*, **45** 241-298.

Parkinson, A. (1996) in *Casarett & Doull's Toxicology: The Basic Science of Poisons*, 5th Edition (ed. C.D. Klaassen), McGraw-Hill Companies, Inc. USA. Chapter 6, Biotransformation of Xenobiotics, pp 113-186.

Pasco, D.S., Boyum, K.W., Merchant, S.N., Chalberg, S.C. and Fagan, J.B. (1988) Transcriptional and post-transcriptional regulation of the genes encoding cytochromes P-450c and P-450d *in vivo* and in primary hepatocyte cultures. *Journal of Biological Chemistry*, **263 (18)** 8671-8676.

Pasco, D.S., Boyum, K.W., Elbi, C., Sin Siu, C. and Fagan, J.B. (1993) Inducer-dependent transcriptional activation of the P4501A2 gene *in vivo* and in isolated hepatocytes. *Journal of Biological Chemistry*, **268 (2)** 1053-1057.

Pichard, L., Fabre, I., Daujat, M., Domergue, J., Joyeux, H. and Maurel, P. (1992) Effect of corticosteroids on the expression of cytochromes P450 and on cyclosporin A oxidase activity in primary cultures of human hepatocytes. *Molecular Pharmacology*, **41** 1047-1055.

Poland, A. and Knutson, J.C. (1982) 2,3,7,8-Tetrachlorodibenzo-*p*-dioxin and related halogenated aromatic hydrocarbons: examination of the mechanisms of toxicity. *Annual Review of Pharmacology and Toxicology*, **22** 517-554.

Poulos, T.L. and Ragg, R. (1992) Cytochrome P450cam: crystallography, oxygen activation and electron transfer. *FASEB Journal*, **6** 674-679.

Powell-Coffman, J.A., Bradfield, C.A. and Wood, W.B. (1998) *Caenorhabditis elegans* orthologs of the aryl hydrocarbon receptor and its heterodimerization partner aryl hydrocarbon receptor nuclear translocator. *Proceedings of the National Academy of Sciences, USA*, **95** 2844-2849.

Prough, R.A., Sherratt, A.J., Banet, D.E., Linder, M.W. (1989) Modulation of the polycyclic aromatic hydrocarbon dependent induction of cytochrome P450IA1 by glucocorticoids. *Drug Metabolism Reviews*, **20 (2-4)** 585-599.

Prough, R.A., Falkner, K.C., Xiao, G.-H. and Lindahl, R.G. (1996a) Regulation of rat ALDH-3 by hepatic protein kinases and glucocorticoids, in *Enzymology and Molecular Biology of Carbonyl Metabolism 6*, (ed. Weiner *et al.*), Plenum Press, NY, pp 29-35.

Prough, R.A., Linder, M.W., Pinaire, J.A., Xiao, G.-H. and Falkner, K.C. (1996b) Hormonal regulation of hepatic enzymes involved in foreign compound metabolism. *FASEB Journal*, **10** 1369-1377.

Quattrochi, L.C., Mills, A.S., Barwick, J.L., Yockey, C.B. and Guzelian, P.S. (1995) A novel *cis*-acting element in a liver cytochrome P450 3A gene confers synergistic induction by glucocorticoids plus antiglucocorticoids. *Journal of Biological Chemistry*, **270 (48)** 28917-28923.

Raney, K.D., Shimada, T., Kim, D.-H., Groopman, J.D., Harris, T.M. and Guengerich, F.P. (1992) Oxidations of aflatoxins and sterigmatocystin by human liver microsomes: significance of aflatoxin Q_1 as detoxification product of aflatoxin B_1. *Chemical Research in Toxicology*, **5** 202-210.

Rannug, U., Rannug, A., Sjöberg, U., Li, H., Westerholm, R. and Bergman, J. (1995) Structure elucidation of two tryptophan-derived, high affinity Ah receptor ligands. *Chemistry and Biology*, **2** 841-845.

RayChaudhuri, B., Nebert, D.W. and Puga, A. (1990) The murine *Cyp1a-1* gene negatively regulates its own transcription and that of other members of the aromatic hydrocarbon-responsive [*Ah*] gene battery. *Molecular Endocrinology*, **4 (12)** 1773-1781.

Roelandt, L., Todaro, A., Thomé, J.P. and Kremers, P. (1995) Effects of PCBs (Arocolor 1254) on cytochrome-P450 expression and monooxygenase activities in cultured foetal rat hepatocytes. *Toxicology*, **98** 95-103.

Roy, N.K., Konkle, B. and Wirgin, I. (1996) Characterization of *CYP1A1* gene regulatory elements in cancer-prone Atlantic tomcod. *Pharmacogenetics*, **6** 273-277.

Schmidt, J.V., Huei-Ting, G., Reddy, J.K., Simon, M.C. and Bradfield, C.A. (1996) Characterization of a murine *Ahr* null allele: involvement of the Ah receptor in hepatic growth and development. *Proceedings of the National Academy of Sciences, USA*, **93** 6731-6736.

Schuetz, E.G. and Guzelian, P.S. (1984) Induction of cytochrome P-450 by glucocorticoids in rat liver II. Evidence that glucocorticoids regulate induction of cytochrome P-450 by a nonclassical receptor mechanism. *Journal of Biological Chemistry*, **259 (3)** 2007-2012.

Schuetz, E.G., Wrighton, S.A., Barwick, J.L. and Guzelian, P.S. (1984) Induction of cytochrome P-450 by glucocorticoids in rat liver I. Evidence that glucocorticoids and pregnenolone 16α-carbonitrile regulate *de novo* synthesis of a common form of cytochrome P-450 in cultures of adult rat hepatocytes and in the liver *in vivo*. *Journal of Biological Chemistry*, **259 (3)** 1999-2006.

Schuetz, J.D., Schuetz, E.G., Thottassery, J.V., Guzelian, P.S., Strom, S. and Sun, D. (1996) Identification of a novel dexamethasone responsive enhancer in the human *CYP3A5* gene and its activation in human and rat liver cells. *Molecular Pharmacology*, **49** 63-72.

Sherratt, A.J., Banet, D.E., Linder, M.W. and Prough, R.A. (1989) Potentiation of 3-methylcholanthrene induction of rat hepatic cytochrome P450IA1 by dexamethasone *in vivo*. *Journal of Pharmacology and Experimental Therapeutics*, **249 (2)** 667-672.

Sherratt, A.J., Banet, D.E. and Prough, R.A. (1990) Glucocorticoid regulation of polycyclic aromatic hydrocarbon induction of cytochrome P450IA1, glutathione S-transferases, and NAD(P)H:quinone oxidoreductase in cultured fetal rat hepatocytes. *Molecular Pharmacology*, **37** 198-205.

Sidhu, J.S. and Omiecinski, C.J. (1995) Modulation of xenobiotic-inducible cytochrome P450 gene expression by dexamethasone in primary rat hepatocytes. *Pharmacogenetics*, **5** 24-36.

Silver, G. and Krauter, K.S. (1988) Expression of cytochromes P-450c and P-450d mRNAs in cultured rat hepatocytes 3-methylcholanthrene induction is regulated primarily at the post-transcriptional level. *Journal of Biological Chemistry*, **263 (24)** 11802-11897.

Silver, G., Reid, L.M. and Krauter, K.S. (1990) Dexamethasone-mediated regulation of 3-methylcholanthrene-induced cytochrome P-450*d* mRNA accumulation in primary rat hepatocyte cultures. *Journal of Biological Chemistry*, **265 (6)** 3134-3138.

Stegeman, J.J. (1993) The cytochromes P450 in fish, in *Biochemistry and Molecular Biology of Fishes, 2 Molecular Biology Frontiers* (eds. P.W. Hochachka and T.P. Mommsen), Elsevier Science Publishers, Amsterdam, The Netherlands.

Stegeman, J.J., Miller, M.R. and Hinton, D.E. (1989) Cytochrome P450IA1 induction and localization in endothelium of vertebrate (teleost) heart. *Molecular Pharmacology*, **36** 723-729.

Stegeman, J.J. and Hahn, M.E. (1994) Biochemistry and molecular biology of monooxygenases: current perspectives on forms, functions, and regulation of cytochrome P450 in aquatic species, in *Aquatic Toxicology Molecular, Biochemical, and Cellular Perspectives* (eds. D.C. Malins and G.K. Ostrander), Lewis Publishers, CRC Press Inc., Boca Raton, FL, USA, pp 87-206.

Stegeman, J.J., Hahn, M.E., Weisbrod, R., Woodin, B.R., Joy, J.S., Najibi, S. and Cohen, R.A. (1995) Induction of cytochrome P4501A1 by aryl hydrocarbon receptor agonists in porcine aorta endothelial cells in culture and cytochrome P4501A1 activity in intact cells. *Molecular Pharmacology*, **47** 296-306.

Thirman, M.J., Albrecht, J.H., Krueger, M.A., Erickson, R.R., Cherwitz, D.L., Park, S.S., Gelboin, H.G. and Holtzman, J.L. (1994) Induction of cytochrome CYPIA1 and formation of toxic metabolites of benzo[*a*]pyrene by rat aorta: a possible role in atherogenesis. *Proceedings of the National Academy of Sciences, USA*, **91** 5397-5401.

Toborek, M., Barger, S.W., Mattson, M.P., Espandiari, P., Robertson, L.W. and Hennig, B. (1995) Exposure to polychlorinated biphenyls causes endothelial cell dysfunction. *Journal of Biochemistry and Toxicology*, **10 (4)** 219-226.

Waxman, D.J., Attisano, C., Guengerich, F.P. and Lapenson, D.P. (1988) Human liver microsomal steroid metabolism: identification of the major microsomal steroid hormone 6β-hydroxylase cytochrome *P*-450 enzyme. *Archives of Biochemistry and Biophysics*, **263 (2)** 424-436.

Waxman, D.J., Lapenson, D.P., Aoyama, T., Gelboin, H.V., Gonzalez, F.J. and Korzekwa, K. (1991) steroid hormone hydroxylase specificities of eleven cDNA-expressed human cytochrome P450s. *Archives of Biochemistry and Biophysics*, **290 (1)** 160-166.

Whitlock, J.P., Jr. (1993) Mechanistic aspects of dioxin action. *Chemical Research in Toxicology*, **6** 754-763.

Whitlock, J.P., Jr., Okino, S.T., Dong, L., Ko, H.P., Clarke-Katzenberg, R., Ma, Q. and Li, H. (1996) Induction of cytochrome P4501A1: a model for analyzing mammalian gene transcription. *FASEB Journal*, **10** 809-818.

Wiebel, F.J. and Cikryt, P. (1990) Dexamethasone-mediated potentiation of P450IA1 induction in H4IIEC3/T hepatoma cells is dependent on a time-consuming process and associated with induction of the *Ah* receptor. *Chemico-Biological Interactions*, **76** 307-320.

Wiebel, F.J. and Singh, J. (1980) Monooxygenase and UDP-glucuronosyltransferase activities in established cell cultures. *Archives of Toxicology*, **44** 85-97.

Wright, M.C., Wang, X.J., Pimenta, M., Ribeiro, V., Paine, A.J. and Lechner, M.C. (1996) Glucocorticoid receptor-independent transcriptional induction of cytochrome P450 3A1 by metyrapone and its potentiation by glucocorticoid. *Molecular Pharmacology*, **50 (4)** 856-863.

Xiao, G.-H., Pinaire, J.A., Rodrigues, A.D. and Prough, R.A. (1995) Regulation of the *Ah* gene battery *via Ah* receptor-dependent and independent processes in cultured adult rat hepatocytes. *Drug Metabolism and Disposition*, **23 (6)** 642-650.

Yang, Y.H., Wang, J.L. and Buhler, D.R. (1995) cDNA cloning and characterization of a novel cytochrome P450 from rainbow trout. *Abstracts of the VII International Congress of Toxicology*, **7 (1)** 10.

Yuan, R., Sumi, M. and Benet, L.Z. (1997) Investigation of aortic CYP3A bioactivation of nitroglycerin *in vivo*. *Journal of Pharmacology and Experimental Therapeutics*, **281 (3)** 1499-1505.

Index